Neurosurgery Explained

A Basic and Essential Introduction

Neurosurgery Explained

A Basic and Essential Introduction

W. Adriaan Liebenberg
MMed Neurosurgery (Stellenbosch), FCS Neurosurg (SA)

With contributions from

Matthew J Tait
MA (Oxon), MRCS (Eng)

J Zakier Hussain
MCh (Neurosurgery) FRCS Ed (SN), MSc (Oxon)

Andreas K. Demetriades
B.Sc (Honours), M.Phil (Cantab)
MRCS (Ed & Eng)

&

Deon Louw
MD, FRCSC

VESUVIUS BOOKS LTD
Published by Vesuvius Books Ltd.
Copyright © Vesuvius Books Ltd, 2005

No responsibility or liability is assumed by either the authors or the publisher for any injury, loss, or damage to persons or property as a matter of products liability, negligence, or otherwise, or from the use or operation of any methods, products, instruments, instructions, or ideas contained in this book. Every effort has been made to ensure that the details given in this book regarding the choice, operation or use of any instrumentation, or the choice, dosage and administration practices relating to pharmaceutical agents, which are mentioned in the text, are in accordance with the recommendations and practices current at the time of publication. However, because new research constantly leads to such recommendations and practices being updated, the reader should obtain independent verification of diagnoses and check the makers' instructions carefully regarding the choice and use of instruments, and regarding the administration practices, doses, indications and contraindications associated with pharmaceutical agents mentioned in this book.

The statements made, and the opinions expressed, in this book are those of the authors and do not necessarily reflect the views of the company or companies which manufacture and/or market any of the instruments or pharmaceutical products referred to, nor do any statement made amounts to an endorsement of the quality or value of such instruments or products, or any claims made by their manufacturers.

ISBN 0-9548813-0-3

'Neurosurgery is no secret - anyone can read it in a book'

Wael Moussa (2004)

Our book is dedicated to the memory of
Nicola Swaysland

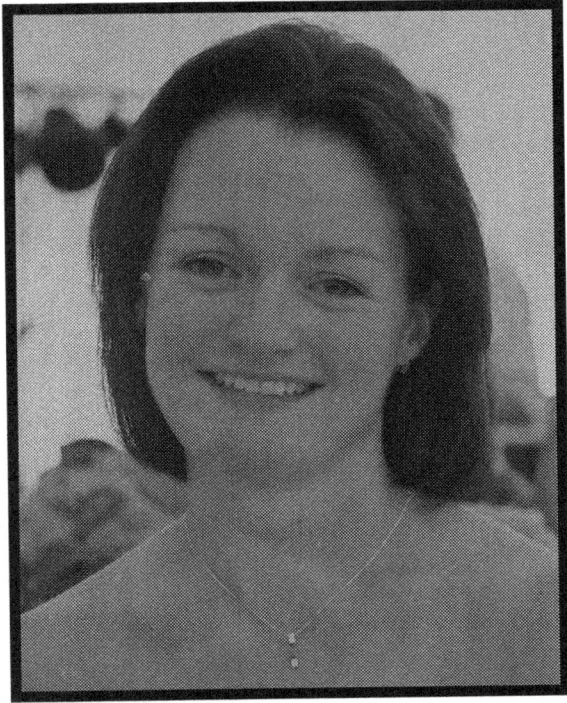

and a dedication from Andreas:

To Christiana, whose inner strength and quiet determination
have never ceased to amaze me.

Professor Al Rhoton Jnr.

This book meets and exceeds its goal of being "a resident's survival guide."

Dr. Liebenberg presents up-to-date concepts in a concise, straightforward, well organized, and easy to understand manner. The book contains material on history, ethics, and the basic sciences, in addition to the essentials of neurosurgical diagnosis and treatment. The book will be especially helpful to trainees in neurosurgery, however, medical students, interns, and multiple other medical specialists will also find it useful. Although designed for trainees, I found the contents interesting, enlightening, and beneficial even after decades of neurosurgical practice.

Albert L. Rhoton, Jr., M.D.
R.D. Keene Family Professor of Neurological Surgery
University of Florida
Department of Neurological Surgery
P.O. Box 100265
Gainesville, Florida 32610-0265

Professor Joanne V Hickey

There is nothing more appreciated and valued by those who seek to master a discipline than a text that provides key information and clinical pearls from experienced practitioners guiding the learner through the maze to understanding and clinical competency. Such is the nature of this well written, well organized, and practical text described by the author as a 'resident's survival guide'. It is a text that will be cherished and revisited often as a beloved friend who provides counsel when needed.

Neurosurgery Explained is designed to support the learner in many of the daily activities of practice. Beginning with the collection of clinical data, the reader is led through the neurological examination, to the correlation of clinical findings with neuroanatomy for localization and generation of a differential diagnosis, arriving at the interpretation of investigations and imaging studies as a basis for clinical reasoning and clinical decision making to support best practice. A major strength of the text is the clarity of explanation about basic principles for interpreting imaging studies, supported by a wealth of excellent radiological images illustrated in the chapters on Interpretation of Cranial CT and MRI Scans, Interpretation of Spinal Imaging, and Neuro Angiography. The chapters on tumours are of remarkable quality and usefulness especially for a book of this size. The text is well illustrated, concise, and substantive.

The author and contributors have created a valuable resource to aid clinical training in neurosurgery. It is also an equally valuable resource for other physicians, nurses, and health professionals dedicated to the care of the neurological and neurosurgical patients. It is my pleasure to recommend this important source of information to all those interested in providing excellent care for neuroscience patients.

Dr. Liebenberg is to be commended for his great effort and success.

Joanne V. Hickey, PhD, RN, FAAN
Professor of Nursing
University of Texas Health Science Center at Houston
Houston, TX
USA

Lizette - jy is my prinses

Niall en Minette - pappa is lief vir julle

Ma en Pa - dankie vir alles

Preface

This project evolved several times as it progressed. I believe that we have created a manuscript that will be a resident's survival guide. It is not an exhaustive reference text and was never meant to be. We have focused on the areas that I believe residents have the most concerns about during their day to day management of patients. Residents frequently have a large radiological duty to perform and interpretation of radiology can be quite taxing. We have included an extensive section on radiology with extensive images, many more than is usually found in a book this size. Knowledge of anatomy is essential in everyday neurosurgery, but is difficult to retain and therefore our anatomy section is fairly complex and is hopefully useful in being a quick reminder of necessary facts. Having a working knowledge of the different tumours of the CNS takes many years to develop and our oncology section contains a broad overview that will allow the reader to be confident about the salient features of most tumours. The rest of the chapters were chosen to be useful whilst entertaining and informative and contain diverse chapters from ethical considerations, to commonly used drugs in neurosurgery to more traditional chapters about the history and examination of the nervous system and chapters on commonly encountered pathology.

You will not find everything about neurosurgery in this book but we believe that this will be an invaluable tool to aid your training in neurosurgery.

Please enjoy the book and please feel free to give feedback so that we may improve on our efforts in the future.

W Adriaan Liebenberg

adriaanlieb@gmail.com

Acknowledgements

Thank you very much to the following staff of Hurstwood Park:

For helping to obtain the images,
Kristina Codling - thank you very much for the efficient, friendly and uncomplaining manner in which you traced those hundreds of X-ray packets and refiled them afterwards.
Liz Hall and **Margot Dormer** - thank you for flagging up interesting cases and helping us obtain images.
Sam Bulled - thank you for the artwork.

For help with the typing of the manuscript,
Margaret van der Neut - thank you for your flawless typing, it is as always a pleasure to work with you.

To our neuroradiologists,
Christina Good - you have been marvellous in your support, thank you for that.
Martin Jeffree - thank you for your help with the neuroradiology chapter

To our intensivists,
Engen Ahmed and **Andrew Elkins** - thank you for your input.

To our neurosurgeons and residents,
John S Norris - this is not the first manuscript that you have helped us with and I hope it will not be the last. Thank you for your support and guidance.
Carl Hardwidge, Lal Gunasekera and **James Akinwunmi** - thank you for your ongoing education.
Sunil Naik and **Sinan Al - Barazi -** thank for your assistance with checking the manuscript, as well as help with the diagrams.
Nigel Page - your detailed check of the manuscript as well as helpful suggestions are greatly appreciated.
Giles R Critchley - thank you for your careful review of our manuscript and invaluable advice. Thank you for making the time, your guidance is greatly appreciated.

&

Deon Lamprecht - thank you for your edit of the anatomy chapter
Professor Richard G Ellenbogen - thank you for making the time in your busy schedule to proof read our manuscript. We are honoured.
Professor Albert L Rhoton - we are honoured to have such a great figure in neurosurgery write a foreword for us.
Professor Joanne V Hickey - we are equally honoured to have a foreword from an icon of neurosurgical nursing care

The greatest thank you must go to **Medtronic's James Blann** and **Leanne Lintula** who have so generously supported the production of this publication. Without you we would not have been able to reach our full potential - thank you very much.

Contents

History
Chapter 1.Historical aspects of neurosurgery

Basic Sciences
Chapter 2.Anatomy
Chapter 3.Physiological aspects

Examination and Investigation
Chapter 4.History and examination
Chapter 5.Interpretation of cranial CT and MRI scans
Chapter 6.Interpretation of spinal imaging
Chapter 7.Neuro angiography

Pathology
Chapter 8.Brain tumours
Chapter 9.Spinal tumours
Chapter 10.Vascular abnormalities
Chapter 11.Hydrocephalus
Chapter 12.Craniospinal trauma
Chapter 13.Infection
Chapter 14.Degenerative conditions
Chapter 15.Congenital neurosurgical conditions

Management
Chapter 16.Monitoring and treatment in neurosurgical ICU
Chapter 17.Drugs commonly used in ICU
Chapter 18.Technology in neurosurgery
Chapter 19.Ethical considerations in neurosurgery

Reading
Chapter 20.Further reading

1

HISTORICAL ASPECTS OF NEUROSURGERY

Andreas K Demetriades

Contents

Prehistoric origins and cranial trepanation
Ancient Egypt
Ancient Greece and Hippocratic medicine
Ancient Rome
Arabic medicine
The Renaissance
Eighteenth and nineteenth centuries
The challenge of localisation
The dawn of modern neurosurgery
Twentieth century, Cushing's influence and beyond

Prehistoric origins and cranial trepanation

The surgery of the nervous system has an interesting place in the history and philosophy of medicine. While neurosurgery as we know it today has recent origins (around the end of the eighteenth and beginning of the nineteenth centuries), it at the same time occupies a distinct position in prehistoric medicine. Trepanation or trephining is probably the oldest recorded operation in history and has been practiced since the Neolithic Age (up to 10,000 years old). Ancient surgeons used a flint scraper in circular motion to remove a portion of the cranium. This practice has been observed in skulls taken from burial grounds of different civilisations on different continents. The predominant explanation is that the procedure was performed to release demonic or bad spirits that presented with convulsions after an accident or battle injury. Possession by demons seems to have been a part of all primitive religions, as suggested by both the continued practice of trepanation into the twentieth century in certain primitive peoples in Africa and the Pacific, and by the fact that priests were also the healers. That the procedure was performed on the living as opposed to a ritual after death is supported by the formation of new bone around the rim of the trepanation hole in archaeological findings.

Bernard de Montfauchon made the first discovery of a trepanned skull in 1685 in Cocherel, France. However, the historical significance was not appreciated until after his death when, in the nineteenth century several other such skulls were discovered in numerous excavation sites in, Spain, Portugal, England, France, Italy, Austria, Sweden, Denmark, Poland, the Caucasus, North Africa, Palestine and the western coast of the Americas. The size of the trepanation on the skull varied from a few centimeters to almost half the skull and the majority were in the parietal region, although frontal and occipital trepanation were also observed. The mode of creation of these sites varied with geography as well as chronology and we know that flints or even shells were used in the Neolithic era as opposed to drills in less

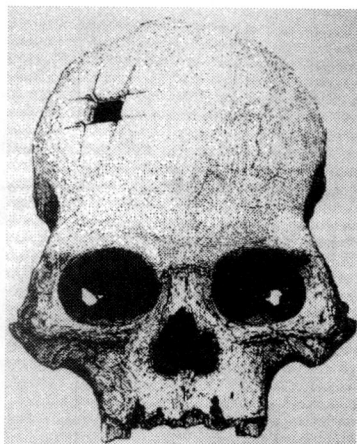

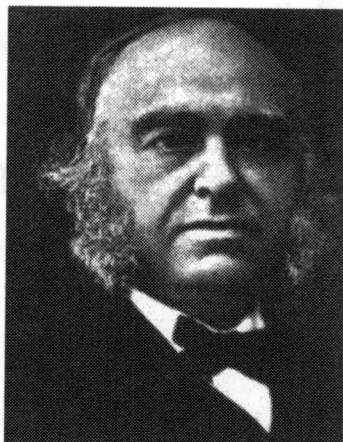

ancient times. The trepanation could have been made using a pointed stone attached to a rotating wooden shaft. The Cuzco region of Peru has a significant place in the history of trepanation. More than 10,000 skulls have been found dating back to 2000-3000 years old. A decent proportion of skulls have more than one hole suggesting an elaborate practice and good survival rates. The instruments found in burial grounds in Peru include sharp obsidian attached to a wooden handle and *tumis*, copper or bronze surgical tools. While theories for the practice of trepanation include rituals and association with tribal superstitions, it has been observed that some trepanned skulls also had fractures, possibly after slingshot, mace or other weapon injuries. This is more the case in the Pre-Columbian Peru region than in the European findings and it signifies a place for trepanation in rational medical practice.

The study of trepanned skulls was popularised by **Paul Broca**, (top right) famous for his studies on the cortical localisation of speech and an eminent physician-anthropologist in 1860's Paris. He first encountered a trepanned Inca skull in 1867 when the US Commissioner to Peru, Ephraim George Squier, had requested a second opinion from the French academic. Squier had previously shown this skull (top left), with cross-hutched cuts in the right fronto-parietal region, to the New York Academy of Medicine in 1866 where the case of trepanation was suggested amidst objection by the audience. Broca agreed that the procedure had been performed while the patient was alive and he subsequently started studying the several trepanned skulls found in France. Although some of Broca's conclusions, like the belief that the procedure was only used in young people, were skewed because of the relative small sample of French skulls, he made significant contributions to the study of cranial trepanation and its popularisation in the medical and anthropological academic circles. The interesting question remains of how so many different civilisations in such remote locations came to develop a very similar surgical procedure.

Ancient Egypt

Ancient Egyptians attributed diseases to evil spirits and sorcery. The early Egyptian medical papyri contain many spells designed to drive the demons out of the sick body and Egyptian healers were therefore a mixture of priests and magicians. Yet even then, according to Herodotus of Halicarnassus, the Greek father of history who had traveled in Egypt about 1000 years after the 2nd dynasty, medicine was practiced according to specialisation. The *Ebers Papyrus*, containing 900 prescriptions in 108 paragraphs in a 65-foot long structure, was discovered in Thebes c.1862 at the feet of a mummy. Dated c. 1555BC it had precise prescriptions for head wounds, such as the anointing of a mixture of the fats from a snake, bird, lion and crocodile. The *Edwin Smith Surgical Papyrus* is the earliest written record dealing with head injuries. Named after its buyer in 1862 in Luxor, part of Thebes, it is dated at around the same time as the Ebers papyrus and seems to contain contributions from three different authors from three different eras: at the time of the pyramids, near the beginning of the Old Kingdom (3000-2500BC); the end of the Old Kingdom; and the 12th dynasty c. 1650BC. The papyrus describes three classes of head injuries - ailments that are to be treated, may be treated, and not to be treated, which seemed to correspond with the observed likelihood of recovery.

Ancient Greece and Hippocratic medicine

The humoral theory of Classical Greek medicine believed that a fine balance of the four bodily humours was essential for good health and that an imbalance was responsible for illnesses. Blood, phlegm, yellow bile and black bile were the corresponding products of air, water, fire and earth. The physician's aim was to re-establish their equilibrium, such as with bloodletting in cases of excess blood, believed responsible for headaches with the signs of bloodshot eyes and a red face. In Hippocrates' *On Diseases II,* we hear of "apoplexy", i.e. stroke or brain haemorrhage, manifesting with sudden pain, loss of speech, rattling in the throat, depressed consciousness and incontinence. The Hippocratic writings identify the presence of fever as a good prognostic sign. The explanation according to the humoral theory was that apoplexy was due to an accumulation of black bile that was allowed to cool down, the presence of fever acting to counteract this imbalance.

Treatments consisted of natural recipes like vapour bathing of the head, purging, and incision of the scalp if all non-invasive measures failed. In addition, the Greek physician, unlike the Egyptian, had in his everyday armamentarium the option of craniotomy. Several instruments could be used such as the *trepanon*, operated by a bow, the *terebra*, spun by a strap wrapped around the centre, or the *prion charactos*, a conical metal with a circular serrated edge at the bottom. A ring of holes were made around the area of cranium to be resected, but there is evidence that such practice was not indicated in areas near major blood vessels and that care was taken not to damage or open the dura. In the Hippocratic text, *On Injuries to the Head* it is clear that closed head injuries were a greater concern to the physician and such cases were more likely to need trepanation than injuries where the skull had been opened, and therefore could allow escape of the excess humours. The head injuries that needed trepanation included *contusion*, whether the bone was laid bare or not; and *fissure*, whether apparent or not and *hedra* (indentation by a weapon). Craniotomies were effective in closed head injuries as they relieved intracranial pressure. The care of the Classical Greek physician not to injure or open the dura must have led to good results, which would explain the increase in the popularity of this treatment.

Ancient Rome

Roman dominance spanned from the 1st century BC to 500AD. With the Roman conquest of Egypt, the medical school at Alexandria faded and the centre of medicine was to shift to the capital. At that time, there were no doctors in Rome as each household practiced its own healing techniques. This allowed Greek physicians, especially via the Greek population dominating Sicily and Southern Italy, to move to Rome and establish themselves, bringing the principles of Hippocratic Medicine. The first Greek physician in Rome was Asclepiades of Bithynia (124BC), who did not believe in the humoral theory of Hippocrates but instead in the balance between contraction and relaxation of body particles. In 30AD Celsus, not a physician himself, wrote his *De Re Medicina*, a compilation of mainly Hippocratic writings that contained descriptions of several surgical instruments, such as trocars, cannulae and specula, as well as several operations. On head injuries, he advocated trepanation and dressing of wounds with oil-and-vinegar soaked wool. He also proposed cautery as a treatment for epilepsy, which would allow the release of excess phlegm and thick bile.

The main influence in Ancient Roman medical times came from **Galen**, (below) who was born in the Greek town of Pergamon and educated in Smyrna and Alexandria, before moving to Rome to practice Hippocratic medicine. As human dissection was forbidden, he studied anatomy on the dog, pig and Barbary ape, adding however a certain degree of misleading speculation and assumption into human anatomical knowledge. However, he had very good understanding of the anatomy of joints from treating gladiator injuries and of the brain, recognising seven of the cranial nerves, the meninges, the cerebral hemispheres, cerebellum, ventricles and corpus callosum. He recognised the contralateral nature of paresis after head injury as well as the resulting paralysis below the level of injury in the spinal cord, and continued to advocate trepanation in his writings.

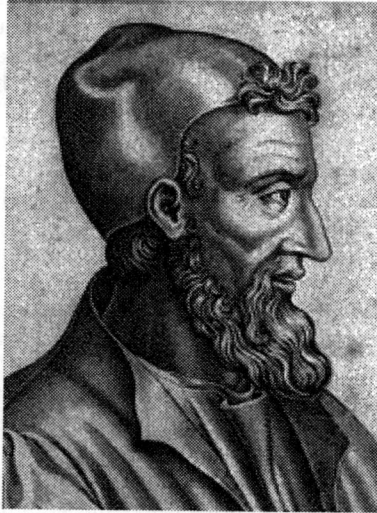

Arabic medicine

Arabian physicians were the most notable successors of Galen. Albucasis (936-1013), or Abul-Quasim Khalif ibn Abbasmal-Zahrawi, was born near Cordoba in Moorish Spain and his writings in Arabic were translated in Latin, Hebrew and Provençal. A prominent surgeon, he relied on the writings of Paul of Aegina, a Byzantine physician of the 7th century, to translate into his work Paul's treatise on hydrocephalus and some of the techniques on trepanation. Albucasis described a non-sinking drill that prevented plunging into the brain during trepanation. He described more than 150 surgical instruments.

Rhazes (c. 900AD) was another influential figure in the golden era of Arabic medicine. He practiced in Baghdad using an amalgamation of Greek, Persian and Indian medical knowledge. His writings were exemplary for this collection of different sources of knowledge, but also for his description of tricks used by charlatans. During trepanation, for instance, quack physicians would pretend to remove a stone from inside the skull. Such growing deceit led to the establishment by the Arabic authorities of a qualifying examination for students of medicine, an event that increased the esteem and reputation of mainstream physicians.

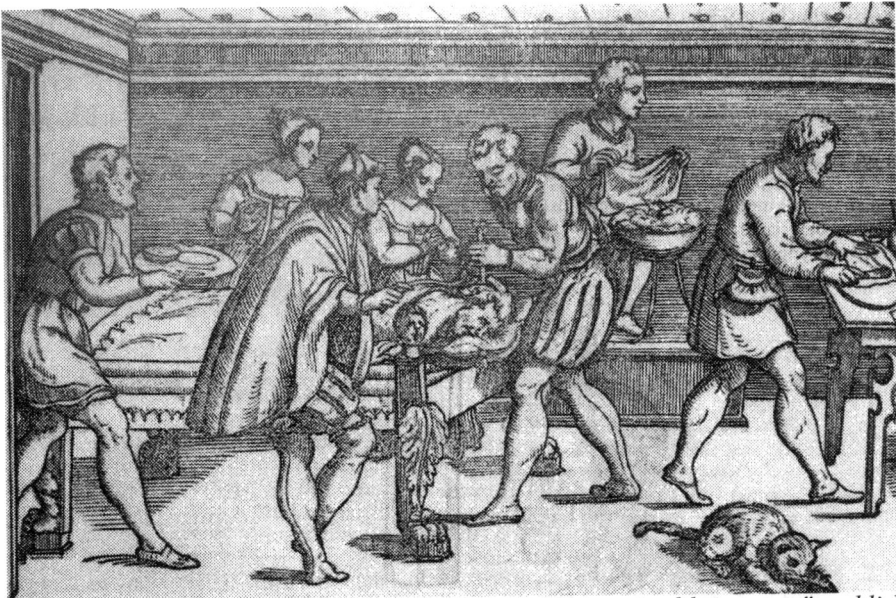

Figure 1. *This picture is from Andrea della Croce's "Chirurgiae libri septem", published in Venice in 1573. Trepanation must have been a common procedure at the time, as this scene depicts how surgeons operated in patients' homes. The surgeon used a brace and drill-stock to which the circular saw or a sharp perforator was fixed with a screw.*

The Renaissance

At the middle of the 14th century, head injuries were still treated by trepanation. Jacopo Berengario da Capri, who published his series of six such patients in Bologna in 1518, promoted the significant step of attempting surgery in patients with dural penetration.

In England, despite the introduction by John Caius in 1546 of the anatomical discoveries of Andreas Vesalius, the actual practice of medicine was still along Hippocratic and Galenic lines. In France, the 16th century military surgeon Ambroise Paré advocated the removal of bone fragments driven into brain and devised several new surgical instruments. He even described a request by a patient to have a brain transplant due to a "rotting brain". In the same century in Berlin, Wilhelm Fabry von Hilden designed a screw-hook-lever instrument that would elevate depressed skull fractures. In addition, a while later Samuel Pepys reported how the French surgeon Moulins performed the same operation on Prince Rupert on 3 February 1677. Advances took place in instrument design and in the undertaking of more difficult surgery, especially of penetrating injury. With time, indications for the procedure were recognised to included obvious fracture, unconsciousness, and haemorrhage from the nose, ear or mouth, seizures and paralysis. Experience and expertise was obtained on the battlegrounds, such as with Joannis Scultetus during the Thirty Years War (1618-1648), who used a *trioploides* (tripod and screw) to elevate skull fractures, and Richard Wiseman, who served in the English, Spanish and Dutch armies and described in his *Severall Chirurgicall Treatises* (1676), 600 different wound cases. Among these, he advised the removal of extradural haematomas and the opening of the dura for subdural haematomas. Interestingly, however, he would not operate unless "the moon was right", showing a persisting influence from the traditions of the past. Baron Larrey, the French surgeon during the Napoleonic wars, amassed a wealth of experience and advised trepanation in depressed skull fractures as well as for the removal of penetrating substances like bullets from the brain. Guthrie, present at the battle of Waterloo, was an advocate of swift trepanation as soon as possible after a skull fracture, admitting, "injuries of the head affecting the brain are difficult of distinction, doubtful in their character, treacherous in their course, and for the most part fatal in their results".

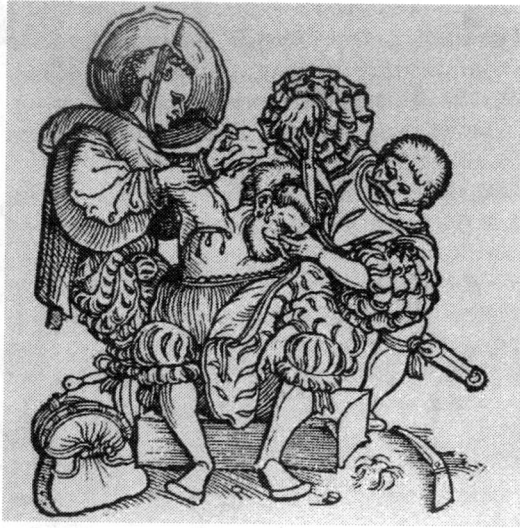

Figure 2. *Sixteenth century treatment by a barber surgeon and his assistant on a military head injury victim (Lanfrancus Mediolanensis 1529)*

Eighteenth and nineteenth centuries

Trepanation for brain injury related epilepsy remained a mainstream operation until the mid nineteenth century. While Percivall Pott from St. Bartholomew's Hospital in London advocated in the eighteenth century that all skull fractures warranted an operation, Astley Cooper believed only compound fractures needed such treatment. Apart from Cooper, John Hunter, and Henry Cline of Guy's Hospital were also frequent users of the technique.

Trepanation went out of fashion rather abruptly. At St. Bartholomew's Hospital, the oldest medical school in London and one of the earliest hospitals to publish annual records, no trepanation took place between 1860 and 1867. It is believed that the widespread avoidance of this operation was due to high mortality rates. A report in the *British Medical Journal* in 1877 mentions that at University College Hospital, for example, 11 out of the 19 trepanned patients died, whereas the mortality rates were 39 out of 51 at Guy's Hospital and 13 out of 16 patients at St. George's Hospital. Similar results were reported elsewhere; in the gunshot wounds needing trepanation during the American Civil War, 125 deaths occurred in 220 operations.

J.S. Billings, however, reported better results. In Cincinnati in 1867, where while 16 out of 72 cases were fatal, 42 were cured, 10 improved and 4 unchanged. Re-awakening of the interest in cranial trepanation occurred in 1877 when Robert Hudson, an unknown surgeon from the mining districts of Cornwall, explained to a meeting of the British Medical Association how Percival Pott's belief on the necessity of trepanation for any injury of the skull had persisted despite the fact that the operation was generally out of favour. His operations gave no problems with infection, which he attributed to the "purity of the Cornish air", but simultaneously suggesting, "the antiseptic system be carried out in the spirit of its apostle". Joseph Lister had introduced antisepsis in surgery and had reported ten years earlier in *The Lancet* a series of 11 patients with long bone compound fractures with only one fatality. In 1880, James West from Birmingham introduced Hudson's views to the Royal Medical and Chirurgical Society of London, the predecessor of the current Royal Society of Medicine, whose influence had a role in the resurgence both of the technique and of its use with Listerian antisepsis.

The challenge of localisation

Trepanning had survived thousands of years and the improved outcome with the introduction of antisepsis gave it new impetus. Another development however was to be the progress in correlating diagnostic signs to intracranial localisation. While operating for a skull fracture was straightforward in terms of position, the localisation of an abscess or tumour was more challenging. Hippocratic and Galenic writings had recognised the effect of brain injury to the opposite of the body, and the attempts at localisation through the ages make a fascinating subject. In modern times, however, it was the Frenchman Dominique Larrey (1776-1842) who first described the constellation of loss of speech, loss of memory and paralysis contralateral to the side of head injury. Another French physician, Jean Cruveilhier (1791-1874), diagnosed a right frontal tumour in a woman with frontal headache, mental impairment, slow speech, left leg weakness and urinary incontinence, which was confirmed on autopsy after her death. Paul Broca presented in 1861 to the Anthropological Society in Paris the brain of a patient who had lost his speech. There was a softening on the left third frontal convolution, which became known as Broca's speech area. Broca's proposal, perhaps the most important clinical presentation in the history of cortical localisation, was confirmed in 1864 by Hughlings Jackson, a physician at the London Hospital in Whitechapel as well as the National Hospital for Nervous Diseases at Queen Square, London.

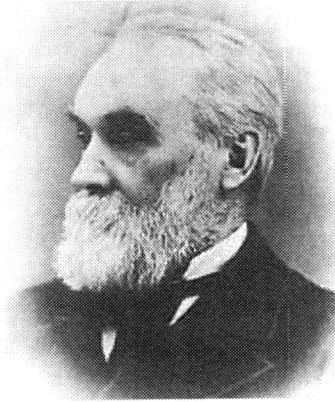

Hughlings Jackson (1835-1911, above) postulated that it would be possible to map the human brain into functionally distinct areas. As proof of concept, this was achieved in 1870 by the Germans Eduard Hitzig (1838-1907) and Gustav Fritsch (1838-1927) who managed to stimulate areas of a canine brain with galvanic current and cause movement on the opposite side of the body. This was the most significant laboratory discovery of cortical localisation. The confirmation of cortical excitability in humans came in 1874 from Roberts Bartholow (1831-1904) in Cincinnati, who electrically stimulated the cortex just behind the Rolandic fissure of Mary Rafferty causing tingling and movement of the contralateral limbs. While Bartholow claimed these observations were made with the patient's consent, he was severely criticised both in the US and Europe.

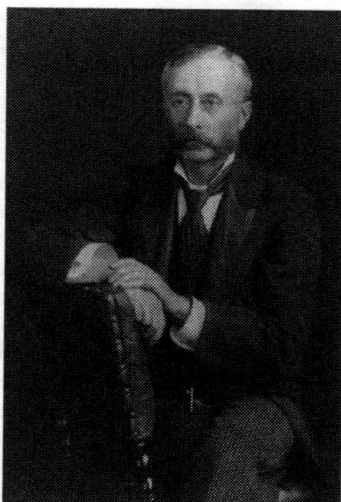

David Ferrier (1843-1928, above) however was the leader of cortical localisation. He was a neurologist at the National Hospital at Queen Square as well as King's College Hospital, London. Ferrier managed in 1873 to map out the cortical areas for the face, arms and legs in apes, using Faradic stimulation. During the seventh International Medical Congress in London in 1881, he exhibited a hemiplegic monkey with a unilateral cortical lesion on the left. It is said that the French neurologist Jean Martin Charcot (1825-1893) exclaimed, "It is a patient!" on seeing the animal limping into the demonstration room. David Ferrier summarised his research findings in *The Functions of the Brain* (1876), which was to have an immense influence on the scientific community and pave the way for modern neurosurgery.

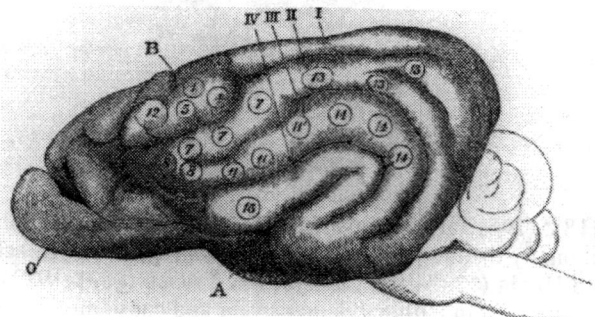

Figure 3. *This figure out of Ferrier's work 'The Functions of the Brain* (1876)' *depicts cortical localisation in a dog's brain.*

The dawn of modern neurosurgery

Broca had himself performed the first trepanation on a patient after localising an intracranial lesion. Although the patient did not survive, he presented in 1861 to the Surgical Society of Paris, a successful case of a child operated on for an intracranial abscess he had diagnosed preoperatively. In Glasgow, William Macewen had also diagnosed an intracranial abscess by localising signs in 1876; the diagnosis was confirmed at post-mortem although the patient never underwent surgery. In 1879, he successfully localised and removed an extradural haematoma in a fourteen-year-old boy, and a left frontal meningioma in a girl of the same age. The girl made a complete recovery and lived for eight more years. This was indeed the first reported successful removal of a brain tumour. By 1893, Macewen had operated on 24 cerebral abscesses with no less than 23 recoveries.

Knowledge of intracranial localisation increased and the work of Broca, Jackson and Ferrier was summarised in 1878 by Lucas-Championnière who published *La Trépanation Guidée par les Localisations Cérébrale*. Operations according to these principles slowly spread through certain centres in Europe and America. In Rome, Francesco Durante removed a meningioma in May 1884 from a 35-year old woman with a 3-month history of anosmia and a lowered and outward-drawn left eye, the physical signs suggesting a left frontal tumour. In London, Rickman Godlee (1849-1925) working at University College Hospital and at the National Hospital at Queen Square, also removed a meningioma in November of the same year. The 25-year old patient had suffered from Jacksonian seizures for three years and had severe headaches, vomiting, left arm and leg weakness and bilateral optic neuritis. David Ferrier and Rickman Godlee diagnosed "a tumour probably of limited size involving the cortex of the brain and situated in the middle part of the fissure of Rolando". As predicted, a hard glioma "about the size of a walnut" was found at operation, where Godlee, Ferrier, Horsley and Jackson were present. The symptoms resolved but unfortunately, the patient died of meningitis 28 days later. Godlee's uncle, Joseph Lister, also operated on a brain tumour six months later that had been diagnosed by David Ferrier. In Baltimore, William Williams Keen successfully removed a meningioma in 1887 and two more in 1888. In Germany, progress was slower as there was opposition by Stromeyer to the theories of localisation, yet von Bergmann did describe operations for brain abscess, tumour and traumatic epilepsy in 1889.

Neurosurgical procedures were at that time part of the spectrum of the skills of a general surgeon. Even though Macewen is considered the first to operate using functional cortical localisation and the first to successfully remove a brain tumour, he remained a general surgeon, as did Godlee. The "first neurosurgical specialist" was Victor Horsley of University College Hospital and The National Hospital at Queen Square. Although initially a general surgeon himself and experienced in other surgical areas such as the thyroid, his particular interest were the brain, spine and nerves. In the 1886 meeting of the British Medical Association in Brighton, he reported three cranial procedures for the treatment of motor epilepsy. One of these cases suffered from traumatic epilepsy from a scar in the superior frontal sulcus, which he had successfully localised using his knowledge of the primate motor cortex. Another was a tuberculous abscess, purely diagnosed on signs and symptoms.

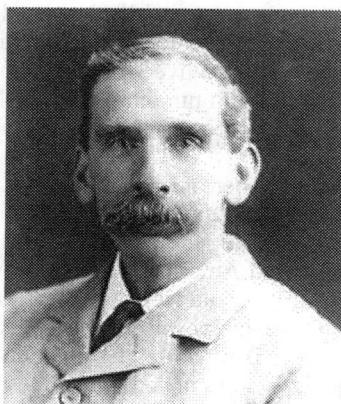

Victor Horsley (top) was the first to successfully remove a correctly localised tumour of the spinal cord (1887), which had been diagnosed by William Gowers. Macewen, however, is the first to have performed a laminectomy (1883). He performed this procedure to relieve the symptoms due to a severe curvature of the spine in a 9-year old suffering from partial paralysis and incontinence. Within three years, Macewen performed six laminectomies with two deaths. Prior to the introduction of this technique, trepanation and partial removal of a vertebra in a case of trauma had been performed by the Irish surgeon McDonnell (1865), on the advice of Brown-Séquard who was visiting Dublin at the time. Astley Cooper had also described such a procedure, previously. Horsley approached each operation with a methodical manner, based on the interpretation of localising signs on examination and sometimes supplemented by animal experiments. Problems of course were still prevalent, as localisation in the pre-imaging era was not perfect, sepsis despite Listerian antiseptic measures was common and control of haemorrhage was often difficult. Mortality rates ranged from 7% for trepanation to anything between 30-80% in craniotomies for abscesses or tumours. However, while the specialty of Neurosurgery had its foundations laid by the contributions of William Macewen and Victor Horsley, the number of dedicated neurosurgeons was very small.

Twentieth century, Cushing's influence and beyond

Macewen and Horsley are indeed pioneers of modern neurosurgery. The honour, however, of founding a school for the specialty goes to **Harvey Cushing** (1869-1939, opposite page) on the legacy of which current practice derives from. Cushing graduated from Harvard Medical School in 1895 and after his house officer year went to work on the surgical team of William Halstead at Johns Hopkins in Baltimore. There he was taught the benefits of speed in operating on the one hand but also of meticulous haemostasis and tissue handling on the other. It was there that Cushing, while helping take the first ever X-ray at his hospital of a patient with a spinal gunshot wound, became interested in neurosurgery. He also met William Osler, who was to have a profound influence on the young surgeon throughout his life. In 1900, the two left for Europe, first to Berne, Switzerland where Cushing worked with Kocher, and then London, where he had hoped to work with Victor Horsley.

The latter arrangement did not work out and Cushing instead went to Liverpool where he spent some time with Charles Sherrington. Upon Cushing's return to Baltimore, he expressed the wish to practice in neurosurgery, a desire that found disapproval from Halstead on the basis that the specialty was not showing promise for the future. Cushing persisted and part of his future success and of the specialty in general, lies in the fact that he had some good results in the treatment of the devastating condition of trigeminal neuralgia.

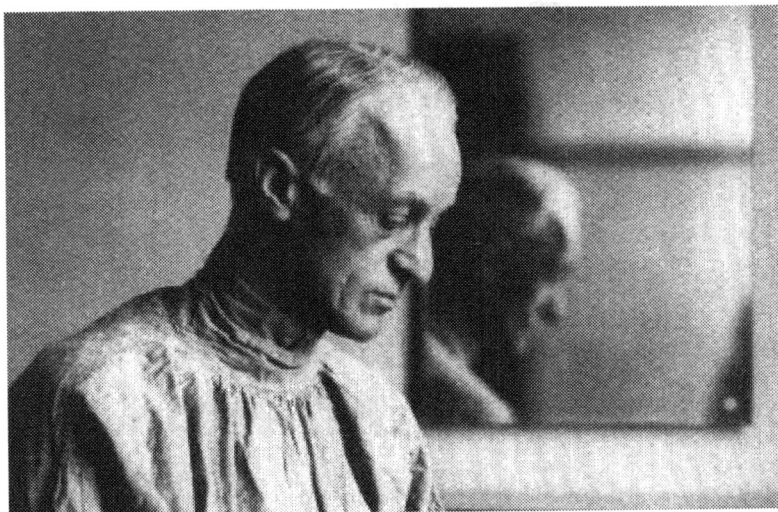

Previous attempts at such treatment included William Rose's removal of the Gasserian ganglion in 1890 at King's College Hospital, London, with a resultant loss of sight in the ipsilateral eye. After Ferrier's suggestion that it would be perhaps safer to section the nerve rather than remove the ganglion, a year later Horsley attempted this only once, after his patient died of shock a few hours later. Another year later (1892) the British surgeon Frank Hartley and the German Fedor Krause returned to the procedure of removing the ganglion. Cushing used the Hartley-Krause technique halving the mortality rate (5%). In 1901, the Philadelphia surgeon Frazer tried again sectioning of the trigeminal nerve, a technique that Cushing eventually adopted in 1907.

Cushing continued to improve on his surgical technique and to attempt other operations on the brain. He quickly realized that better care was necessary than tearing tumours out with one's fingers, so he developed a gentler dissection technique using gentle pressure with the use of swabs. He developed silver clips to occlude meningeal and cerebral vessels; introduced the use of suction to deal with haemorrhage and controlled scalp bleeding with adrenalin infiltration and traction with a series of artery forceps to the skin edges. True to the mark of a good surgeon, he knew when not to operate; when localisation was difficult he avoided extensive craniotomies with their associated blood loss and instead used the principle of palliative decompression, in effect simple trepanning. By 1905, he was the first full time neurosurgeon and had improved greatly on Horsley's mortality rates of 40%. After he moved to take up a Chair at Boston's Peter Bent Brigham hospital, he dedicated his time to cerebral tumour work, reaching a mortality of only 8% in 130 cases by 1915.

Between 1915 and 1919, he volunteered his services to a military ambulance unit in France during World War I, where he amassed a large experience in head injuries. Upon his return to Boston, he set up a team of interested surgeons who wanted to learn neurosurgery. To this date, many neurosurgical programs in the US and abroad have their roots in that original team of doctors around Cushing. One such person was Hugh Cairns, who was later to set up the mobile neurosurgical units of World War II as well as the neurosurgical department at Oxford. A story goes that Cairns, present at the first demonstration of another of Cushing's innovations, the use of diathermy (1928), fainted with the smell of coagulating brain tissue. Cushing's contribution to neurosurgery was multi-faceted; he operated on more than 2000 brain tumours, described Cushing's syndrome, introduced careful observations during anesthesia, and apart from advances against blood loss he practiced strict asepsis and encouraged the use of sulphonamides and penicillin. Further advances in 20th century neurosurgery were to follow with the advent of imaging techniques.

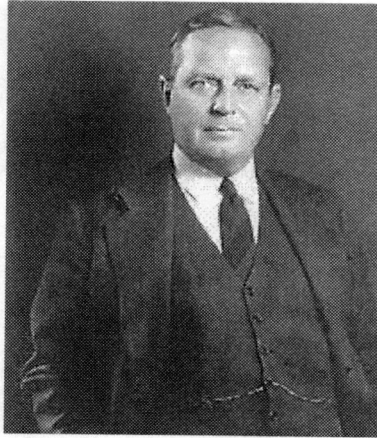

Walter Dandy (1886-1946, above) introduced the diagnostic process of pneumoencephalography (or ventriculography) at Johns Hopkins in 1918 using X-rays after injecting air into the brain ventricles. Sicard in Paris used injection of another contrast, Lipiodol, for spinal localisation. Both these methods were dangerous and became obsolete but heralded the era of neuro radiological diagnosis.

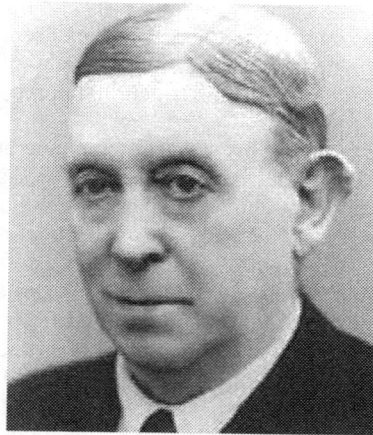

Antonio de Egas Moniz (above) introduced further diagnostic advances with cerebral angiography; and with Berger in 1929 the Electroencephalogram (EEG), which revolutionised the diagnosis of epilepsy. Both these are still in mainstream use today. He was also responsible for the introduction of prefrontal leucotomy (1935), an operation for obsessional or melancholic states that later fell into disrepute. Psychosurgery, however, is still used today in a highly selected manner. Walter Dandy, on his part, also pioneered the treatment for hydrocephalus, diverting cerebrospinal fluid from the ventricles of the brain to the peritoneum, ureter or bowel. A revolutionary step in this rationale came in 1956 by Spitz, a surgeon in Philadelphia, and Holter, an engineer whose son suffered from the condition; the Spitz-Holter valve allowed one-way drainage away from the ventricles.

Currently, technological advances are incorporated in the practice of neurosurgery. Computed Tomography, pioneered by Godfrey Hounsfield and James Ambrose, introduced cross-sectional imaging and was first used on a human patient to diagnose a brain tumour at

London's Atkinson Morley Hospital in 1972. Magnetic Resonance Imaging followed with the first clinical images taken in 1980 after research at Nottingham and Aberdeen. CT and MRI have totally revolutionised diagnostic localisation, while further advances are engineered continuously. Currently, computerised intra-operative image guidance allows real-time navigation during surgery. Advances in basic sciences, furthermore, allow the translation from theory to bedside, as is the case with stereotactic neurosurgery, a technique actually used by Horsley in 1908 but currently employed for the pioneering treatment of functional disorders like Parkinson's disease by deep brain stimulation. Probably the biggest advances have been the development of microneurosurgical techniques and the operating microscope.

Modern neurosurgery has come a long way in the last 100 years, long after its humble beginnings with trepanation. More than ever before, it continues to combine diagnostic accuracy, surgical skill and innovative technological advance, making it one of the most exciting and challenging medical specialties.

2

ANATOMY

Matthew J Tait

Contents

The Scalp
Bones of the Cranial Vault
The Cranial Meninges
The Surfaces of the Brain
Surface anatomy of the brainstem.
Surface anatomy of the cerebellum.
The Ventricular System
The Suprasellar region or Anterior Incisura
The Pituitary Gland
The Cavernous sinus
Structures passing over the Petrous Ridge

The Cerebellopontine Angle

This chapter is not intended to be a general review of neuroanatomy. It therefore contains some areas of particular relevance to neurosurgeons. Vascular neuroanatomy is covered in chapter 7.

The Scalp
The scalp consists of five layers. Fortunately for ease of memory these spell the word SCALP when arranged in order.

Skin
Connective tissue
Aponeurosis (galea aponeurotica)
Loose connective tissue
Pericranium

Skin. The skin of the scalp is usually hair bearing.
Connective tissue. The skin is supported by an underlying layer of dense connective tissue, which helps it withstand minor trauma. This layer contains the neurovascular plane of the scalp. The larger scalp vessels tend to be found just superficial to the aponeurosis. This is therefore a good place to search for scalp bleeders and to place haemostatic clips. Due to the

density of this layer, arterial contraction in response to section is inhibited and bleeding may be copious.

Galea aponeurotica. The aponeurosis is an expanded tendon which runs from the paired frontalis muscles anteriorly to the occipitalis muscles posteriorly. In neurosurgery, this aponeurosis is referred to as the galea. The galea provides the scalp with its tensile integrity and therefore is the most important layer to repair when closing the scalp to avoid dehiscence.

Loose connective tissue. This is below the galea. It acts like a bursa, allowing the aponeurosis to move over the pericranium. It is this layer which is opened when raising a scalp flap or if a patient is 'scalped' by trauma. As the vascular plane is superficial to the loose connective layer, the flap remains well supplied with blood.

Pericranium. The pericranium is the deepest layer. It is the periosteum of the bones of the skull. As such, it passes into the sutures and may be adherent at these points.

Muscles of the scalp

Frontalis muscle. This paired muscle attaches anteriorly to the facial muscles (corrugator supercilii and orbicularis oculi) and the skin of the forehead. Posteriorly its fascia is continuous with the galea. It thus sits between the two connective tissue layers of the scalp. When raising a frontal flap, the loose connective tissue layer is opened and *frontalis* is reflected with the flap. Innervation is by the temporal branch of the facial nerve. *Frontalis* is an important muscle of facial expression - it raises the ipsilateral eyebrow. Denervation gives an obvious cosmetic deformity.

Occipitalis muscle. The fascia of this muscle is also continuous with the galea. It inserts onto the highest nuchal line of the occiput and mastoid temporal bone. It provides countertraction to the frontalis muscle. Innervation is by the posterior auricular nerve.

Temporalis muscle. This muscle arises from a large area of the temporal fossa (although not the zygomatic part). The most superior point of attachment is the superior temporal line. This line runs in a smooth arc arising from just behind the anterior attachment of the zygomatic arch. The fibres run in a fan shape, converging into a tendon and passing under the zygomatic arch. Inferior attachment is to the coronoid process of the mandible and the anterior border of the mandibular ramus. *Temporalis* is enclosed within the thick temporalis fascia, which is immediately inferior to the galea. The fascia and the galea ought to be closed separately.

The action of *temporalis* is to elevate the mandible, closing the jaw. The most posterior portions of the muscle have fibres that are horisontal. These retract the jaw from protrusion. Lateral, grinding actions of the jaw are also executed by temporalis.

The fibres of *temporalis* pass immediately inferiorly from their attachments to the temporal bone. Thus, if the muscle is to be stripped from the bone (e.g. when forming a free bone flap for pterional craniotomy) it is much easier to strip upwards from the zygomatic arch towards the superior temporal line. This results in less trauma and so less bleeding.

Innervation is by deep temporal branches of the mandibular nerve (V)

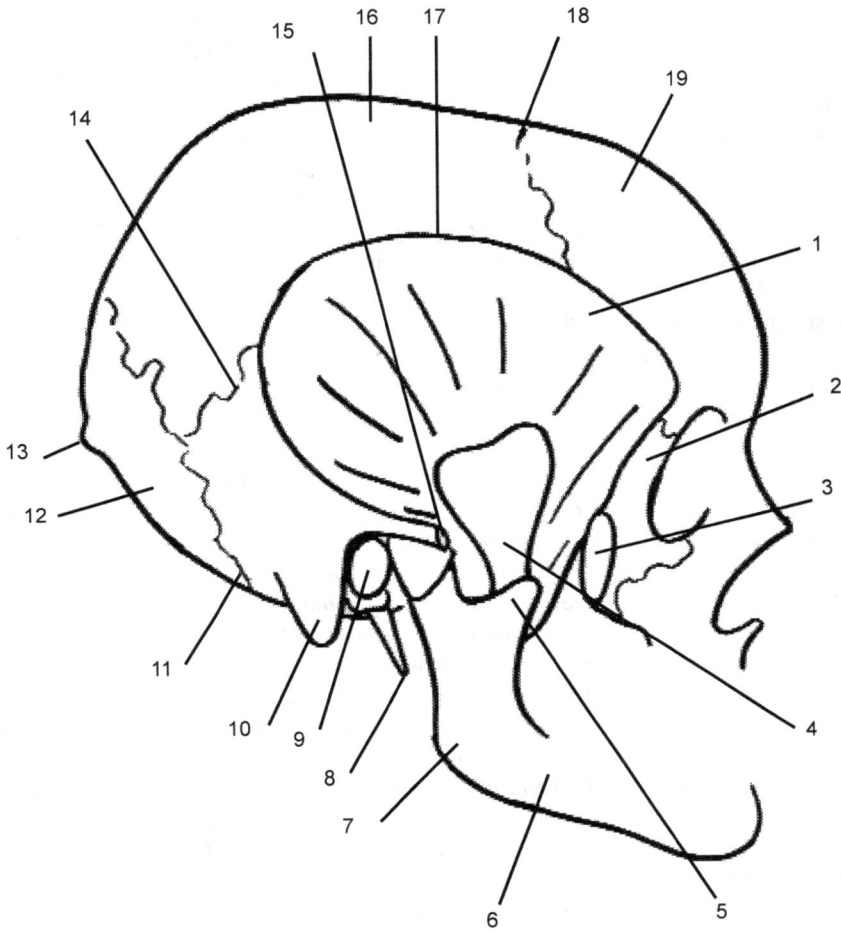

Figure 1. *Temporalis muscle. This is a lateral view of the skull. The zygomatic arch has been removed. 1. Fibres of temporalis muscle 2. Zygomatic bone 3. Cut end of temporal process of zygomatic bone 4. Tendon of temporalis muscle 5. Coronoid process of mandible 6. Mandible 7. Angle of mandible 8. Styloid process of temporal bone 9. External acoustic meatus 10. Mastoid process of temporal bone 11. Lambdoid suture 12. Occipital bone 13. External occipital protuberance 14. Temporoparietal suture 15 .Cut end of zygomatic process of temporal bone 16. Parietal bone 17. Superior temporal line 18. Coronal suture 19. Frontal bone*

Vessels of the scalp

The frontal portion of the scalp is supplied by the *supraorbital and supratrochlear arteries* as well as the *superficial temporal artery*. The *supraorbital and supratrochlear arteries* are branches of the *ophthalmic artery*. They exit the orbit superiorly and pass through the scalp to anastomose with the *superficial temporal artery*.

The side of the scalp is supplied by the *superficial temporal artery (STA)*. This is a terminal branch of the *external carotid artery*. It arises in the parotid gland and passes over the posterior root of the zygomatic arch before dividing into anterior and posterior branches to supply the scalp. The *STA* is palpable anterior to the tragus. The *STA* may be preserved by placing skin incisions immediately anterior to the tragus. Although preservation of the vessel is generally not vital, it is essential if subsequent *STA* bypass surgery may be required.

The posterior scalp supply is from the *occipital artery* (a branch of the *external carotid artery*) and the *occipital branch* of the *posterior auricular artery* (again from the *external carotid artery*). It is worth noting that the *posterior auricular artery* also supplies the facial nerve (via the stylomastoid artery) and that endovascular embolisation of meningiomas (with particles of less than 150μm in diameter) may result in a facial nerve palsy if the particles used scatter down the stylomastoid artery.

Veins of the scalp are named as for the arteries and follow a similar course. They drain into both the *internal* and *external jugular veins*. The scalp lymphatics run with the veins to the submental, submandibular, parotid, mastoid and occipital nodes.

Innervation of the scalp

The sensation of the scalp is supplied anteriorly by the *supraorbital* and *supratrochlear nerves*. These are the terminal branches of the *frontal nerve*, which is the largest branch of the *ophthalmic division* of the *trigeminal nerve*. Both the *supraorbital* and *supratrochlear nerves* arise within the orbit. They leave via the superior border of the orbit and pass towards the vertex. Sensory distribution is variable but the *trigeminal nerve* generally supplies the scalp almost as far back as the lambdoid suture. A bicoronal skin incision will therefore denervate a variable area of scalp behind the flap due to the section of these nerves.

Sensation to the posterior aspect of the scalp is via the *greater* and *lesser occipital nerves*, which are branches of the dorsal ramus of the second cervical nerve. Sensation to the lateral aspect is by *zygomaticotemporal nerve (V2)* and *auriculotemporal nerve (V3)*.

Motor supply of the frontalis muscle is via *temporal branch* of *facial nerve*. The main trunk of the facial nerve exits the cranial vault via the stylomastoid foramen, just behind the base of the styloid process. It then passes anteriorly to enter the parotid gland where it divides into its five branches. The main trunk and the lower four branches are all inferior to the zygomatic arch. The *temporal branch* crosses the arch and passes anteriorly and superiorly to *frontalis, orbicularis oculi* and *corrugator*.

Bones of the Cranial Vault

External aspect of the cranial vault

The bony casing of the brain consists of several bones, fused together by sutures. Anteriorly, the *frontal bone* forms the forehead. It passes posteriorly over the frontal lobes of the brain to the coronal suture, which is its border with the paired *parietal bones*. The *parietal bones* are separated in the midline by the sagittal suture. Posteriorly, the *parietal bones* terminate at the parieto-occipital suture, which is the boundary with the *occipital bone*. The parieto-occipital suture is often referred to as the lambdoid suture. The *occipital bone* passes round under the cerebellum to terminate against the *temporal* and *sphenoid bones*.

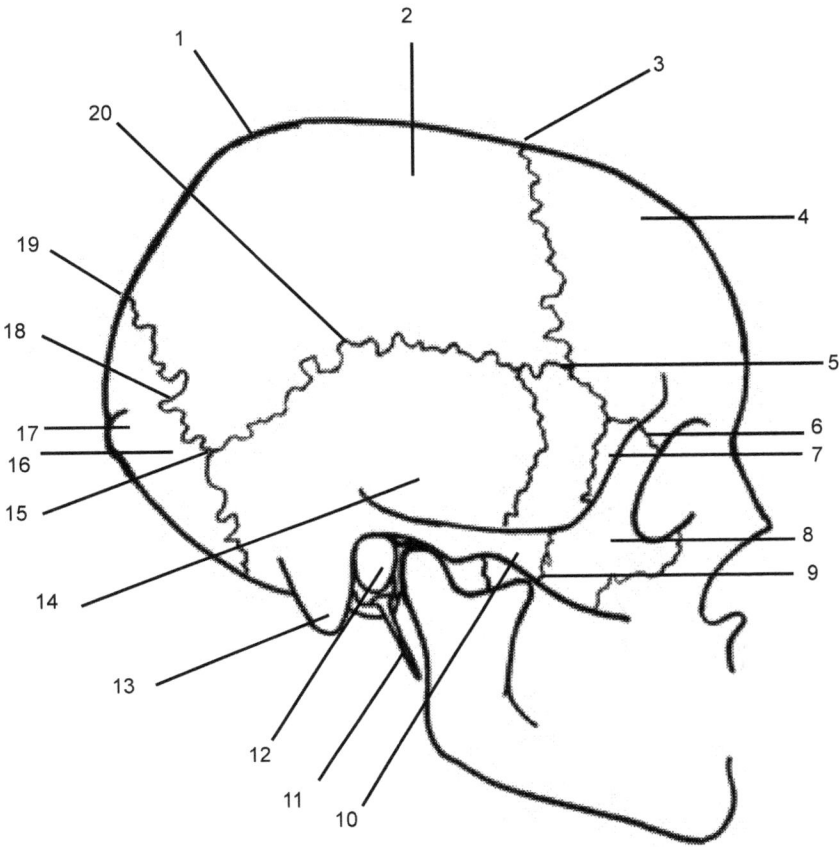

Figure 2. *The lateral aspect of the skull. 1 Vertex 2. Parietal bone 3. Bregma 4. Frontal bone 5. Pterion 6. Frontozygomatic suture 7. Zygomatic bone 8. Zygomatic bone 9. Temporozygomatic suture 10. Zygomatic arch 11. Styloid process of the temporal bone 12. External auditory meatus 13. Mastoid process of the temporal bone 14. Squamous temporal bone 15. Asterion 16. Occipital bone 17. Inion or external occipital protuberance 18. Lambdoid suture 19. Lambda 20. Temporoparietal suture*

Two other bones are visible on the external surface of the cranial vault. The *sphenoid bone* is composed of the greater and lesser wings and a central body. The lateral aspect of the greater wing is visible inferior to the *frontal* and *parietal bones*. Anteriorly is the *zygomatic bone* and posteriorly is the *squamous temporal bone*.

The *temporal bone* is visible on the lateral aspect of the vault. It consists of a thin, plate like squamous portion and a complex petrous part, which contains the apparatus of the middle ear and inner ear. The *squamous temporal bone* borders the *parietal bone* superiorly and the *sphenoid bone* anteriorly. Medially and posteriorly the *petrous temporal bone* borders the *occipital bone*. The zygomatic process of the *temporal bone* forms most of the zygomatic arch and joins with the zygomatic bone of the face anteriorly. The fibres of the temporalis muscle overlie the *squamous temporal bone* and the greater wing of the *sphenoid bone*. The *squamous temporal bone* is the thinnest part of the cranial vault. This region should be avoided when placing cranial fixation pins at surgery to avoid piercing the bone and damaging the underlying dura or even the middle meningeal artery.

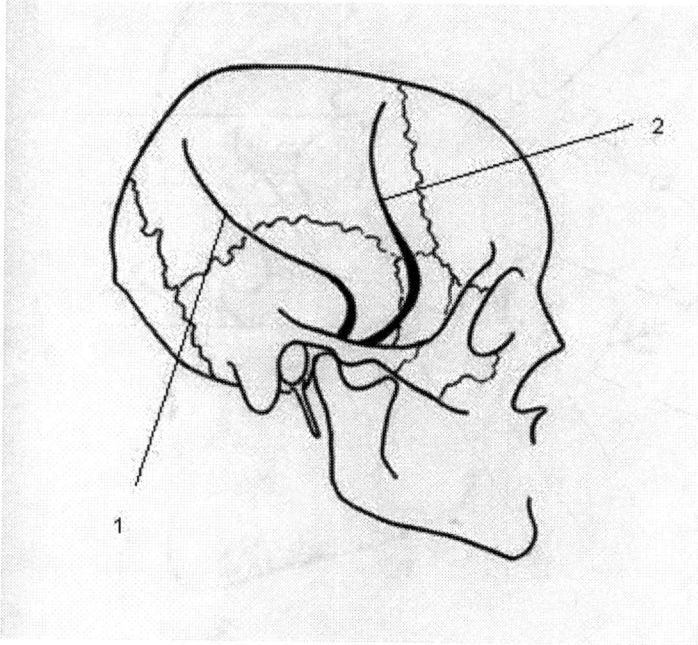

Figure 3a. *The middle meningeal artery. 1. Posterior branch of middle meningeal artery 2. Anterior branch of middle meningeal artery*

Important landmarks of the external aspect of the cranial vault

The structure of the sphenoid and temporal bones give rise to two further confluences of sutures. These are named the pterion and the asterion.

The pterion. This is the area in which the *frontal, sphenoid, parietal and temporal bones* meet. The *pterion* is one thumb's breadth behind the frontal process of the zygoma and two finger breadths above the zygomatic arch. It is related internally to the lateral aspect of the sphenoid wing and thus the Sylvian fissure also. The anterior branch of the *middle meningeal artery* passes in its groove behind the *pterion*. Pterional craniotomy and removal of the lateral aspect of the sphenoid wing allows access to the suprasellar CSF spaces via the Sylvian fissure.

The asterion. This is at the junction of the *parietal, occipital and temporal bones*. On the internal surface of the skull it is posterior and slightly inferior to the lateral extent of the petrous ridge. It is within the angle at which the *transverse sinus* meets the *superior petrosal sinus* and bends inferiorly, becoming the *sigmoid sinus*.

Inion. The *external occipital protuberance* of the *occipital bone* (also called the *inion*) is in the midline below the *lambda*. It overlies the *internal occipital protuberance* on the internal aspect of the *occipital bone*. The *inion* marks position of the *torcular* as well as the superior aspect of the posterior fossa in the midline.

The Keyhole. The keyhole is about 3cm anterior to the *pterion*, behind the most anterior point of attachment of the *temporalis muscle*. A burr hole at this point gives access to the lateral aspect of the floor of the anterior fossa. If placed to inferiorly, the burr hole will enter the orbit.

The external occipital protuberance. This raised hump or spur of bone is found in the midline on the *occipital bone*. It marks the location of the *internal occipital protuberance* on the internal aspect of the skull. The confluence of the dural sinuses (torcular) is situated against the *internal occipital protuberance*.

Other landmarks. The point at which the coronal sutures and the sagittal sutures meet is the *bregma*. There is another three-way confluence of sutures where the sagittal suture and parieto-occipital sutures meet. This is called the *lambda*.

Measured landmarks. A point halfway between the nasion and the inion will be about 2cm in front of the central sulcus. It will also be 2cm behind the *bregma*. The motor strip can therefore be avoided by staying anterior to the coronal suture. The Sylvian fissure is orientated towards a point three quarters of the way from the nasion to the inion.

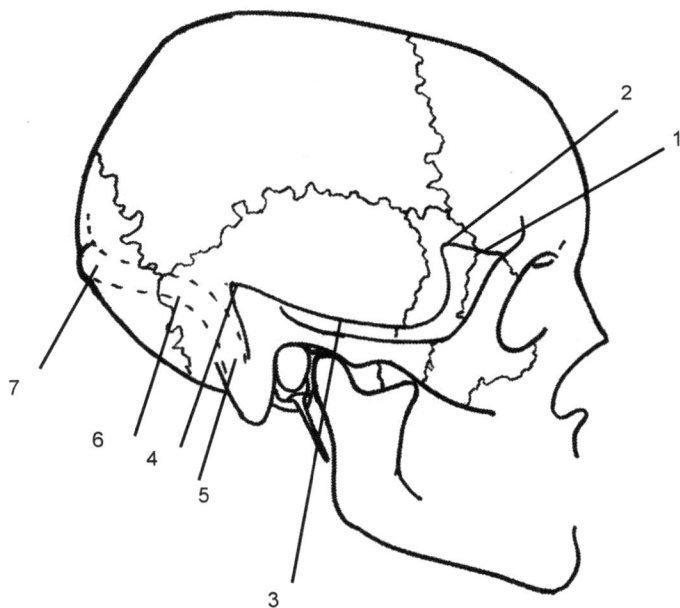

Figure 3b. *The lateral aspect of the skull base. 1. Floor of anterior fossa 2. Sphenoid wing 3. Floor of middle fossa 4. Petrous ridge 5. Torcular 6. Transverse sinus 7. Sigmoid sinus*

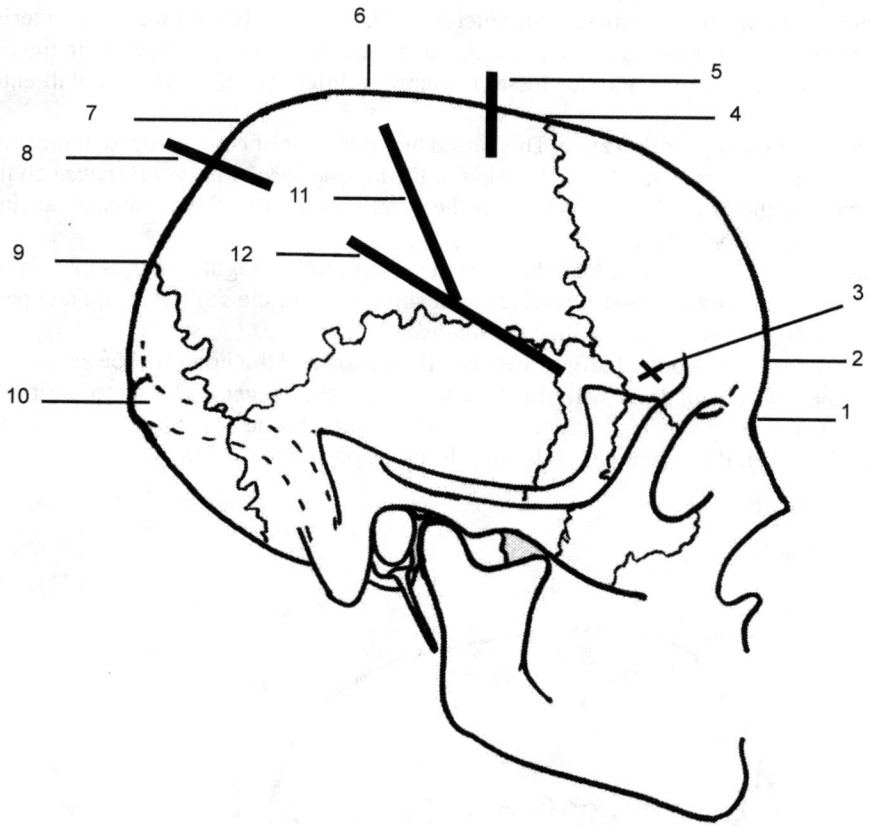

Figure 3c. *Surface markers. 1. Nasion 2. Glabella 3. Keyhole 4. Bregma 5. Midpoint between nasion and inion 6. 2cm posterior to midpoint 7. Vertex 8. Three quarters of the distance from the nasion to the inion 9. Lambda 10. Inion (external occipital protuberance) 11. Central sulcus 12. Sylvian fissure*

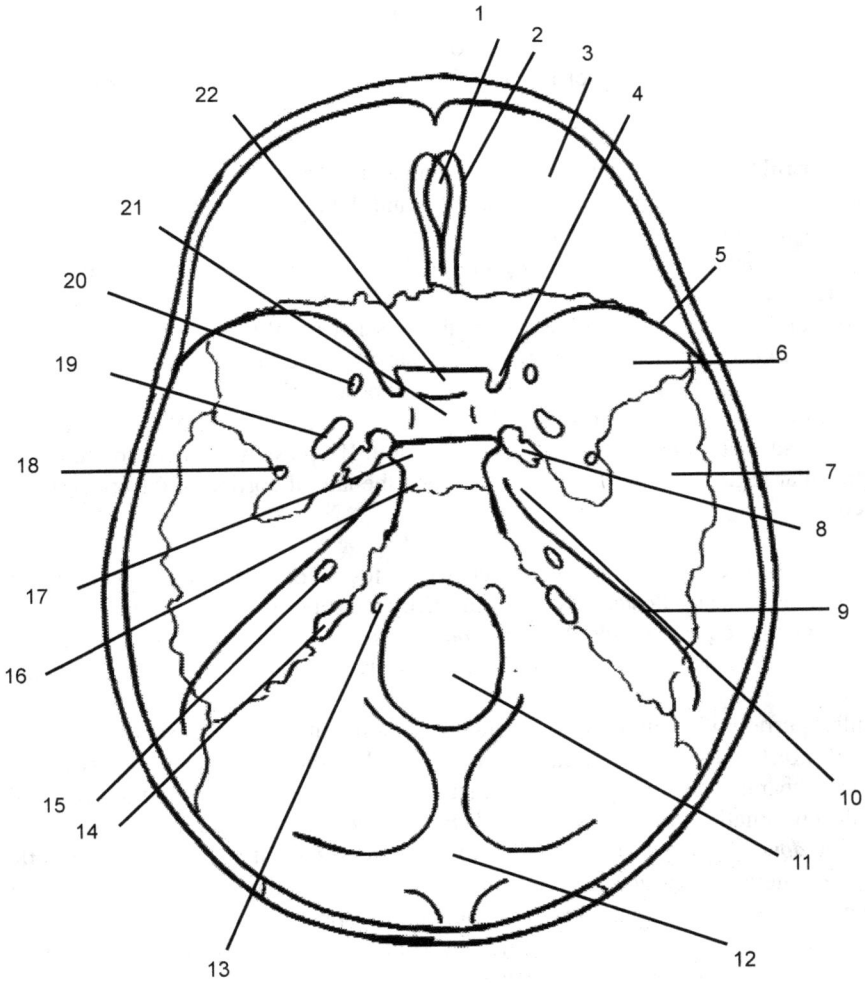

Figure 4. *Internal aspect of the skull base. 1.Crista galli (ethmoid) 2. Cribriform plate (ethmoid) 3. Floor of anterior fossa (frontal) 4. Anterior clinoid process (sphenoid) 5. Sphenoid wing 6. Floor of middle fossa (sphenoid) 7. Floor of middle fossa (temporal) 8. Foramen lacerum 9. Petrous ridge 10. Petrous apex 11. Foramen magnum 12. Internal occipital protuberance 13. Hypoglossal canal 14. Jugular foramen 15. Internal acoustic meatus 16. Clivus (basisphenoid) 17. Posterior clinoid process (sphenoid) 18. Foramen spinosum 19. Foramen ovale 20. Foramen rotundum 21. Pituitary fossa 22. Chiasmatic sulcus*

The internal aspect of the cranial vault.

The floor of the internal aspect of the cranial vault is referred to as the skull base. The skull base consists of three major concave areas on each side. These are called the anterior fossa, the middle fossa and the posterior fossa. It is important to note that each fossa is at a different level to those adjacent to it.

Anterior cranial fossa. The anterior fossa contains the frontal lobes of the brain. The anterior part is formed by the *frontal bone* laterally and the *ethmoid bone* medially. The *frontal bone* forms the roof of the orbit and the *ethmoid bone* the roof of the nasal cavity. The *ethmoid bone* contains the *cribriform plate* and the midline *crista galli*. Anterior to *crista galli* is the *foramen caecum*.

The posterior aspect of the fossa consists of the lesser wing of the *sphenoid bone*. The sphenoid wing marks the border between the anterior and middle fossae. The most medial part of the sphenoid wing gives rise to the anterior clinoid process. The sphenoid wing sits between the frontal lobe in the anterior fossa and the temporal lobe in the middle fossa. It terminates on the inner surface of the skull close to the pterion. If access is required to the contents of the suprasellar region via the Sylvian fissure then the lateral portion of the sphenoid wing is removed.

Middle cranial fossa. The anterior border of this fossa consists of the sphenoid wing and anterior clinoid process. Posteriorly, it is limited by the superior border of the *petrous temporal bone* (called the petrous ridge) and the *dorsum sellae* of the *sphenoid bone*. The floor is formed by the greater wing of the sphenoid anteriorly and the *petrous temporal bone* posteriorly.

The central portion of the middle fossa contains the structures of the dorsal aspect of the body of the *sphenoid bone*. The optic canal opens medial to the anterior clinoid. The two optic canals are separated by the chiasmatic sulcus (which does not contain the optic chiasm). Below the chiasmatic sulcus is the *tuberculum sella*. Next comes the pituitary fossa and, posteriorly, the *dorsum sellae*. The posterior clinoid processes are at the lateral extent of the *dorsum sellae*. Lateral to the *sella turcica* is a groove containing the *internal carotid artery*. The middle clinoid process is a raised area on the medial aspect of that groove.

The orbit is anterior to the middle fossa. They are connected by the superior orbital fissure, which is a large, oblique opening. Near the inferior extent of the superior orbital fissure is the round *foramen rotundum*. Continuing in a gentle curve, is the oval *foramen ovale* and then the *foramen spinosum*. The *foramen lacerum* is at the posterior end of the carotid groove. This foramen is unique in having a cartilaginous cuff, which is the source of skull base chondrosarcomas. Posterior and lateral to the *foramen lacerum*, on the medial aspect of the petrous ridge, is *Meckel's cave*.

Posterior cranial fossa. This portion of the skull base stretches from the petrous ridge and *dorsum sellae* to the back of the skull. At the *dorsum sellae*, the body of the sphenoid falls rapidly inferiorly before joining the *occipital bone*, which has risen to meet it. This sloping structure between the *dorsum sellae* and the *foramen magnum* is the clivus and it consists of the basisphenoid and the basiocciput. More laterally, the fossa consists of the remainder of the *petrous temporal bone* although the major part of the posterior fossa is formed by the occipital bone. Below the petrous ridge (lateral to Meckel's cave) is the internal auditory meatus. Further inferior is the *jugular foramen* (at the posterior end of the petro-occipital fissure) and then the hypoglossal canal and finally the *foramen magnum*.

The *transverse, sigmoid and inferior petrosal sinuses* form grooves in the inner surface of the posterior fossa. The internal *occipital protuberance* is situated in the midline of the occipital bone.

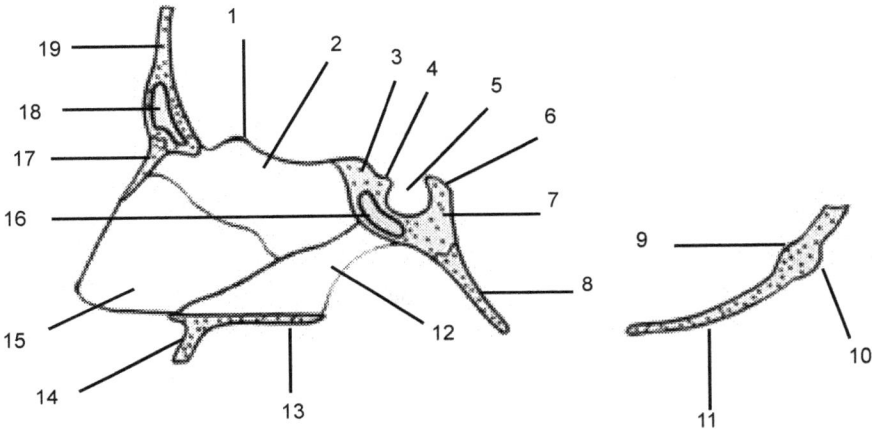

Figure 5. *Cross section of the skull base in the midsagittal plane. 1. Crista galli 2. Perpendicular plate of ethmoid 3. Chiasmatic sulcus 4. Tuberculum sellae 5. Pituitary fossa 6. Dorsum sellae 7. Basisphenoid 8. Basiocciput (7&8 make up clivus) 9. Internal occipital protuberance 10. External occipital protuberance 11. Occipital bone 12. Vomer 13. Palatine bone 14. Maxilla 15. Septal cartilage 16. Sphenoid sinus 17. Nasal bone 18. Frontal sinus 19. Frontal bone*

Anterior Fossa

Foramen caecum	Ethmoid	Empty/ draining vein from nasal mucosa that enters SSS
Cribriform plate	Ethmoid	Olfactory nerve

Middle Fossa

Optic canal	Sphenoid	Optic nerve
		Ophthalmic artery
		Central retinal vein
Superior orbital fissure	Sphenoid	Lacrimal nerve
		Frontal nerve
		Trochlear nerve
		Oculomotor nerve
		Nasociliary nerve
		Abducens nerve
		Ophthalmic veins
		Sympathetic fibres
Foramen rotundum	Sphenoid	Maxillary nerve
Foramen ovale	Sphenoid	Mandibular nerve
		Accessory meningeal artery
Foramen spinosum	Sphenoid	Middle meningeal artery and vein
		Meningeal branch of the mandibular nerve
Foramen lacerum		Meningeal branches of ascending pharyngeal artery
		Internal carotid artery
		Sympathetic nerves
		Deep and greater petrosal nerves/ nerve of pterygoid canal

Posterior fossa

Internal acoustic meatus	PT	Facial nerve
		Superior and inferior vestibular nerves
		Cochlear nerve
		Nervus intermedius
		Labarynthine vessels
Jugular foramen	PT/ Occipital	Glossopharyngeal nerve
		Sigmoid sinus/ internal jugular vein
		Accessory nerve
		Vagus nerve
Mastoid foramen	PT	Emissary vein
		Meningeal branch of occipital artery
Hypoglossal canal	Occipital	Hypoglossal nerve
Foramen magnum	Occipital	Medulla
		Meninges
		Vertebral arteries
		Anterior and posterior spinal arteries
		Spinal accessory nerve
		Sympathetic nerves

Table 1. *Foramina of the skull base and their contents. The second column denotes the bone which contains the foramen. PT - petrous temporal bone.*

The Cranial Meninges

The meninges are the membranous structures that surround the central nervous system. They have three layers. From outside to inside they are the dura mater, the arachnoid mater and the pia mater.

Dura mater. The dura is a tough, fibrous, membraneous covering. It consists of two layers. The outer layer is the internal periostium of the cranial vault. It therefore closely follows the contours of the internal surface of the vault and passes into the sutures to join the pericranium. As the body ages the outer layer of the dura becomes more adherent to the skull. The clinical implications of these anatomical features are listed below:

The pressure required to strip the dura from the skull is fairly high. As a result an extradur al haematoma that does so bulges. It is described as lentiform (lens shaped). Extradural haematomas are less common with age as the extradural space requires higher pressures to open it. Extradural haematomas rarely cross suture lines because of the passage of the dura into the suture, which restricts further spread. Extra care should be taken when performing craniotomies on older patients as tearing of the dura is more common.

The inner layer of the dura is generally fused to the outer layer. The two layers diverge in key places to form the venous sinuses and the deep extensions of the dura. These deep extensions form four septa that partially divide the cranial vault (see below).
The two layers of the dura are referred to as the pachymeninges

Arachnoid mater. The next meningeal layer is the delicate arachnoid mater. It is loosely applied to the surface of the brain but does not enter the sulci or fissures (except the inter-hemispheric fissure). The arachnoid has many folds that attach to nerves and vessels during their intradural course and to the underlying pia. These folds give the appearance of a spider's web. An important fold is *Liliequist's membrane*. This passes from the arachnoid covering of the posterior clinoid processes and *dorsum sellae* and joins the pia over the posterior edge of the *mamillary bodies*. It marks the divide between the supratentorial and infratentorial spaces anterior to the brainstem.
Between the dura and arachnoid is the subdural space. This is a potential space containing a film of serous fluid. Multiple bridging vessels cross the meninges. These may become stretched if the brain atrophies with age, leaving them prone to haemorrhage after minor trauma. This bleeding will occupy the subdural space. Only low pressures are required to open the subdural space. As a result, a subdural haematoma is convex, following the contour of the brain. It is unimpeded by the skull sutures but tends not to cross the falx or tentorium.
The subarachnoid space lies between the arachnoid mater and the pia mater. This contains CSF that has already left the ventricular system. At certain points there are large gaps between the arachnoid and the pia forming the CSF cisterns of the skull (and spinal cord). The major vessels of the circle of Willis are invested with arachnoid and run through the CSF cisterns of the suprasellar region. Haemorrhage from these vessels will therefore spread through the subarachnoid space.
Pia mater. The pia is also thin and delicate. It is the only layer to faithfully follow the surface of the brain, even so far as to pass down into the sulci. It also follows arteries as they pass into the brain parenchyma.

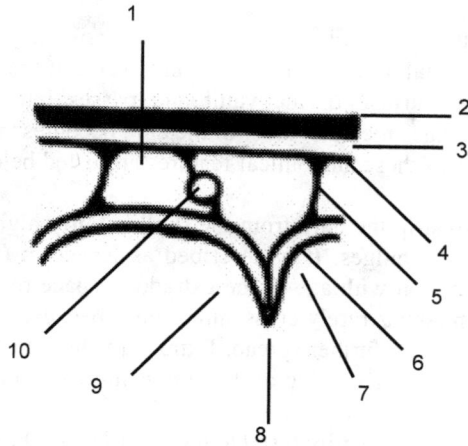

Figure 6. *Relationships of the meninges. 1. Subarachnoid space, containing CSF 2. Dura mater 3. Subdural space (potential space) 4. Arachnoid mater 5. Arachnoid trabecula 6. Pia mater 7. Brain 8. Sulcus 9. Gyrus 10. Vessel running in the subarachnoid space*

Septa of the Dura Mater and the Venous Sinuses

The dura forms four septa within the cranial vault

Falx cerebri. This sickle shaped dural fold projects vertically from the midline of the cranial vault. It sits between the cerebral hemispheres in the interhemispheric fissure. Anteriorly it is attached to the crista galli and is narrow. As it arches back through the cranial vault it becomes progressively broader before inserting into the midline of the tentorium cerebelli. The narrow anterior section of the falx is less able to prevent subfalcine herniation than the broader posterior section. This is why midline shift is more prominent anteriorly on CT scans. The falx is associated with the superior sagittal sinus above and the inferior sagittal sinus below. The straight sinus runs within the attachment of the falx and the tentorium.

Tentorium cerebelli. The tentorium or 'tent' stretches over the cerebellum, supporting the occipital lobes of the hemispheres. It divides the vault into the supratentorial and infratentorial spaces. Posteriorly, the tent is formed by dural reflections either side of the internal occipital protuberance and the transverse sulci of the occipital bone. Laterally it arises either side of the superior border of the petrous bone. Medially, the tentorium has a free edge. At its anterior extent, the free edge passes over the petrous apex to insert into the anterior clinoid process. The attached edge of the tent, by contrast makes a small leap from the petrous apex to attach to the posterior clinoid process (passing under the free edge in the process).

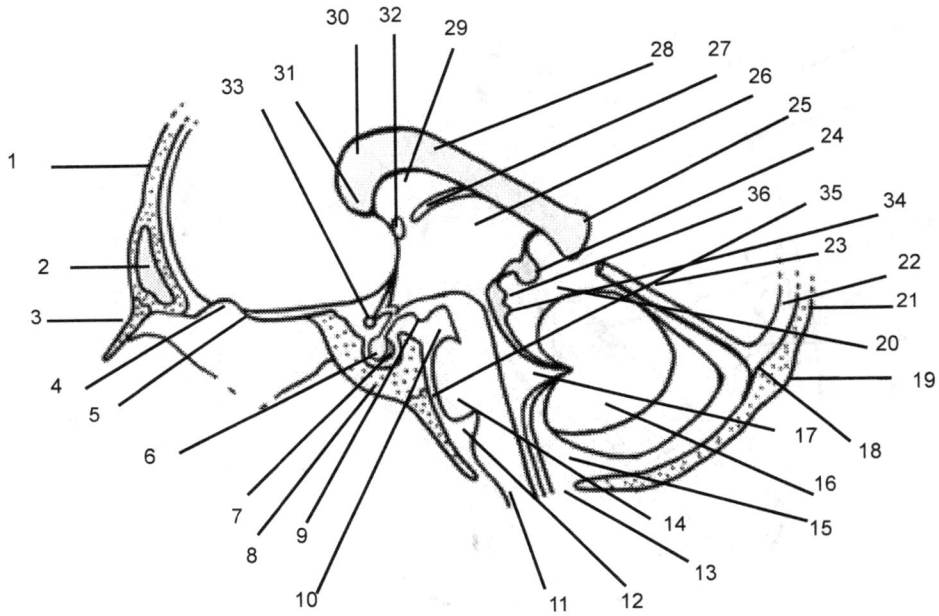

Figure 7. *Basal CSF cisterns. 1. Frontal bone 2. Frontal air sinus 3. Nasal bone 4. Crista galli 5. Floor of the anterior fossa 6. Anterior lobe of pituitary gland 7. Posterior lobe of pituitary 8. Sphenoid bone 9. Mamillary body 10. Interpeduncular cistern 11. Medulla oblongata 12. Pre medullary cistern 13. Foramen magnum14. Pons 15. Cisterna magna 16. Midsagittal section of the cerebellum 17. Fourth ventricle 18. Internal occipital protuberance 19. External occipital protuberance 20. Quadrigeminal cistern 21. Occipital bone 22. Terminal portion of superior sagittal sinus 23. Straight sinus 24. Pineal gland 25. Third ventricle 26. Splenium of corpus callosum 27. Fornix 28. Body of corpus callosum 29. Septum pellucidum 30. Genu of corpus callosum 31. Rostrum of corpus callosum 32. Anterior commissure 33. Optic chiasm 34. Inferior colliculus 35. Prepontine cistern 36. Superior colliculus*

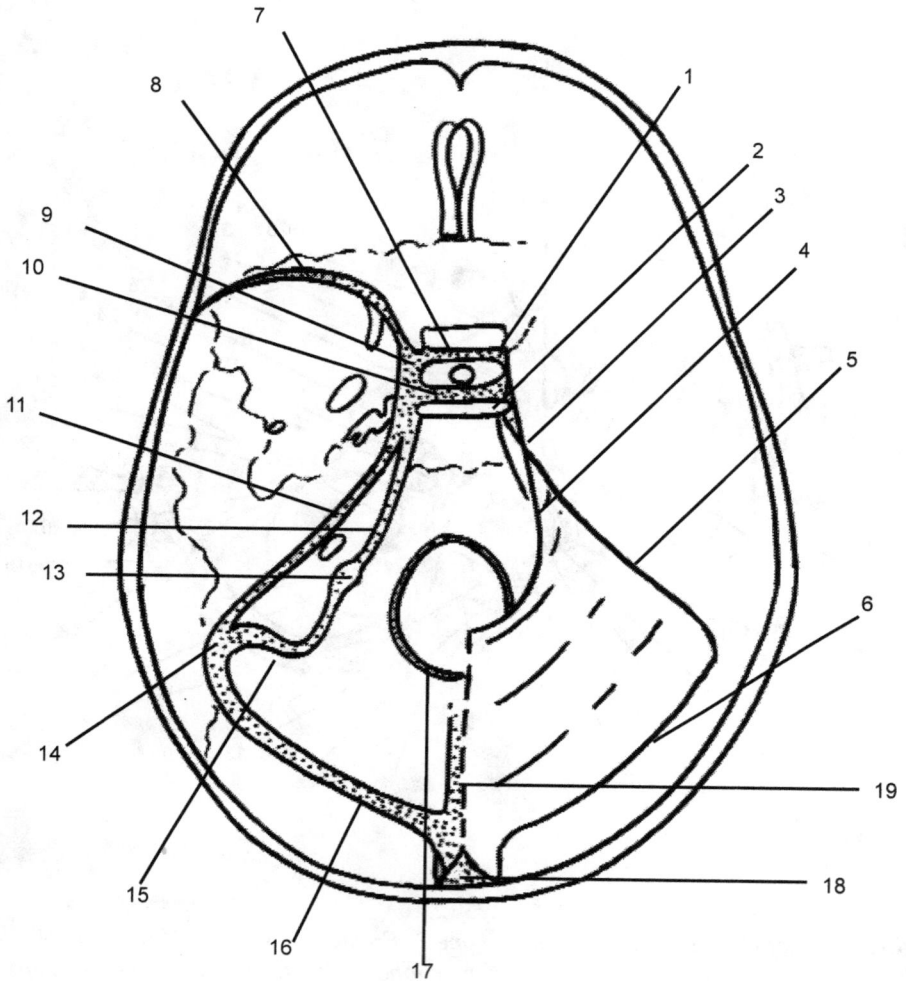

Figure 8. *Venous sinuses and tentorium cerebelli. 1. Attachment of free edge of the tentorium to the anterior clinoid 2. Attachment of the attached edge of the tentorium to the posterior clinoid 3. Free edge passing over the attached edge 4. Free edge of the tentorium 5. Tentorium adherent to the petrous ridge, forming the superior petrosal sinus*
6. Tentorium adherent to the inner table of the skull forming the transverse sinus 7. Anterior intercavernous sinus 8. Sphenoparietal sinus 9. Cavernous sinus 10. Posterior intercavernous sinus 11. Superior petrosal sinus 12. Inferior petrosal sinus 13. Jugular foramen 14. Junction of the transverse and sigmoid sinus 15. Sigmoid sinus
16. Transverse sinus 17. Marginal sinus 18. Cross section of the superior sagittal sinus 19. Straight sinus (running along midline of the tentorium)

The space left by the free edge of the tent is called the tentorial incisure. The midbrain sits in this space but is far too small to fill it. Thus there are CSF spaces anterior to and posterior to the midbrain. These are called the anterior and posterior tentorial incisura or the suprasellar and pineal regions.

The petrous apex contains an indentation for the trigeminal (Gasserian) ganglion called Meckel's cave. At this point the bottom layer of the tentorium passes anterolaterally under the superior petrosal sinus (which passes along the superior border of the petrous temporal bone). This forms a recess between the inner and outer layers of the dura, which contains the trigeminal ganglion. The torcular, transverse sinuses and superior petrosal sinuses are all contained in the tentorial attachment.

Falx cerebelli. This thin dural infolding attaches superiorly to the posterior part of the tentorium in the midline and posteriorly either side of the internal occipital crest. At its base runs the occipital sinus.

Diaphragma sellae. The diaphragma is a small disc of dura that stretches over the roof of the pituitary fossa, dividing the pituitary fossa and its contents from the suprasellar region. There is a midline aperture for the infundibulum of the pituitary gland. The dura also lines the inside of the pituitary fossa. Within the pituitary fossa, the meningeal layers are fused. Thus there is no visible arachnoid and no CSF within the pituitary fossa.

Superior sagittal sinus (SSS). The division of the two layers of the dura mater over the midline interhemispheric fissure, forming the falx, results in a triangular space at the base of the falx. This is the superior sagittal sinus.

The sinus begins just behind the frontal air sinuses (although there may be a connection with the nasal veins via the foramen caecum of the anterior fossa floor). Blood flows from anterior to posterior so the sinus gets larger as it progresses back towards its termination at the internal occipital protuberance. At the internal occipital protuberance it drains into the transverse sinus, via the torcular Herophili. The SSS may drain into either transverse sinus or both equally although most commonly it drains to the right. The SSS drains the convexities as well as the anterior part of the basal surface of the frontal lobe.

Drainage into the sinus is via a network of superficial cortical veins. These veins (referred to as bridging veins) either empty directly into the SSS or join a meningeal sinus before draining into the lateral angle of the SSS. Bridging veins rarely enter the SSS in the 4-6cm prior to its insertion into the torcular.

As well as the sinus, the midline space between the two dural layers contains venous lacunae, lateral to the sinus. These receive drainage mainly from the meningeal veins and are most prominent near the frontal and parietal lobes. The cortical veins typically pass beneath the lacunae. These lacunae increase in size with age.

Arachnoid granulations are protrusions of the arachnoid mater into the venous lacunae (less commonly they project into the superior sagittal sinus). They are also found in the other major sinuses.

Inferior sagittal sinus. The inner layer of the dura, which passes inferiorly, forming the lateral wall of the SSS and the falx, meets with its contralateral counterpart to form the free edge of the falx inferiorly. There is another sinus running in the free edge, called the inferior sagittal sinus. The sinus arises over the anterior part of the body of corpus callosum, enlarging as it goes and terminates on the straight sinus. Drainage anteriorly is from the falx, corpus callosum and cingulate gyrus. The main tributaries are the pericallosal veins.

Straight sinus. The straight sinus is formed by the union of the great vein of Galen and the inferior sagittal sinus. This occurs posterior to the splenium of corpus callosum. The sinus is straight and runs obliquely, inferiorly and posteriorly towards the torcular. It is contained within the attachment of the falx to the tentorium. At the torcular it may drain into either transverse sinus but most usually the left side.

Transverse sinus. These are paired structures arising at the torcular, which drain the superior and inferior sagittal sinuses and the straight sinus. They run in a cranial groove on the occipital bone and are formed by the division of the two dural layers to form the tentorium cerebelli. When the transverse sinus reaches the petrous ridge, it projects inferiorly as the sigmoid sinus. This is also the point at which the transverse sinus meets the superior petrosal sinus. Tributaries of the transverse sinus include the small tentorial sinuses, cortical veins from the lateral aspect of the temporal lobe (via the tentorial sinuses), emissary veins passing through the skull from the extracranial veins and the vein of Labbé.

Sigmoid sinus. The sigmoid sinus is the continuation of the transverse sinus after it has left the base of the tentorium. It follows an 'S' shaped course inferiorly, running in a groove on the mastoid temporal bone. The sinus terminates by exiting the jugular foramen and becoming the internal jugular vein. Along its course it receives emissary veins from the pericranial veins.

Superior petrosal sinus. This sinus is contained within the tentorial attachment to the petrous ridge. Laterally, it joins the transverse sinus at the posterior extent of the petrous ridge at the point where it becomes the sigmoid sinus. Medially it is continuous with the cavernous sinus. Drainage is from the brainstem and cerebellum.

Inferior petrosal sinus. These drain the cavernous sinuses directly to the internal jugular vein. They pass either side of the clivus, running along the suture between the petrous temporal bone and the occipital bone.

Cavernous sinus. These are paired structures, situated either side of the sella turcica. They are connected across the midline by the anterior and posterior intercavernous sinuses. Anterior inflow is via the sphenoparietal sinus and ophthalmic veins. Posterior drainage is into the basilar sinus then the superior and inferior petrosal sinuses.

The inside dura of the floor of the middle cranial fossa ascends to form the lateral wall of the cavernous sinus. This fold passes up until it joins the anterior section of the free edge of the tentorium (on its way to the anterior clinoid). At the free edge it projects medially to form the roof of the cavernous sinus. At its medial extent it is continuous with the diaphragma sellae.

External bony landmarks of the dural venous sinuses

In order to avoid tearing the sinuses with the craniotome it is important to know where they are likely to be before opening the skull.

The superior sagittal sinus is marked by the sagittal suture for the middle portion of its course. Extrapolation of this line to behind the frontal sinuses anteriorly and to the external occipital protuberance posteriorly gives the remainder of the course. Associated venous lacunae can bleed heavily and may be 2cm from the midline. Wider lacunae are more common in the elderly.

The torcular sits over the internal occipital protuberance, which is marked externally by the external occipital protuberance.

The transverse sinus runs in a straight line from the external occipital protuberance towards the root of the temporal zygomatic process. A landmark for the lateral extent of the transverse sinus is the mastoid groove, which is palpable behind the external acoustic meatus. The sigmoid sinus then passes inferiorly beneath the posterior part of the mastoid process.

The retrosigmoid approach to the cerebellopontine angle requires good lateral exposure and therefore should involve the asterion, extending into the angle of the transverse and sigmoid sinuses.

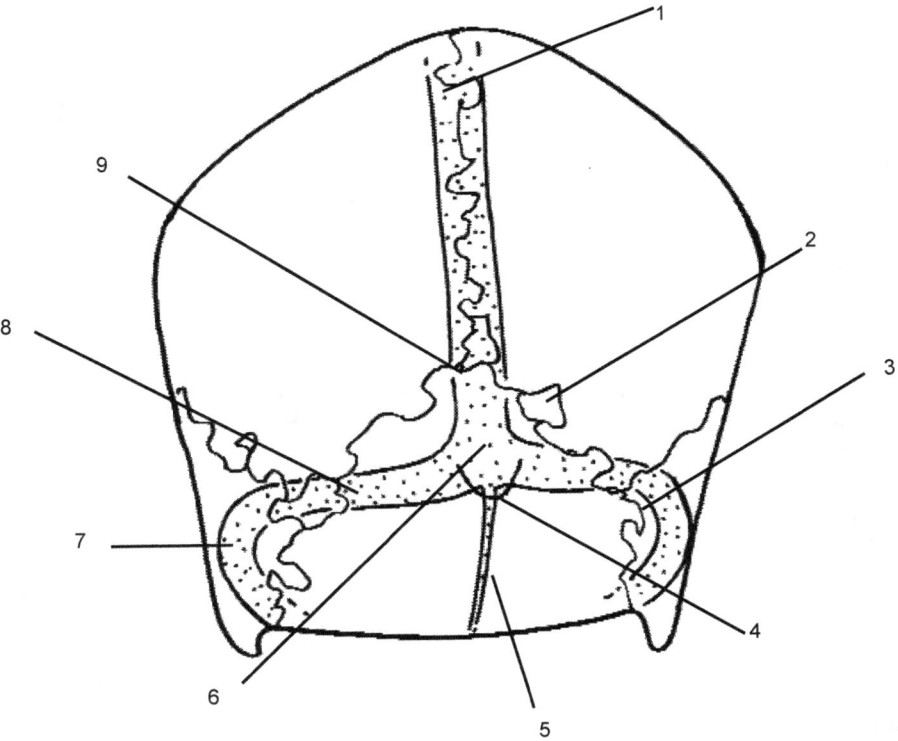

Figure 9. *External markings of the major posterior fossa sinuses. 1. Superior sagittal sinus 2. Interparietal bone (os incae) 3. Lambdoid suture 4. External occiptal protuberance 5. Occipital sinus 6. Torcula 7. Sigmoid sinus 8. Transverse sinus 9. Lambda*

Blood supply to the dura

Arteries to the dura are numerous, giving it an excellent blood supply. By far the most relevant is the *middle meningeal artery*. This vessel arises from the *maxillary branch* of the *external carotid artery* and enters the cranial vault via the foramen spinosum of the middle cranial fossa floor. As it runs over the surface of the dura (in the extradural space) it may sit in a bony sulcus. The artery divides into *anterior and posterior branches*.

The *anterior branch* sits behind the pterion and is a common source of bleeding at pterional craniotomy. Fractures of the thin squamous temporal bone may tear the *middle meningeal artery*. Contraction of the vessel in response to damage is inhibited by the bony sulcus. The resultant haemorrhage pushes the temporal lobe medially causing uncal herniation.

Innervation of the dura

The dura is innervated by all three branches of the *trigeminal nerve,* the first three *cervical spinal nerves* and the *cervical sympathetic trunk*. The role of sympathetic outflow is unknown but may be related to autoregulation of cerebral blood flow. Sensory nerves mediate the pain of meningeal irritation e.g. due to meningitis or subarachnoid haemorrhage.

The Surfaces of the Brain

Surface Anatomy of the Cerebral Lobes.

The frontal lobe.

The frontal lobe extends from the frontal pole anteriorly to the central sulcus at its posterior extreme. The lateral aspect is divided from the medial face by the superior hemispheric border. It consists of four principle gyri. The most posterior is the *precentral gyrus*, which runs parallel to the central sulcus. This gyrus passes over the superior hemispheric border onto the medial aspect of the lobe and reaches the Sylvian fissure laterally. In front of the *precentral gyrus* is the *precentral sulcus*. This sulcus divides the *precentral sulcus* from the three *horizontal gyri* that form the remainder of the lateral surface. These gyri run parallel to the superior hemispheric border and are called the *superior, middle and inferior frontal gyri*. They are divided by the *superior and inferior frontal sulci*. The *inferior frontal gyrus* abuts the Sylvian fissure. The *superior frontal gyrus* wraps around the superior hemispheric border to from the superior portion of the medial aspect of the lobe.

The medial aspect of the frontal lobe will be described alongside that of the parietal lobe.

The parietal lobe.

The lateral surface of the parietal lobe is divided into three major areas. The first is the *postcentral gyrus*, which runs parallel to the *central sulcus*. It is divided from the rest of the lobe by the *postcentral sulcus*. Posterior to the *postcentral sulcus* the lobe is divided into *superior and inferior lobules* by the *intraparietal sulcus*, which passes horisontally across the lobe. The *superior parietal lobule* is the area between the *intraparietal sulcus* and the superior hemispheric border.

The *inferior parietal lobule* contains the *supramarginal gyrus* anteriorly and the *angular gyrus*. The *supramarginal gyrus* wraps around the posterior extreme of the, and is continuous with, the *superior temporal gyrus*. The *angular gyrus* is posterior to the *supramarginal gyrus* and arches over the posterior extreme of the superior temporal sulcus, which turns upwards as it terminates.

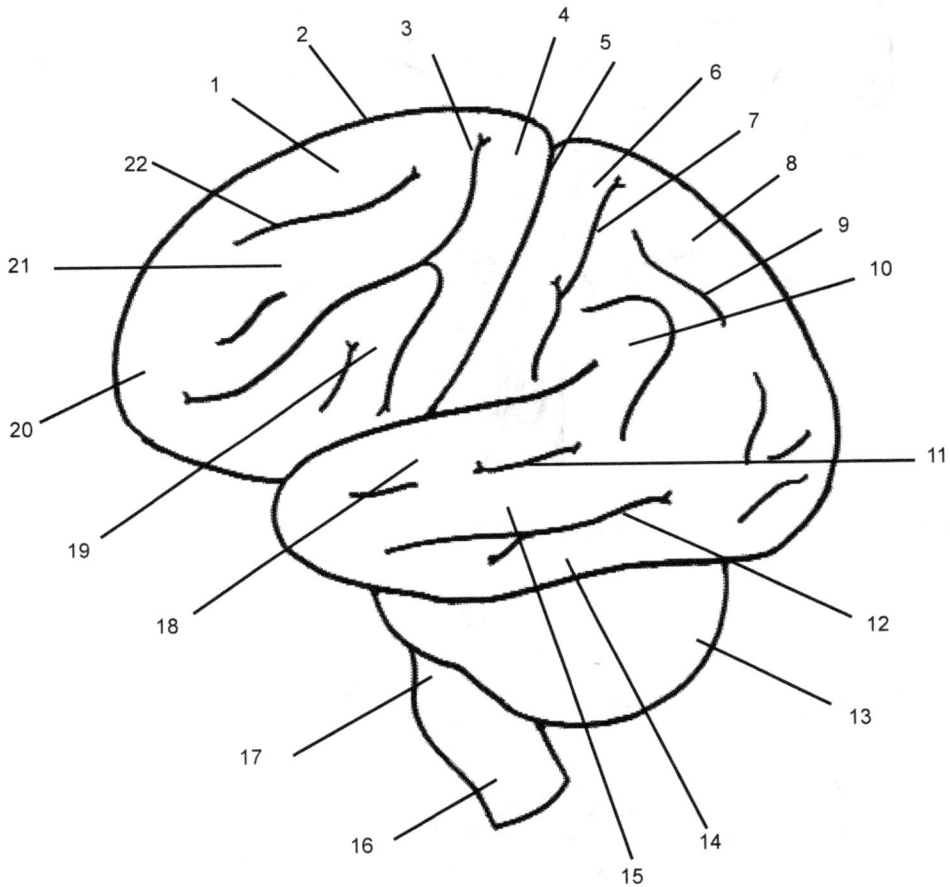

Figure 10 a. *Lateral aspect of the cerebral hemispheres. 1. Superior frontal gyrus 2. Superior hemispheric border 3. Precentral sulcus 4. Precentral gyrus 5. Central sulcus 6. Postcentral gyrus 7. Postcentral sulcus 8. Superior parietal lobule 9. Intraparietal sulcus 10. Supramarginal gyrus 11. Superior temporal sulcus 12. Inferior parietal sulcus 13. Cerebellum 14. Inferior temporal gyrus 15. Middle temporal gyrus 16. Medulla oblongata 17. Pons 18. Superior temporal gyrus 19. Inferior frontal gyrus 20. Frontal pole 21. Middle frontal gyrus 22. Superior frontal sulcus*

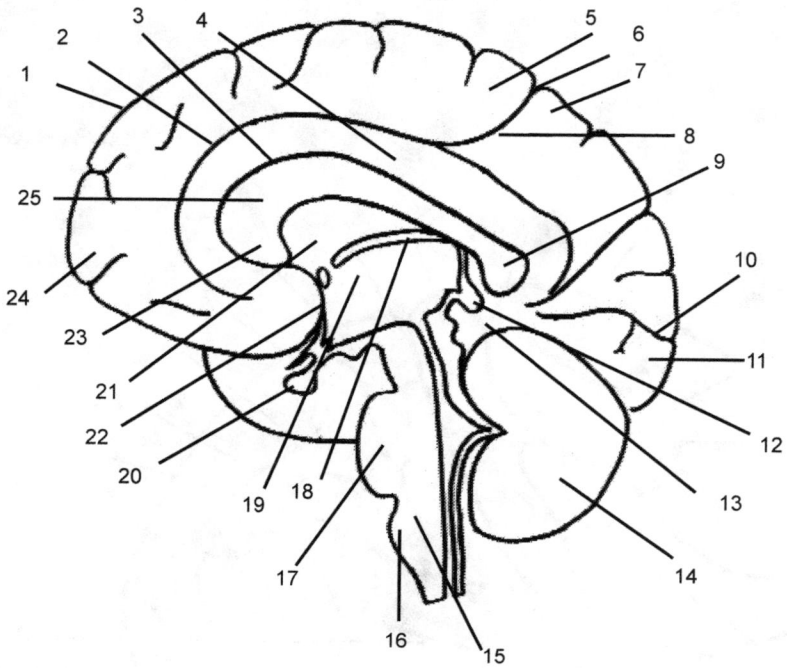

Figure 10b. *See legend on opposite page*

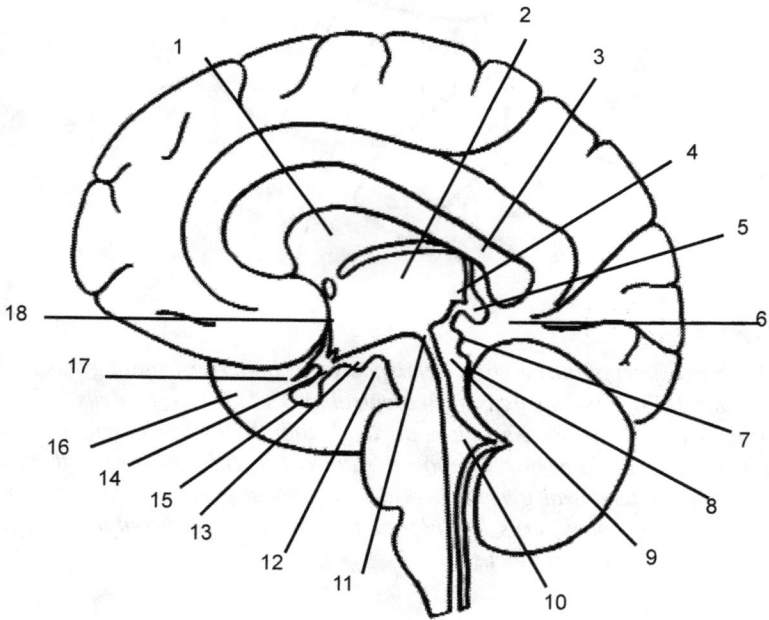

Figure 10c. *See legend on opposite page*

Figure 10b. *Medial brain structures. 1. Superior hemispheric border 2. Cingulated sulcus 3. Sulcus of the corpus callosum 4. Body of the corpus callosum 5. Precentral gyrus 6. Central sulcus 7. Postcentral gyrus 8. Pars marginalis 9. Splenium of corpus callosum 10. Calcarine fissure 11. Occipital pole (primary visual cortex) 12. Pineal gland 13. Quadrigeminal cistern 14. Cerebellum 15. Medulla oblongata 16. Pontomedullary sulcus 17. Pons 18. Fornix 19. Third ventricle 20. Pituitary gland 21. Septum pellucidum 22. Lamina terminalis 23. Rostrum of corpus callosum 24. Frontal pole 25. Genu of corpus callosum*

Figure 10c. *Medial brain structures. 1. Septum pellucidum 2. Third ventricle 3. Corpus callosum 4. Pineal recess 5. Pineal gland 6. Quadrigeminal cistern 7. Superior colliculus 8. Inferior colliculus 9. Tectal plate 10. Fourth ventricle 11. Aqueduct of Sylvius 12. Interpeduncular cistern 13. Mamillary bodies 14. Tuber cinereum 15. Pituitary gland 16. Temporal lobe 17. Optic chiasm 18. Lamina terminalis*

The medial surfaces of the frontal and parietal lobes share characteristics. Both face the falx and terminate inferiorly at the corpus callosum, from which they are divided by the *callosal sulcus*. The *cingulate gyrus* arises in the frontal lobe inferior to the rostrum of the corpus callosum and curves round the corpus callosum to pass behind the splenium and terminate as a narrow bridge (the isthmus of the cingulate gyrus) connecting with the *parahippocampal gyrus* of the temporal lobe. The *cingulate gyrus* is seperated from the *superior gyri* by the *cingulate sulcus*. This sulcus gives off a consistent ramus superiorly, termed the *marginal ramus*.

The remainder of the medial side of the frontal lobe consists of the *superior frontal gyrus*, which folds over the superior hemispheric border, and the *paracentral lobule*. The *paracentral lobule* is the medial fold of the *pre- and postcentral gyri*, which also fold over the superior hemispheric border. The posterior part of the *paracentral lobule* is in the parietal lobe. The *marginal ramus* passes posterior to the *paracentral lobule*. It can be seen on MRI and is an important radiological landmark for identification of the central sulcus. Posterior to the *marginal ramus* is the *precuneus*, which occupies the space between the *cingulate gyrus* inferiorly, the superior hemispheric border superiorly and the *parieto-occipital sulcus* posteriorly.

The occipital lobe.
On its lateral surface, the occipital lobe is separated from the parietal and temporal lobes by an imaginary line extending from the *preoccipital notch* to the superior extent of the *parieto-occipital sulcus*. The gyri and sulci in this area show considerable anatomical variability. The most consistent feature is the *lateral occipital sulcus*, which divides the *superior and inferior occipital gyri*. The most important feature of the medial aspect of the occipital lobe is the *calcarine fissure*. It runs anteriorly from the occipital pole towards the splenium of the corpus callosum at about 45 degrees.

The temporal lobe.
The lateral surface of the temporal lobe is separated from the anterior portion of the parietal lobe and the frontal lobe by the *Sylvian fissure*. Posteriorly it is separated from the parietal lobe by a line representing a continuation of the *Sylvian fissure*, called the extended Sylvian line. The lateral surface contains three gyri: the *superior, middle and inferior temporal gyri*.

51

These run parallel to the *Sylvian fissure* and are separated by the *superior and inferior temporal sulci*. The *superior temporal gyrus* is continuous medially with the *transverse temporal gyri* of the *Sylvian fissure* and posteriorly with the a*ngular gyrus*. The *middle temporal gyrus* overlies the temporal horn of the lateral ventricle as well as the *crural and ambient cisterns*.

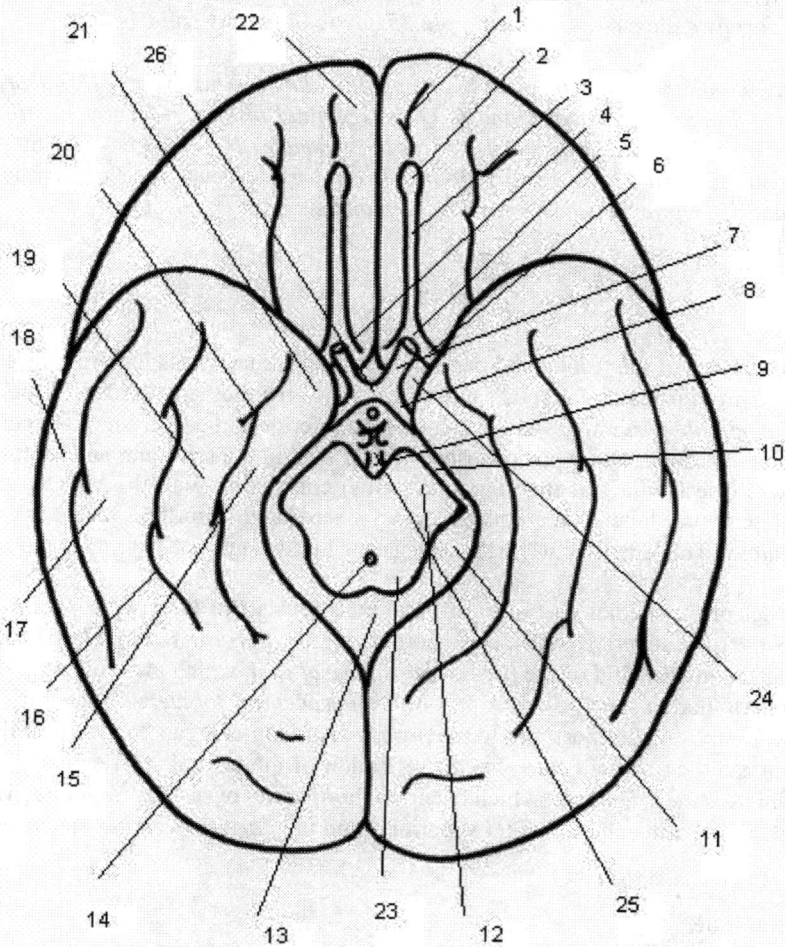

Figure 11d. *Basal aspect of the cerebral hemispheres. 1. Olfactory sulcus 2. Olfactory bulb 3. Olfactory tract 4. Medial olfactory stria 5. Olfactory nerve 6. Lateral olfactory stria 7. Optic nerve (cut) 8. Optic tract 9. Interpeduncular cistern 10. Crural cistern 11. Ambient cistern 12. Midbrain (basis pendunculi) 13. Quadrigeminal cistern 14. Aqueduct of Sylvius 15. Parahippocampal gyrus 16. Occipitotemporal sulcus 17. Temporal lobe 18. Inferior temporal gyrus 19. Occipitotemporal gyrus 20. Collateral sulcus 21. Uncus 22. Gyrus rectus 23. Left superior colliculus 24. Anterior perforated substance 25. Posterior perforated substance 26. Optic chiasm*

The Sylvian fissure, insula and operculum

The *Sylvian fissure* is not simply a cleft in the side of the brain. The superficial part begins near the anterior clinoid process of the skull base and passes along the sphenoid ridge, separating the frontal and temporal lobes. Behind the pterion it passes posteriorly and superiorly along the lateral aspect of the hemisphere to separate the parietal and temporal lobes before turning upwards into the *supramarginal gyrus*.

Deeper within the hemisphere is the *Sylvian cistern*, which is divided into the sphenoidal and operculoinsular compartments. The sphenoidal segment is the section of the fissure that separates the anterior temporal lobe entirely from the frontal lobe. It arises basally from the *carotid cistern*. Thus the fissure emerges on both the basal and lateral aspects of the hemisphere.

The operculoinsular compartment is formed of two clefts. The opercular cleft is between the cortex of the frontal and parietal lobes above and the temporal lobe below. The floor of the cleft includes Heschl's gyrus (the site of the primary auditory cortex).

At the base of the opercular cleft is the insular compartment. As the cortex of the roof and floor of the opercular cleft run medially they again reflect, this time to be face to face with the insula, which they then turn towards and form. The insular compartment therefore has a superior and a posterior limb.

The insula is continuous with the frontal, parietal and temporal lobes. It is delineated by the *circular sulcus*. It is triangular in shape with its anterior apex at the limen insula (a process overlying the uncinate fasciculus). The putamen lies deep to the insula.

Important cortical regions.
The motor strip contains the premotor cortical areas and the primary motor cortex.

The primary motor cortex occupies the posterior aspect of the *precentral gyrus* laterally and the full width of the gyrus medially. It folds around the superior hemispheric border medially and extends inferiorly to the *cingulate sulcus*. The organisation of the *primary motor cortex* is somatotopic: different areas of cortex are associated with different body parts. Those body areas that are involved in fine movement, such as the hand and face, have a correspondingly larger area of cortex ascribed to them. The representation of the body in the motor cortex is called the motor homunculus. Beginning at the inferior aspect of the medial end of the primary cortex and progressing laterally the arrangement is: lower limb (medial aspect and superior hemispheric border), trunk, upper limb, hand, face and mouth (close to the Sylvian fissure) then tongue and larynx.

There are two important consequences of this arrangement. Different areas of motor cortex are supplied by different arteries and so ischaemic strokes will lead to predictable patterns of weakness. The *anterior cerebral artery* supplies the medial aspect and the superior portion of the convexity. The remainder is supplied by the *middle cerebral artery*. The other consequence is that different areas of the homunculus contribute to different output projections.

The premotor areas consist of the premotor cortex, supplementary motor area and cingulate motor area. The premotor cortex and supplementary area are within the anterior part of the *precentral gyrus* on the frontal convexity laterally but spread further anteriorly at their medial extent. The premotor area is more lateral than the supplementary motor area. The supplementary motor area stretches from the medial aspect of the frontal convexity and folds round the superior horisontal border to occupy part of the medial aspect of the frontal lobe as far inferiorly as the cingulate motor area. The cingulate motor area is a thin strip between the inferior aspect of the supplementary motor cortex and the cingulate sulcus.

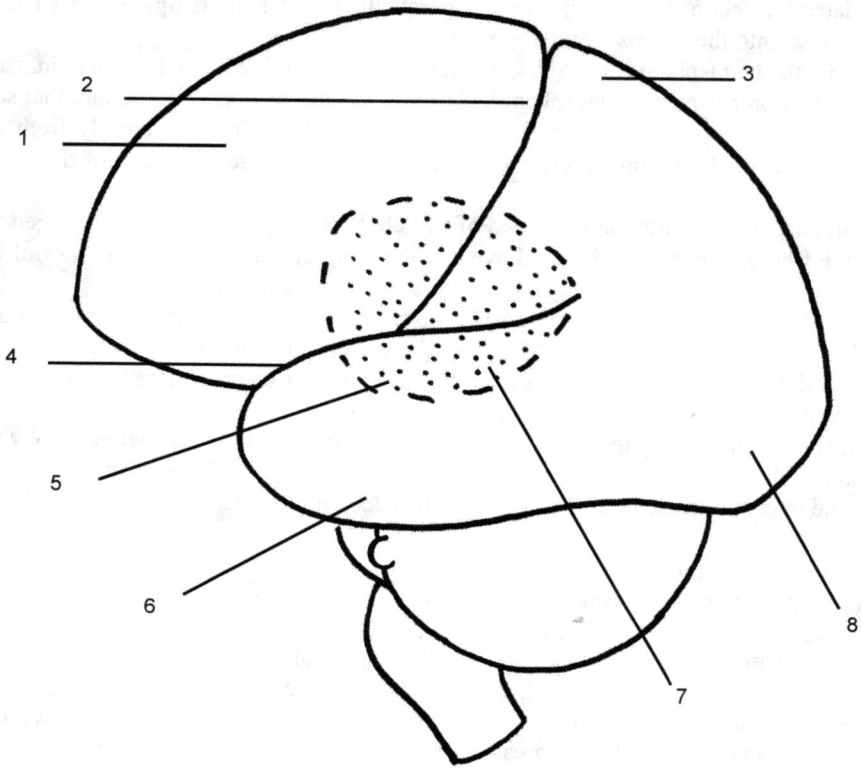

Figure 12. *Insula (deep to the lateral aspect of cortex). 1. Frontal lobe 2. Central sulcus 3. Parietal lobe 4. Sylvian fissure 5. Insula 6. Temporal lobe 7. Circular sulcus 8. Occipital lobe*

The primary visual cortex is situated predominantly in the calcarine fissure of the temporal lobe. It also extends posteriorly onto the occipital pole. The primary visual cortex contains a map of the retina. The occipital pole and posterior aspect of the *calcarine fissure* process information from the macula, more anteriorly are the perimacular regions, then, at the anterior aspect of the fissure lies the peripheral field representation. The superior lip of the *calcarine fissure* represents the inferior portion of the field and vice versa. Surrounding the primary visual cortex are the visual association areas.

The speech area of *Broca* has been linked to articulation of speech and to semantic processing. Semantic processing has been linked to the upper portion of the area and articulation in the center of Broca's area. Broca's area controls not only spoken, but also written and signed language production. *Wernicke's* area is a semantic processing area and is most often associated with language comprehension, or processing of incoming language written as well as spoken. Structures around the sylvian fissure mediate auditory language repetition. Auditory signals are processed by Heschl's gyrus (primary auditory cortex), and analysis takes place in the adjacent auditory association cortex (Wernicke's area).

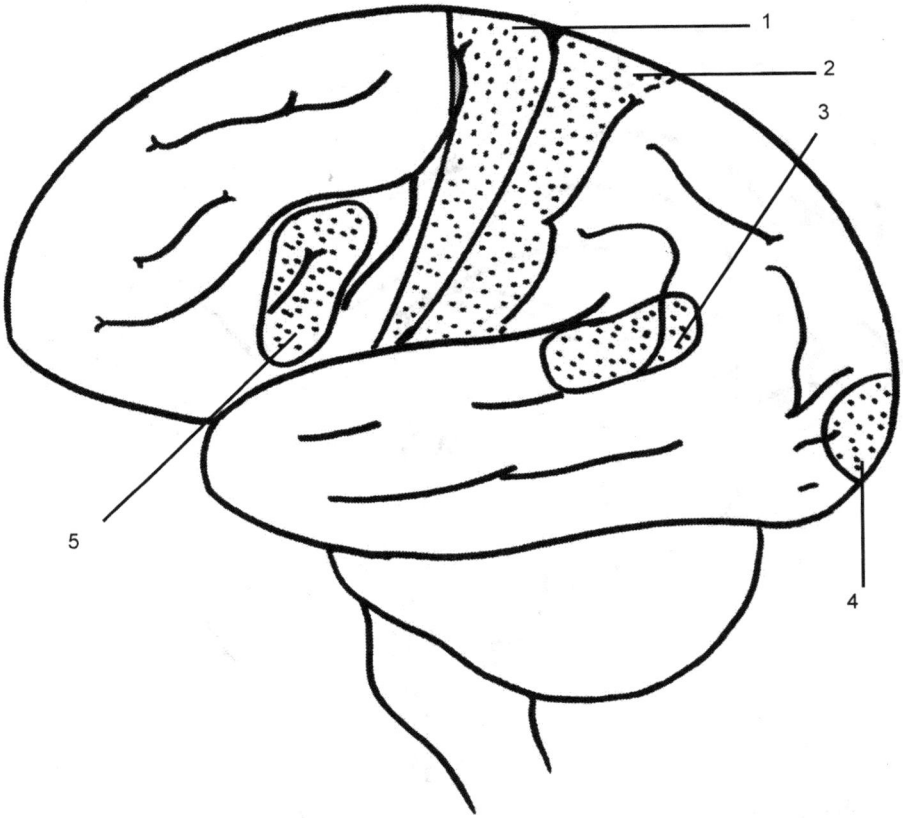

Figure 12 . *Important areas of the lateral cortex. 1. Motor cortex 2. Somatosensory cortex 3. Wernicke's area 4. Visual cortex 5. Broca's area*

Anterior regions encode speech (Broca's area and others), and these regions direct the motor cortex adjacent to produce the movements needed to produce speech. The hallmark of peri-sylvian damage is impaired speech repetition. Language comprehension is completed by communication of the analysed information with association areas like the angular gyrus.

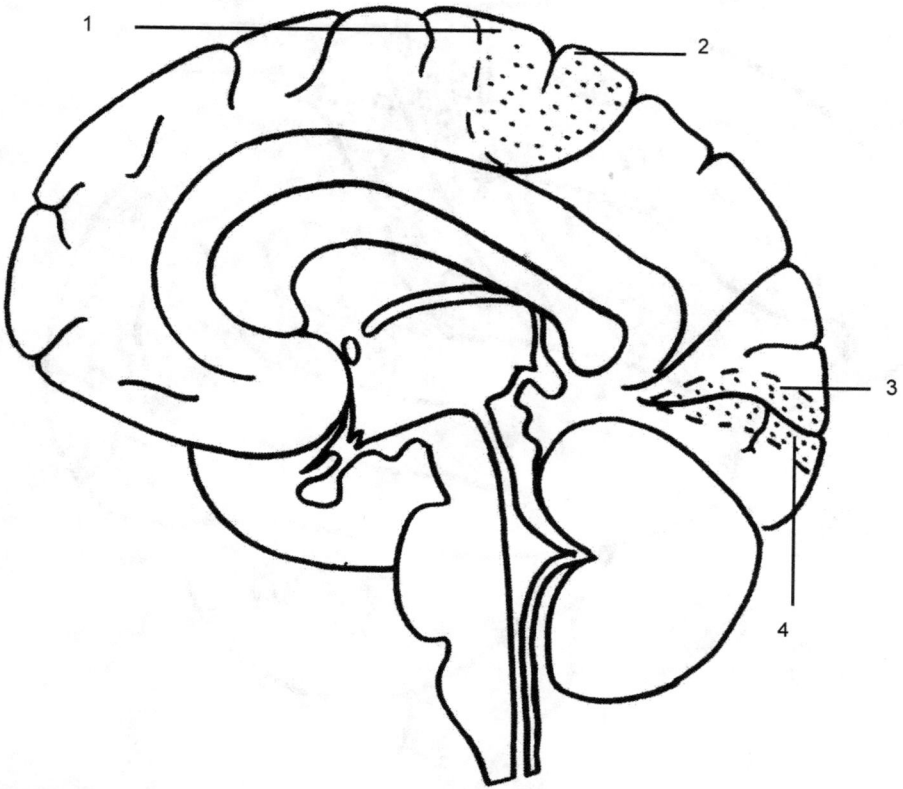

Figure 13. *Important areas of the medial cortex 1. Motor cortex 2. Somatosensory cortex 3. Visual cortex (macula region) 4. Visual cortex (perimacula region)*

Surface anatomy of the brainstem.

The brainstem consists of the midbrain, pons and medulla oblongata.

The midbrain is the junction between the cerebral hemispheres and the pons. Posteriorly, the four bulges of the *colliculi* are the most obvious feature. The *superior colliculi* are uppermost. They receive projections from most sensory modalities via the brachium of the *superior colliculus*, which is seen laterally. Below are the *inferior colliculi* and their brachia. The four colliculi make up the *tectal plate* of the midbrain, which sits posterior to the *aqueduct of Sylvius*. Lateral to the colliculi is the *pulvinar* of the *thalamus* and its associated *medial and lateral geniculate bodies*. The *pineal gland* sits between the *superior colliculi*. The *pineal gland* and colliculi face out into the *quadrigeminal cistern*.

Within the midbrain, the *aqueduct of Sylvius* runs centrally (anterior to the tectal plate). Anterior to the aqueduct, in the midline are the *oculomotor nucleus* (at the level of the superior colliculus) and the *trochlear nucleus* (at the level of the inferior colliculus). These are connected to the *vestibular and abducens nuclei* (in the pons) by the medial longitudinal fasciculus. Adjacent to the oculomotor nucleus is the *Edinger-Westphal nucleus*. Compression of the posterior aspect of the midbrain by a pineal tumour causes obstructive hydrocephalus and Parinaud's syndrome. Parinaud's syndrome is a loss of vertical gaze, nystagmus on attempted convergence and pseudo-Argyll-Robertson pupils (large pupils with sluggish reaction to light) caused by compression of the oculomotor apparatus.

The anterior aspect of the midbrain is dominated by the cerebral peduncles. The *oculomotor nerve* leaves the midbrain near the midline, between the peduncles. The *trochlear nerve* decussates deep to the *inferior colliculi* and exits the midbrain dorsally, below the *inferior colliculi*.

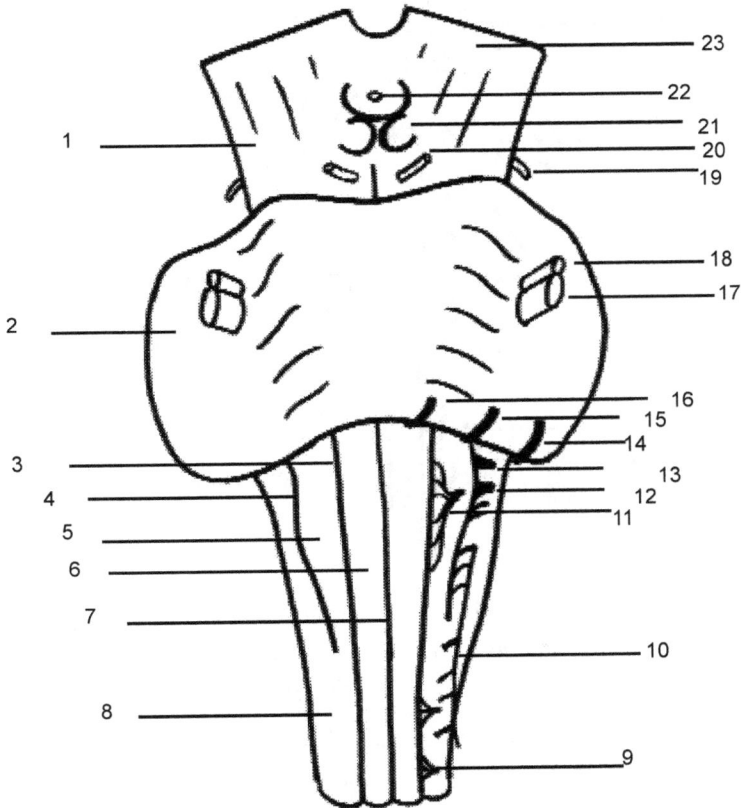

Figure 14. *The anterior surface of the brainstem. 1. Midbrain 2. Pons 3. Pre-olivary sulcus 4. Post-olivary sulcus 5. Olive 6. Pyramid 7. Ventral median fissure 8. Medulla oblongata 9. Rootlets of cervical nerves 10. Rootlets of spinal accesory nerve 11. Rootlets of hypoglossal nerve 12. Rootlets of vagus nerve 13. Origin of glossopharyngeal nerve. 14. Vestibulocochlear nerve 15. Facial nerve 16. Abducens nerve 17. Trigeminal sensory branch 18. Trigeminal motor branch 19. Trochlear nerve 20. Occulomotor nerve 21. Mamillary body 22. Tuber cinereum 23. Crus cerebri of midbrain (cut).*

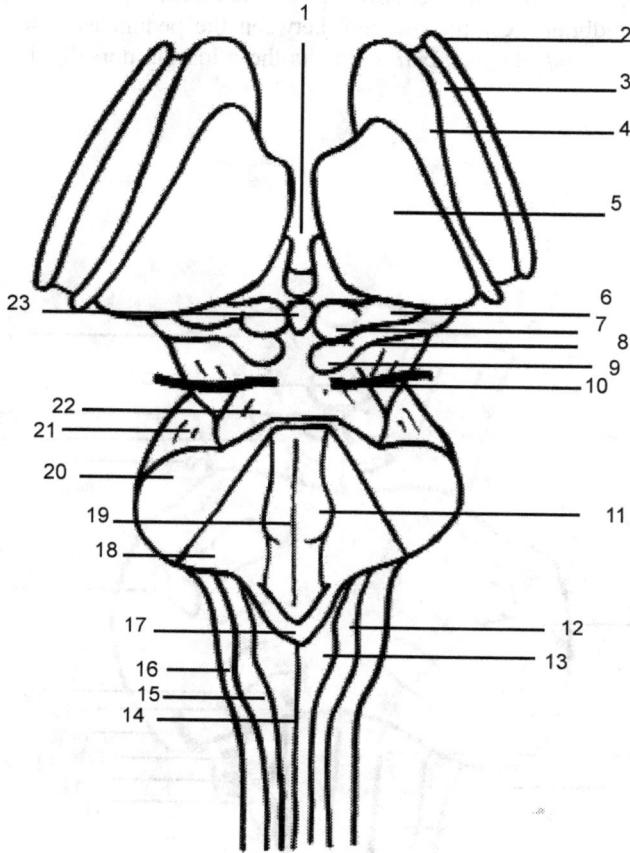

Figure 15. *Posterior surface of the midbrain. 1. Third ventricle 2. Basal ganglia 3. Internal capsule 4. Basal ganglia 5. Thalamus 6. Brachium of superior colliculus 7. Superior colliculus 8. Brachium of inferior colliculus 9. Inferior colliculus 10. Trochlear nerve 11. Facial colliculus 12. Tuberculum gracilis 13. Tuberculum cuneatum 14. Dorsal median sulcus 15. Dorsal intermediate sulcus 16. Dorsolateral sulcus 17. Obex 18. Inferior cerebellar peduncle 19. Median sulcus 20. Middle cerebellar peduncle 21. Middle cerebellar peduncle 22. Superior cerebellar peduncle 23. Pineal gland*

The pons connects the midbrain and the medulla. It is also connected to the cerebellum by the superior, middle and inferior cerebellar peduncles bilaterally. Anteriorly, the pons bulges forwards. The *trigeminal nerve* has separate motor and sensory roots. They arise on the lateral aspect of the pons near the shoulder of the middle cerebellar peduncle. The motor root is superior to the sensory root. Posteriorly and laterally the pons gives rise to the cerebellar peduncles. It also forms the floor of the forth ventricle. The boundary between the pons and the medulla is marked by the *pontomedullary sulcus*. This sulcus contains the origin of three cranial nerves. Most medial is the *abducens nerve*. The *facial nerve* is more lateral, sitting over the superior extent of the *pre-olivary sulcus* (see below). The *vestibulocochlear nerve* arises in the lateral extent of the pontomedullary sulcus, over the superior extent of the post-olivary sulcus.

The medulla oblongata runs between the pons and the spinal cord. Anteriorly, the midline is marked by the *ventral median sulcus*. At the head of the ventral median sulcus (i.e. at the base of the forth ventricle) is the *obex*. Either side of the sulcus runs the pyramids (the pyramidal decussation is at the rostral end of the medulla). Lateral to the pyramid is the *olivary nucleus* which is delineated by the *pre-olivary sulcus* anteriorly and the *post-olivary sulcus* posteriorly. The lateral aspect of the medulla is simply called the lateral medulla. Posteriorly, in the midline, runs the *dorsal median sulcus*. Either side of this are the dorsal columns: the *fasciculus gracilis* medially and the *fasciculus cuneatus* laterally. The two fassicule are separated by the *dorsal intermediate sulcus*.

The origins of the *glossopharyngeal* (IX), *vagus* (X) and *accessory nerves* (IX) arise from the *post-olivary sulcus*, as a line of fine nerve rootlets. The *glossopharyngeal* and *vagus* nerves are adjacent to the superior section of the olive. The *glossopharngeal nerve* is most superior and generally arises as one or two roots just below the *facial nerve* origin. Next comes the *vagus nerve*, which begins as a line of nerve roots that rapidly coalesce. The widely spaced roots that form the *spinal accessory nerve* run within the *post-olivary sulcus* from adjacent to the inferior section of the olive (just below the vagus roots) to the first segments of the cervical spine.

The *hypoglossal nerve* emerges from the *pre-olivary sulcus*. This sulcus is continuous with the exit points of the ventral spinal roots. The roots of the hypoglossal nerve do not coalesce until they have entered the hypoglossal canal.

Surface anatomy of the cerebellum.

Two grooves run over the dorsal surface of the cerebellum in the sagittal plane near the midline. They divide the cerebellum onto the midline vermis and the cerebellar hemispheres on either side.

The cortex is highly corrugated to give it a larger surface area. These folds are called folia. The folia are further subdivided into lobules. There are ten lobules in all, divided by fissures. In the midsagittal plane these lobules radiate from the centre of the cerebellum in a stellate array. The individual lobules are grouped into lobes by two fissures that are deeper than the others. The primary fissure separates the anterior lobe (lobules I-V) from the posterior lobe (lobules VI-IX). Lobule X contains the nodulus of the vermis and the flocculus of each hemisphere on either side. Lobule X is called the *flocculonodular lobe* and is separated from the posterior lobe by the *posterolateral fissure*.

Input and output to and from the cerebellum run in three paired peduncles: the superior, middle and inferior peduncles (also termed the brachium conjunctivum, brachium pontis and restiform body respectively).

The cerebellar tonsils are paired structures that are located on the inferior aspect of the cerebellum. These are the structures that herniate into the foramen magnum in Chiari malformations.

The Ventricular System

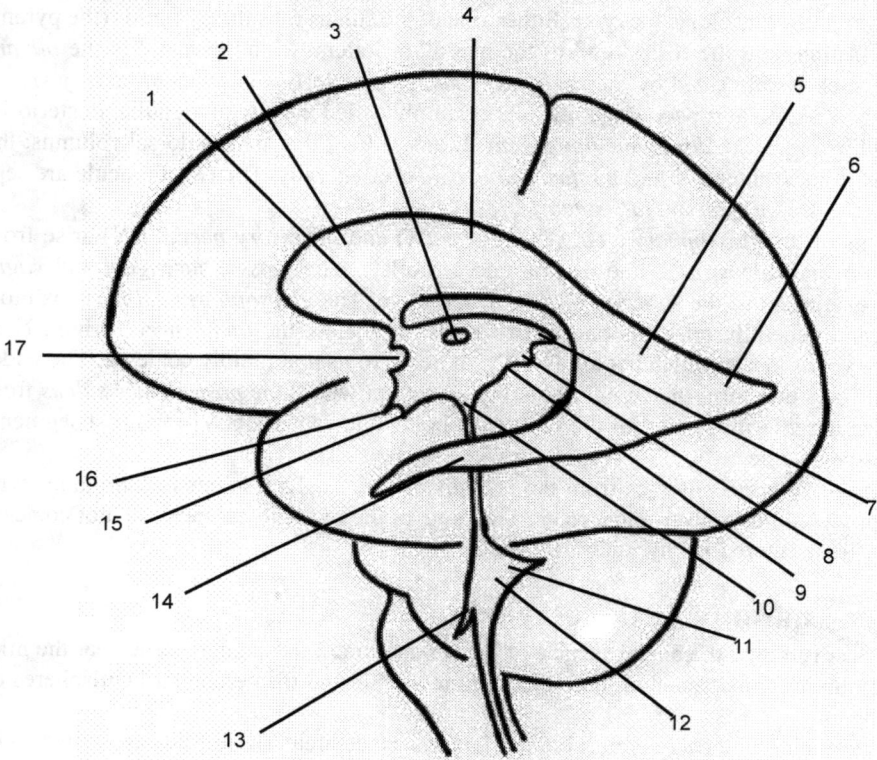

Figure 15. *The ventricles. 1. Foramen of monroe 2. Anterior horn of lateral ventricle 3. Massa intermedia 4. Body of lateral ventricle 5. Atrium of lateral ventricle 6. Occipital horn of lateral ventricle 7. Suprapineal recess 8. Pineal recess 9. Posterior commissure 10. Sylvian aqueduct 11. Median dorsal recess 12. Fourth ventricle 13. Foramen of Luschka 14. Temporal horn of lateral ventricle 15. Infundibular recess 16. Optic recess 17. Anterior commisure*

General structure of the ventricular system

The ventricles are a system of chambers and channels, lying deep within the brain, which allow the passage of cerebrospinal fluid (CSF).

The lateral ventricles are paired structures within the cerebral hemispheres. They have a 'C' shaped structure in common with the other deep hemispheric structures. Each ventricle is divided into five parts. There are three horns (named after the lobe that contains them): the frontal, occipital and temporal horns as well as a body and an atrium. The lateral ventricles open medially into the third ventricle via the interventricular foramen (foramen of Monroe). The third ventricle is a midline structure, which can be thought of as a flat rhombus, lying in the sagittal plane. At the base of the third ventricle is the cerebral aqueduct (also called the aqueduct of Sylvius). The aqueduct is in the midline at the posterio-inferior aspect of the third ventricle. It passes inferiorly through the midbrain and rostral pons before enlarging into the fourth ventricle. The fourth ventricle sits posterior to the pons and rostral medulla. It is continuous with the central canal of the medulla and the subarachnoid space. Communication with the subarachnoid space is either through the midline foramen of Magendie or the paired lateral foramina of Luschka.

The Lateral Ventricles

The lateral ventricles are the only paired ventricles. They each consist of three horns, an atrium and a body. The relations of each are different and so will be considered in turn.

The frontal horn is the section of the lateral ventricle that is anterior to the foramen of Monroe. It is separated from its contralateral fellow by the thin septum pellucidum. The septum pellucidum is a non-neural structure (although inferiorly it is closely related to the septal nuclei of the limbic system). In cases of ventriculomegaly the septum becomes stretched and may tear spontaneously. Operative fenestration of the septum pellucidum puts the two lateral ventricles in communication with one another. This is of benefit if one foramen of Monroe is blocked or (more likely) if both foramina are blocked and one lateral ventricle contains a shunt.

The frontal horns are situated immediately below the corpus callosum. Thus the roof of the frontal horn is formed by the genu of the corpus callosum, which continues inferiorly and also forms the anterior wall of the frontal horn. The rostrum of the corpus callosum then forms the floor of the horn. Laterally, the frontal horn is indented by the large bulge of the head of the caudate nucleus.

The body of the lateral ventricle runs from the foramen of Monroe to the point at which the fornix and corpus callosum meet and the septum pellucidum ends. The roof again consists of the corpus callosum. The septum pellucidum runs from the midline of the corpus callosum superiorly to the body of the fornix inferiorly. Thus the medial wall is formed by the septum pellucidum and the fornix (inferiorly). At the posterior aspect of the body, the fornix is in contact with the corpus callosum and the septum pellucidum terminates. Lateral to the body of the third ventricle is the body of the caudate nucleus. The floor is formed by the thalamus.

The atrium is the junction of the lateral ventricle. It is situated posterior to the pulvinar of the thalamus. The atrium opens anteriorly into the body of the ventricle above the thalamus and into the temporal horn below the thalamus. Posteriorly it opens into the occipital horn. The anterior wall of the atrium therefore consists of the pulvinar. The pulvinar also forms part of the wall of the quadrigeminal CSF cistern. The boundary between the atrium (laterally) and the cistern (medially) is marked by the fornix which loops around the thalamus.

In common with the frontal horn and body, the roof of the atrium is formed by the corpus callosum. The lateral wall comprises the caudate nucleus anteriorly. The tapetum and corpus callosum form the posterior part of the lateral wall. The collateral trigone forms the floor of the atrium. It is a triangular area made up of the posterior end of the collateral sulcus.

The occipital horn extends posteriorly from the atrium. The distance it passes into the occipital lobe is variable (even between the two hemispheres of the same brain). The tapetum forms the roof and lateral wall and the trigone forms the floor.

The temporal horn is the inferior of the two anterior continuations of the atrium (the other being the body of the lateral ventricle). It begins at the posterior border of the pulvinar of the thalamus.

     Anterior wall: amygdala

     Floor: hippocampus

     Roof: thalamus and caudate tail

     Lateral: wall tapetum

Medial: wall choroidal fissure

The choroid plexus of the lateral ventricle is attached to the choroidal fissure. The thalamus and the fornix form the two lips of the choroidal fissure. The fissure runs in a 'C' shape from the inferior choroidal point (just behind the head of the hippocampus) around the inferior, posterior and superior aspects of the thalamus to the foramen of Monroe. As the fornix passes around the thalamus (forming the choroidal fissure) it marks the division between the lateral ventricle and the quadrigeminal cistern posteriorly and the lateral ventricle and the third ventricle superiorly. The choroid plexus follows the choroidal fissure from the inferior choroidal point and exits through the foramen of Monroe at the other end. The choroid plexus from each lateral ventricle is continuous with the ipsilateral of the two choroid plexus strands that run on the underside of the roof of the third ventricle. Within the atrium is a tuft of choroid called the glomus.

As a result of this overall arrangement there is no choroid plexus anterior to the foramen of Monroe (i.e. none in the frontal horn). Some surgeons therefore aim to place the tips of shunt catheters within the frontal horn to reduce the likelihood of blockage of the catheter perforations by choroid plexus fronds. When viewing the inside of the ventricle, the choroid plexus aids with orientation as it is reliably found on the medial aspect of the ventricle and leads to the foramen of Monroe.

The foramen of Monroe is the aperture connecting the lateral and third ventricles. It is normally crescent shaped but becomes round when the ventricles are enlarged. It marks the boundary of the frontal horn and body of the lateral ventricle and is situated at the lateral aspect of the junction of the roof and anterior wall of the third ventricle. The roof and anterior wall of the foramen are formed by the fornix. The posterior aspect is formed by the thalamus. Passing instruments through the foramen may potentially damage the fornix, which (particularly if both fornices are damaged) may cause profound short-term memory loss.

If a rigid endoscope is used to perform third ventriculostomy then the placement of the initial burr hole has anatomical constraints. If it is too anterior the endoscope will stretch the fornix. If too posterior there is risk of damage to the areas of motor cortex.

The structures that pass through the foramen are the choroid plexus, branches of the medial posterior choroidal arteries, the septal, thalamostriate and superior choroidal veins. The septal and thalamostriate veins are relatively consistent indicators of the foramen.

The Third Ventricle.

The third ventricle is a flat, midline structure. It is slit-like when viewed from an anterior perspective. From the lateral aspect it has an irregular shape. The ventricle sits between the two thalami.

The lateral walls of the third ventricle consist of the thalamus superiorly. The inferior section of the lateral wall consists of the hypothalamus (specifically the periventricular nuclei of the hypothalamus, which control the anterior pituitary lobe). The border between the hypothalamus and thalamus is indicated by the hypothalamic sulcus (which passes from the foramen of Monroe to the opening of the aqueduct). The foramina of Monroe are found bilaterally at the superior anterior border of the lateral wall. The massa intermedia (or thalamic adhesion) crosses the third ventricle in its superior half, joining the two thalami. It is not always present.

62

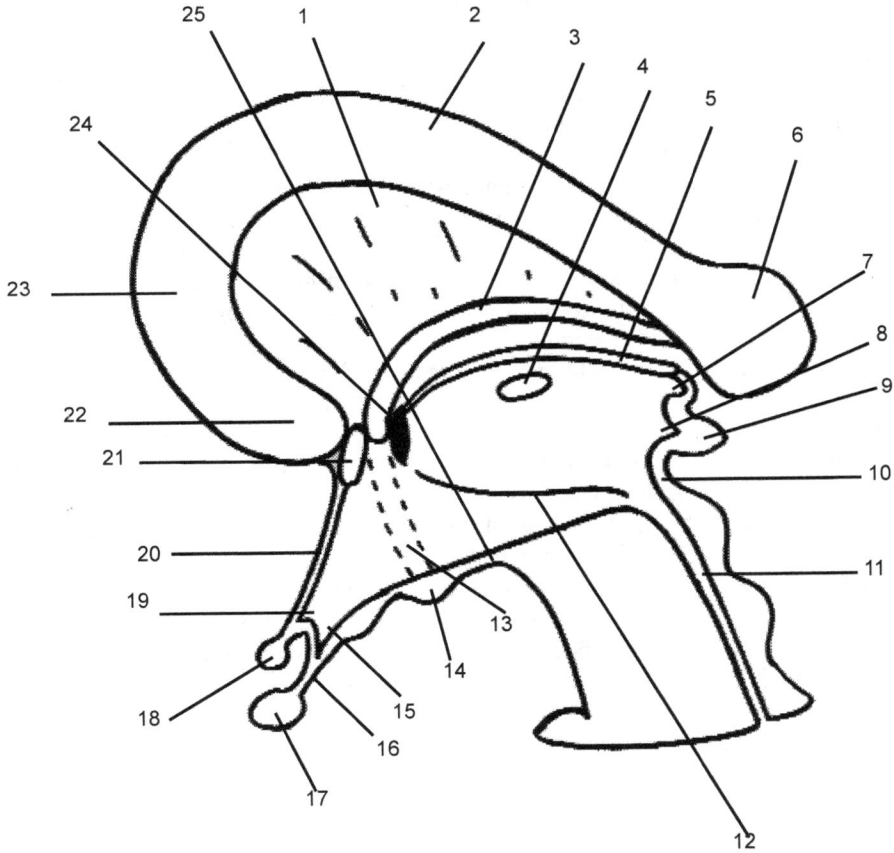

Figure 17. *The third ventricle. 1. Septum pellucidum 2. Body of corpus callosum 3. Fornix 4. Massa intermedia 5. Tela choroidea 6. Splenium of corpus callosum 7. Suprapineal recess 8. Pineal recess 9. Pineal gland 10. Posterior commissure 11. Aqueduct of Sylvius 12. Hypothalamic sulcus 13. Continuation of fornix running lateral to the third ventricle 14. Mamillary body 15. Infundibular recess 16. Infundibulum 17. Pituitary gland 18. Optic chiasm 19. Optic recess 20. Lamina terminalis 21. Anterior commissure 22. Rostrum of corpus callosum 23. Genu of corpus callosum 24. Foramen of monroe*

Inferiorly the third ventricle is closely related to the suprasellar region. The most anterior point of the floor of the third ventricle consists of the optic chiasm. Continuing in a posterior direction, the remainder of the floor of the ventricle consists of the infundibulum, the tuber cinereum, the mamillary bodies, the posterior perforated substance and the midbrain tegmentum. The floor terminates at the opening of the aqueduct. The aim of third ventriculostomy is to create a CSF channel between the third ventricle and the prepontine cistern, thus circumventing the aqueduct of Sylvius (a common site of obstructive hydrocephalus). The new passage is made in the floor of the third ventricle (which is also the roof of the suprasellar region) anterior to the mamillary bodies. Complications therefore include damage to the basilar bifurcation.

The anterior wall of the third ventricle consists of the lamina terminalis for the inferior two thirds. The lamina terminalis is a sheet of grey matter and pia that stretches from the top of optic chiasm to rostrum of corpus callosum. More superiorly, the anterior commissure and fornix form the anterior wall. The anterior commissure is a horisontal band of fibres, which connects the anterior temporal lobe and the amygdala to their contralateral counterparts.

The roof of the third ventricle passes from the foramina of Monroe anteriorly to the suprapineal recess posteriorly. It is formed of four layers. The superior layer is the fornix. Below the fornix are two layers of tela choroidea. The fourth layer consists of vascular structures and is between the two layers of tela choroidea. It is called the velum interpositum. The inferior layer of tela choroidea gives rise to two lines of choroid plexus, either side of the midline. These hang down into the anterior part of the third ventricle. The velum interpositum runs from the foramina of Monroe anteriorly to the superior surface of the pineal gland inferiorly. It stretches between the two thalami and attaches to the inferior aspect of the fornix in the midline. Within the velum interpositum the draining veins of the frontal horn and body coalesce to form the internal cerebral veins. These exit the velum posteriorly, pass over the pineal gland and join the great cerebral vein of Galen. Also within the velum is the medial posterior choroidal artery and its branches, which supply the choroid.

The posterior wall of the third ventricle consists of the suprapineal recess, the habenular commissure, the pineal recess and pineal body and the aqueduct. The pineal gland is supported by the upper and lower lamina. The habenular commissure is situated in the upper lamina and the posterior commissure is in the lower lamina.

Potential complications of surgery in the third ventricle include hypothalamic dysfunction (causing disturbances of homeostasis and pituitary function), visual impairment due to the proximity of the chiasm and short-term memory loss due to damage to the fornix.

The Fourth Ventricle

The cerebral aqueduct drains into the fourth ventricle inferiorly. The fourth ventricle sits posterior to the pons and superior half of the medulla. The area of the ventricle which lies on the posterior aspect of the pons and medulla is diamond shaped and is referred to as the floor of the fourth ventricle or the rhomboid fossa. Posterior to the fourth ventricle is the cerebellum. The ventricle extends posteriorly into the white matter of the cerebellum as the median dorsal recess. Thus in the midsagittal plane the ventricle is a triangle with the base facing the pons and medulla and the apex pointing into the cerebellum. Either side of the median dorsal recess are the lateral dorsal recesses, which also extend into the cerebellum. At the inferior base, the ventricle is continuous with the central canal of the medulla and spinal cord.

The lateral extent of the fourth ventricle is marked superiorly by the cerebellar peduncles and inferiorly by the gracilis and cuneate fassicule. The lateral recesses of the fourth ventricle extend laterally from the mid-level of the ventricle passing below the inferior cerebellar peduncles to communicate with the subarachnoid space via the lateral apertures (foramina of Luschka). The foramen of Luschka contains some choroid plexus, which spills into the subarachnoid space forming an important operative landmark (see below).

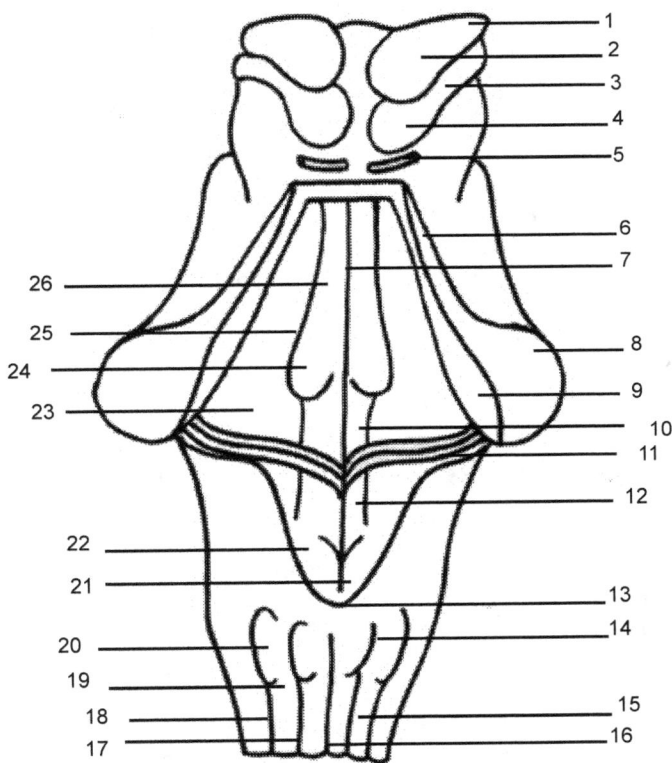

Figure 17. *Relations of the floor of the fourth ventricle. 1. Brachium of superior colliculus 2. Superior colliculus 3. Brachium of inferior colliculus 4. Inferior colliculus 5. Trochlear nerve 6. Superior cerebellar peduncle 7. Median sulcus 8. Middle cerebellar peduncle 9. Inferior cerebellar peduncle 10. Median eminence 11. Striae medullares 12. Hypoglossal triangle 13. Obex 14. Tuberculum cuneatum 15. Fasciculus cuneatus 16. Dorsal median sulcus 17. Dorsal intermediate sulcus 18. Dorsolateral sulcus 19. Fasciculus gracilis 20. Tuberculum gracilis 21. Area postrema 22. Vagal triangle 23. Superior fovea 24. Facial colliculus 25. Sulcus limitans 26. Median eminence*

The roof consists of the superior cerebellar peduncles and the superior medullary velum (which runs between the peduncles) on its superior aspect. Inferiorly it is formed of the ventricular ependyma, and the tela choroidea. The tela choroidea of the fourth ventricle is a double layer of pia mater containing the choroid plexus of the fourth ventricle. Inferiorly the roof is continuous with the obex which overlaps the inferior angle of the ventricle. Dorsally, the roof merges with the median dorsal and lateral dorsal recesses. The inferior portion of the roof contains the median aperture (foramen of Magendie), which lets CSF out of the ventricle and into the subarachnoid space.

Floor of the fourth ventricle.
The floor of the fourth ventricle consists of the posterior wall of the pons and upper half of the medulla. Like the remainder of the ventricular system, it is covered by ependyma. The floor is divided vertically by the median sulcus, which marks the midline. The two medial eminences run either side of the median sulcus. The lateral extent of the medial eminence is marked by the sulcus limitans. The facial colliculus forms the mid-section of the medial eminence. This colliculus is formed by the abducens nucleus and the fibres of the facial nerve as they pass around the abducens nucleus. Inferiorly, the medial eminence contains the hypoglossal triangle, which is formed of the hypoglossal nucleus and the nucleus intercalatus. Below the hypoglossal triangle is the vagal triangle (corresponding to the dorsal vagal nucleus) and below that the area postrema.
The sulcus limitans widens into the superior fovea above the facial colliculus and the inferior fovea below. The locus coeruleus is related to the superior fovea. This nucleus is an important site of origin of noradrenergic neurones. Lateral to the inferior fovea is the vestibular area, which corresponds to the dorsal cochlear nucleus and cochlear nerve. The striae medullares run from the inferior cerebellar peduncle, passing across the vestibular area and median eminence to enter the median sulcus.

The Suprasellar region or Anterior Incisura

Neural relations of the region
In the midline, the roof of the suprasellar region is made up of the inferior relations of the third ventricle. From posterior to anterior these are the posterior perforated substance (in the roof of the interpeduncular fossa), the mamillary bodies, tuber cinereum and the pituitary infundibulum then the subcallosal region.
Laterally, the uncus of the temporal lobe protrudes medially over the free edge of the tent. The uncus forms an arrow pointing laterally with an anterior and a posterior surface. The relations of these two surfaces are important considerations during temporal lobectomy. The anterior surface of the uncus contains the amygdala and faces the anterior portion of the suprasellar region. It is lateral to the internal carotid artery and is crossed above by the middle cerebral artery. The anterior choroidal artery arises from the internal carotid artery and passes over the medial aspect of the anterior surface. The apex of the uncus faces the oculomotor nerve and the posterior communicating artery.
The posterior surface contains the head of the hippocampus and faces towards the broad edge of the cerebral peduncle. The space between the posterior surface of the uncus and the cerebral peduncle is the crural cistern. This contains the posterior cerebral artery, the superior cerebellar artery, the anterior choroidal artery and the basal vein of Rosenthal. The optic tract runs in its roof. Posteriorly, the crural cistern is continuous with the ambient cistern and then the quadrigeminal cistern.
Both the amygdala and hippocampus are visible in the wall of the temporal horn when approached from the lateral aspect in temporal lobectomy. The notch that can be seen between them in the wall of the temporal horn is the uncal recess. The uncal recess is directly lateral to the uncal apex and therefore allows early orientation to the medial structures.

Uncal herniation caused by a unilateral space occupying lesion leads to compression of the oculomotor nerve (causing an ipsilateral blown pupil) and the posterior cerebral artery (causing contralateral blindness)

Anterior and superior to it is the anterior perforated substance of the basal forebrain. The basal forebrain marks the start of the Sylvian fissure, which is continuous laterally with the suprasellar region. The superior relations of the basal forebrain are the head of the caudate nucleus and anterior limb of the internal capsule. The posterior extent of the space is formed of the cerebral peduncles and interpeduncular fossa as well as being continuations with the crural cisterns. The interpeduncular cistern communicates with the crural cisterns laterally but is separated from the chiasmatic cistern anteriorly by the membrane of Liliequist. Anteriorly, the chiasmatic cistern communicates with the cisterna laminae terminalis, which is anterior to the lamina terminalis.

Nerves and tracts of the suprasellar region

Olfactory tract. The *olfactory tract* runs posteriorly from the *olfactory bulb* (over the cribriform plate) lateral to the gyrus rectus and splits above the anterior clinoid process into the medial and lateral olfactory striae. It therefore forms an important landmark for aneurysm surgery via the pterional approach. Once the olfactory tract is encountered, it can be followed posteriorly to its bifurcation which is closely related to the *optic nerve* and hence the internal carotid artery.

Optic nerve. The *optic nerves* arise from the orbit via the optic canal (which they share with the ophthalmic artery and the central retinal vein). The nerve is covered by all three layers of the meninges throughout its course within the canal. The meninges fuse with the sclera of the globe and contain the central retinal vein. This arrangement underpins the development of papilloedema (the mechanism of which is considered in the chapter on physiology).

On leaving the canal it is covered by a dural fold called the falciform ligament. This passes over the nerve from the anterior clinoid process. The *optic nerve* is separated from the sphenoid sinus by bone but this may be absent, allowing the nerve to protrude into the sinus. The *optic nerves* then pass posteriorly, medially and superiorly to meet, forming the optic chiasm. The *optic nerve* passes under the bifurcation of the *olfactory tract*.

Optic chiasm. The chiasm is beneath the anterior border of the third ventricle. The tuber cinereum is therefore superior and posterior to the chiasm and the infundibulum runs behind it, passing into the pituitary fossa via the central hole in the diaphragma sellae. The chiasmatic recess of the third ventricle points towards the chiasm.

In the majority of cases, the chiasm is positioned over the sella turcica. The infundibulum, therefore, runs slightly anteriorly as it descends. In less than a third of cases, however, the chiasm may be prefixed (situated over the tuberculum) or postfixed (situated over the dorsum sellae).

Optic tract. The optic tracts arise from the chiasm and pass posteriorly and laterally either side of the cerebral peduncles, in the roof of the crural cisterns. They terminate on the lateral geniculate nucleus of the thalamus.

The clinical effects of compression of the optic apparatus are detailed in the chapter on clinical examination.

Oculomotor nerve. From its origin on the anterior aspect of the midbrain, the *oculomotor nerve* runs between the posterior cerebral artery (above) and the superior cerebellar artery (below), through the lateral wall of the interpeduncular cistern to pass medial to the uncus of the temporal lobe. During its course it gives off multiple arachnoid folds, including an attachment of Liliequist's membrane. It passes into the roof of the cavernous cistern.

The *oculomotor nerve* runs almost parallel to the *posterior communicating artery* and is therefore prone to compression by *posterior communicating artery* aneurysms. This results in a painful, pupil involving, third nerve palsy. Aneurysms of the *posterior cerebral artery* and *superior cerebellar artery* are less common causes of third nerve palsies (they compress the nerve near its origin as it passes between the two vessels).

Trochlear nerve. This nerve arises dorsally from the midbrain just below the inferior colliculus. It is unusual in two respects, being the only cranial nerve to either fully decussate or arise from the dorsal aspect of the brainstem. From its origin it then passes around the cerebral peduncles and runs between the *posterior cerebral artery* and *superior cerebellar artery* (as does III) before entering the free edge of the tentorium. It continues anteriorly to enter the cavernous sinus.

Arterial relationships of the suprasellar region

The *internal carotid artery* enters the suprasellar region by piercing the roof of the cavernous sinus, adjacent to the anterior clinoid process. The cerebral segment of the artery runs superiorly, posteriorly and laterally towards the anterior perforated substance, where it bifurcates. It begins inferior to the optic chiasm and *optic nerve* and terminates lateral to the *optic nerve*.

The *ophthalmic artery* arises after the *internal carotid artery* has left the cavernous sinus and courses inferior to the *optic nerve* to enter the optic canal, again below II. The *posterior communicating artery* passes from its origin on the posterior wall of the *internal carotid artery* and runs posteriorly and medially to join the *posterior cerebral artery* in the interpeduncular fossa. It runs below the *optic tracts* and above the *oculomotor nerve* (which is almost parallel). The *anterior choroidal artery* arises from the posterior surface of the *internal carotid artery* and passes posteriorly and laterally below the optic tract and enters the crural cistern (between the cerebral peduncle and posterior surface of the uncus) before entering the choroidal fissure.

The *anterior cerebral artery* arises from the carotid bifurcation below the anterior perforated substance. It then passes anteromedially over the optic nerve before entering the interhemispheric fissure. A triangle is therefore formed in the space between the optic nerve and the internal carotid artery passing underneath the chiasm and the *anterior cerebral artery* passing above the optic nerve more anteriorly. Perforating branches from the *internal carotid artery* to the optic apparatus and floor of the third ventricle may hinder access through this triangle.

The *anterior communicating artery* is usually above the optic chiasm. The recurrent branch *(recurrent artery of Heubner)* of the *anterior cerebral artery* usually arises from the *anterior cerebral artery* after the origin of the *anterior communicating artery* and then passes back across the *optic nerve*, running superior to the first section of the *anterior cerebral artery* before passing over the carotid bifurcation and entering the anterior perforated substance.

More posteriorly, the basilar bifurcation is below the posterior part of the third ventricle, anterior to the midbrain, in the interpeduncular cistern. The bifurcation gives off the two *posterior cerebral arteries*. These arteries run over the origin of the *oculomotor nerve* to pass round the midbrain in the crural cistern to enter the quadrigeminal cistern.

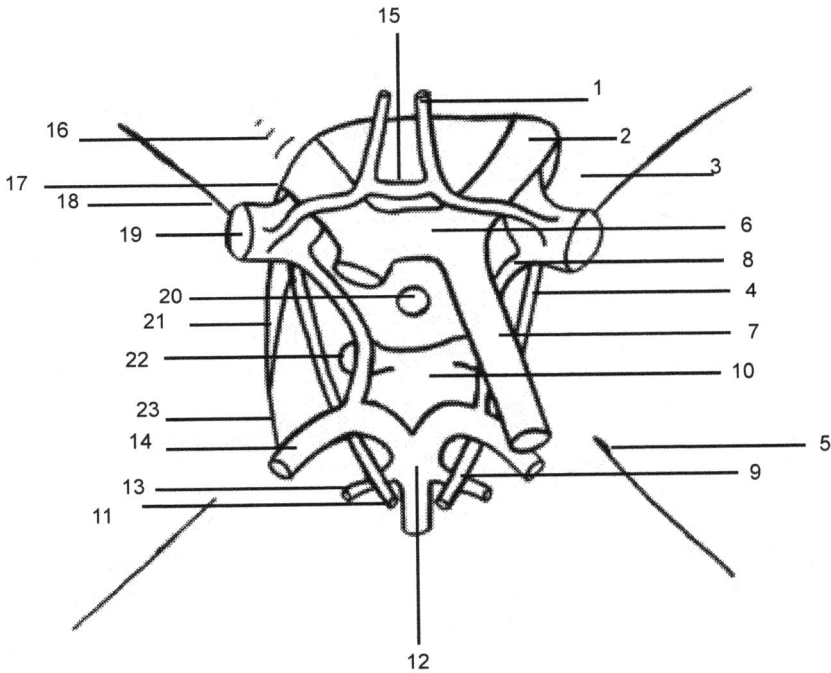

Figure 18. *The contents of the suprasellar region. Viewed from above and behind. The brainstem and right side of the tentorium have been removed. 1. Right anterior cerebral artery (A2) 2. Optic nerve 3. Anterior clinoid process 4. Right oculomotor nerve 5. Petrous ridge 6. Optic chiasm 7. Optic tract 8. Posterior communicating artery 9. Right oculomotor nerve 10. Clivus 11. Left oculomotor nerve 12. Basilar artery 13. Superior cerebellar artery 14. Posterior cerebral artery 15. Anterior communicating artery 16. Falciform ligament 17. Left anterior cerebral artery (A1) 18. Sphenoid wing 19. Cut end of internal carotid artery 20. Pituitary stalk 21. Trochlear nerve 22. Posterior clinoid process 23. Free edge of tentorium*

The Pituitary Gland

Structure of the pituitary gland

The pituitary has two functionally distinct lobes called the anterior lobe (or adenohypophysis) and the posterior lobe (or neurohypophysis). The infundibulum or pituitary stalk connects the tuber cinereum of the hypothalamus (which lies just below the infundibular recess of third ventricle) to the posterior lobe of the pituitary gland. It also passes anteriorly as it descends behind the optic chiasm such that the body of the pituitary is inferior to the chiasm.

The anterior lobe produces most of the pituitary hormones: growth hormone, luteinising hormone, follicle stimulating hormone, prolactin, melanocyte stimulating hormone, adrenocorticotrophic hormone and thyroid stimulating hormone. Control of these hormones is by direct feedback loops and by hypothalamic neurones in the periventricular nuclei. The neurones of the periventricular nuclei are collectively termed the parvocellular system. They terminate on the capillaries of the pituitary portal circulation. This system of capillaries runs from the median eminence of the proximal section of the infundibulum down the stalk (as portal veins) and forms another capillary bed in the anterior lobe. The parvocellular hypothalamic cells release their hormones into the pituitary portal circulation and they are then delivered to their target.

Most of the hormones delivered in this way are excitatory. Corticotropin releasing hormone (CRH), for example, is released by the periventricular nuclei. It arrives in the anterior pituitary lobe via the portal venous system and stimulates production of adrenocorticotropin (ACTH). This in turn stimulates the zona fasciculata of the adrenal gland to produce cortisol. Each step of the process is under negative feedback control.

Control of prolactin production by the adenohypophysis is, by contrast, inhibitory in nature. Prolactin production by the anterior pituitary lobe occurs without stimulus from the hypothalamus. The amount of prolactin released is controlled by dopamine, which reduces the rate of prolactin production by the pituitary. High circulating prolactin levels lead to an increase in dopamine (from the hypothalamus) and therefore reduced prolactin production and a fall in circulating levels. Compression of the pituitary stalk prevents dopamine from reaching the anterior pituitary gland. As a result, a tumour with no endocrine function can cause a rise in prolactin levels. This is called ' stalk effect' and produces a smaller rise in prolactin levels than a prolactinoma. The distinction between hyperprolactinaemia due to stalk compression and hyperprolactinaemia due to a prolactinoma is important as the latter often responds well to medical management.

The posterior lobe produces anti-diuretic hormone and oxytocin. These hormones are produced in the paraventricular and supraoptic nuclei of the hypothalamus. These are found lateral to the periventricular nuclei and form the magnocellular system. The axons of neurones in these nuclei project down the pituitary stalk and terminate on the capillaries of the posterior lobe. Thus the posterior lobe hormones are produced in the hypothalamus and released in the posterior pituitary by the same cells. Axonal transport is used to move the hormones from the hypothalamus to the pituitary.

Location and relations of the pituitary gland

The pituitary fossa is situated in the midline on the superior aspect of the body of the sphenoid bone. Anterior is the tuberculum sellae and posteriorly the dorsum sellae, which is continuous with the clivus behind. The anterior clinoid processes are at the medial end of the lesser sphenoid wing. The middle clinoid processes are lateral to the tuberculum sellae. The posterior clinoid processes are lateral to the dorsum sellae. In sagittal section, the tuberculum sellae, pituitary fossa and dorsum sellae resemble a Turkish saddle and are called the sella turcica (lat. Turkish saddle). The terms pituitary fossa and sella turcica are often used interchangeably.

The floor and walls of the sella turcica are lined with dura. This divides superiorly to form the roof of the sella turcica, called the diaphragma sellae. This thin layer of dura separates the pituitary gland from the CSF spaces above. It has a central hole, through which the infundibulum passes. The diaphragma is not sturdy enough to protect the suprasellar structures from trauma during transphenoidal hypophysectomy if the instruments are inserted too far. The diaphragma is continuous laterally with the roof of the cavernous sinus.

Within the pituitary fossa, the layers of the meninges are fused. As a result there is no separate arachnoid mater and no CSF containing subarachnoid space. This is why initial opening of the dura during transphenoidal hypophysectomy does not cause egress of CSF. In up to half of cases, however, there is a loop of arachnoid passing through the central hole into the pituitary fossa. This loop is hard to avoid and may be a common cause of CSF leak following transphenoidal hypophysectomy.

Anterior and inferior to the pituitary fossa are the sphenoidal air sinuses. These paired sinuses are lined with mucous membrane and are continuous with the nasal cavity via paired apertures in the anterior wall that open posterior to the superior nasal conchae. The two sphenoid sinuses are separated by a vertical septum. The septum often deviates laterally or (less commonly) is duplicated, giving three sinuses. It is therefore not a very reliable indicator of the midline for pituitary surgeons.

Pneumatisation of the sphenoid sinus occurs at puberty and is also variable. Extensive sphenoid sinuses may extend into the sphenoid wings. They may also allow the optic nerve to prolapse into the sinus if the usual bony division is absent. Smaller sinuses tend to be anterior (as opposed to inferior) to the pituitary fossa. Complete failure of pneumatisation is less common but makes the transphenoidal approach difficult. Image guidance techniques are used to maintain the midline.

The perpendicular plate of the ethmoid and the vomer attach to the anterior aspect of the sphenoid sinus in the midline and these are fractured and displaced to one side to give access to the full extent of the sphenoid sinus at transphenoidal hypophysectomy.

The Cavernous sinus

Either side of the sella turcica are the cavernous sinuses. The sinuses are also lateral to the sphenoid air sinus. These venous sinuses are formed by the division of the two layers of dura of the floor of the middle cranial fossa. The inner layer rises vertically to meet the free edge of the tent (which is passing anteriorly to the anterior clinoid process) and then runs horisontally and medially becoming continuous with the diaphragma sellae. The outer layer runs along the body of the sphenoid to meet the inner layer. It forms the lateral wall of the pituitary fossa.

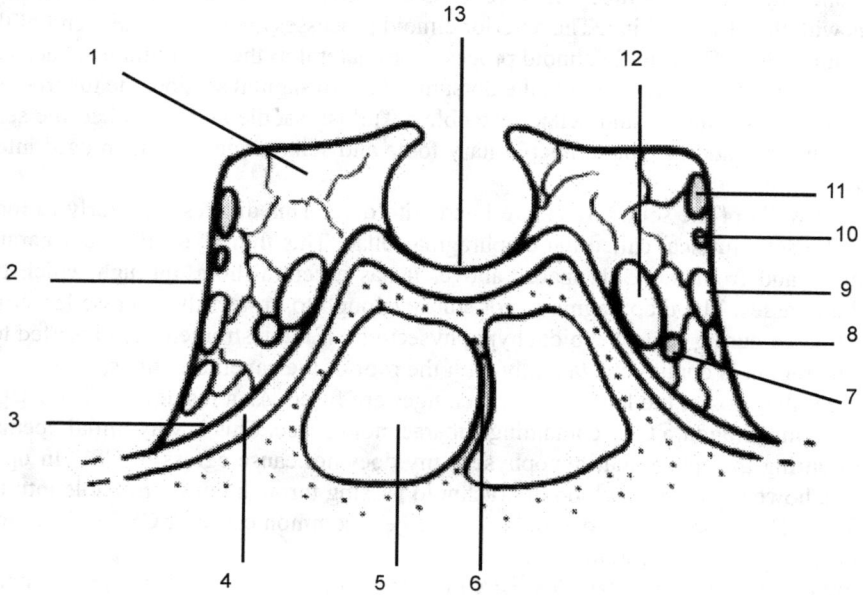

Figure 20. *Coronal section of the cavernous sinuses. 1. Cavernous sinus showing trabeculations 2. Inner layer of dura 3. Outer layer of dura 4. Cortex of the skull 5. Right side of sphenoid air sinus 6. Septum of sphenoid air sinus 7. Abducens nerve 8. Maxillary nerve 9. Ophthalmic nerve 10. Trochlear nerve 11. Oculomotor nerve 12. Intracavernous portion of ICA 13. Pituitary fossa*

The cavernous sinus drains the superior and inferior ophthalmic veins and is therefore in communication with the facial vein. It is also in communication with the pterygoid venous plexus inferiorly. The facial vein has no valves and therefore, if flow is retrograde, it drains into the cavernous sinus. Thus thrombophlebitis of the facial vein caused by infection can cause cavernous sinus thrombosis. The cavernous sinus also drains the lateral aspects of the cerebral hemispheres (via the sphenoparietal sinus) and the pituitary gland. The two cavernous sinuses are in communication via the anterior and posterior intercavernous sinuses, which pass in front of and behind the infundibulum. Drainage of the cavernous sinus is by the superior and inferior petrosal sinuses.

The space within the cavernous sinus is unique in that it contains multiple subdivisions. It is unclear whether these are trabeculations or the walls of a bunched up venous plexus. Other contents are either arterial or nervous.

The *internal carotid artery (ICA)* enters the cranial vault via the foramen lacerum, lateral to the posterior clinoid process. It then turns anteriorly and enters the cavernous sinus. It runs forward for about 2cm before turning again, this time superiorly to pierce the roof of the cavernous sinus next to the anterior clinoid process. This section of the *internal carotid artery* is called the *intracavernous segment*. It normally runs in the carotid groove on the lateral aspect of the body of the sphenoid. The degree of separation between the *ICA* and the pituitary gland

72

is variable. In about a quarter of cases, the *carotid artery* passes through the wall of the cavernous sinus and indents the pituitary gland, distorting it. The two *ICAs* may pass extremely close to one another in the midline of the sella, termed 'kissing carotids'.

The *intracavernous carotid* gives off the *meningohypophyseal trunk* (which gives rise to the *inferior hypophyseal artery*) and *McConnell's capsular arteries*. The *inferior hypophyseal artery* passes medially to supply the sella contents.

The cavernous sinus contains the *oculomotor (III), trochlear (IV), ophthalmic (V1), maxillary (V2) and abducens nerves (VI)*. The *oculomotor and trochlear nerves* enter the roof of the sinus anterolateral to the dorsum sella and pass between the dural leaves of the lateral sinus wall. The *ophthalmic nerve* enters inferiorly and also runs in the lateral wall of the sinus. The *maxillary nerve* runs for a short length within the lateral wall before exiting inferolaterally to pass to the foramen rotundum. From superior to inferior, the nerves are arranged in numerical order in the lateral wall. The *abducens nerve* enters posteriorly and runs within the sinus itself. It is medial to the *ophthalmic nerve* and adherent to the *carotid artery* laterally. The nerves (except the *maxillary nerve*) exit via the superior orbital fissure into the orbit.

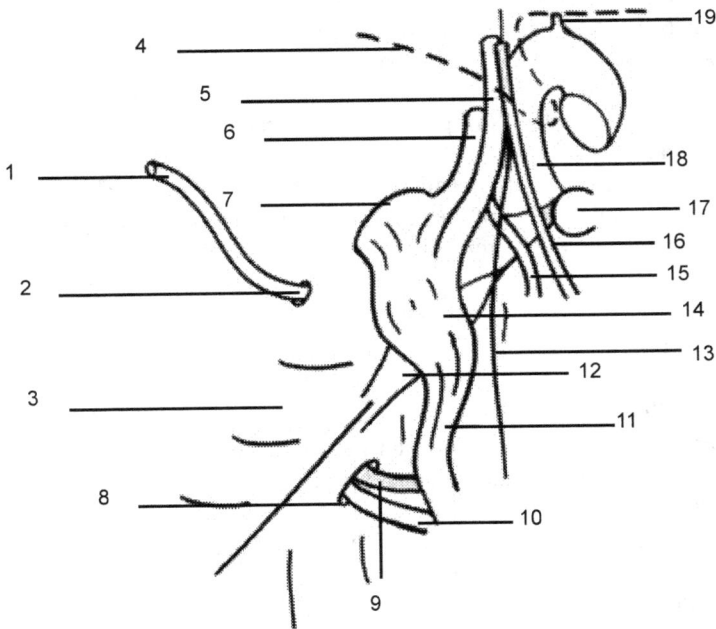

Figure 21. *Superior view of the structures entering the cavernous sinus and structures crossing the petrous ridge. Dural structures have been removed. 1. Middle meningeal artery 2. Foramen spinosum 3. Floor of middle cranial fossa 4. Sphenoid wing 5. Ophthalmic nerve 6. Maxillary nerve 7. Mandibular nerve 8. Internal acoustic meatus 9. Facial nerve 10. Vestibulocochlear nerve 11. Trigeminal nerve 12. Meckel's cave 13. Trochlear nerve 14. Trigeminal ganglion (Gasserian) 15. Abducens nerve 16. Oculomotor nerve 17. Posterior clinoid process 18. Internal carotid artery 19. Ophthalmic artery*

Structures passing over the Petrous Ridge

The petrous ridge runs anteriorly and medially from its lateral extent anterior to the asterion and behind the mastoid groove. The most medial aspect of the ridge is called the petrous apex. Just lateral to this is Meckel's cave, a narrow indentation containing the trigeminal or gasserian ganglion of the trigeminal nerve. The tentorium is attached to the apex throughout its length. Medially, the edge of the tent passes from the petrous apex to the posterior clinoid process. The base of the tentorial attachment contains the superior petrosal sinus.

The two principle structures crossing the petrous ridge are the *trigeminal and abducens nerves*. Both pass underneath the *superior petrosal sinus*. The *trigeminal nerve* is considered more carefully in the section on the upper neurovascular complex of the cerebellopontine angle.

The *abducens nerve* nuclei are found in the floor of the forth ventricle. They are either side of the *medial longitudinal fasciculus*. The fibres of the *facial nerve* loop round the *abducens nuclei* forming the facial colliculi in the floor of the forth ventricle. The *abducens nerve* fibres run anteriorly and exit from the medial end of the pontomedullary junction. The nerve then runs anteriorly and superiorly crossing the petrous ridge medial to Meckel's cave at the petrous apex. It passes under the attached edge of the tent as it passes to the posterior clinoid process (the petroclinoid ligament) in Dorello's canal. It then enters the *cavernous sinus* where it runs alongside the *carotid artery* and enters the orbit via the superior orbital fissure. The *abducens nerve* may be damaged by lesions involving the petrous apex. Gradenigo's syndrome (otorrhea, retro-orbital pain and sixth nerve palsy) is the result of mastoiditis with diffuse inflammation of the petrous bone. The *facial and vestibulocochlear nerves* and the *superior petrosal sinus* may also be involved. Nasopharyngeal or paranasal sinus carcinomas may present with a *abducens* palsy.

Abducens nerve palsies are a classical 'false localising' sign of hydrocephalus. This is thought to be caused by downwards displacement of the brainstem (due to ventriculomegaly), which stretches the abducens nerves over the petrous tips, causing unilateral or bilateral palsies.

The Cerebellopontine Angle

Boundaries of the cerebellopontine angle.
The cerebellopontine angle is situated in the posterior fossa between the lateral aspect of the cerebellum, the lateral pons and the petrous ridge and petrous temporal bone. The superior boundary is the *trigeminal nerve*, which passes from the pons anteriorly to the petrous ridge, and the inferior aspect is marked by the passage of the *glossopharyngeal nerve* from the medulla towards the jugular foramen. As such the area is a shallow triangle with its blunt angle at the cerebellopontine fissure.

Bony relations of the cerebellopontine angle.
The cerebellopontine angle faces the basisphenoid and basiocciput of the clivus anteriorly. The vertical surface of the petrous temporal bone and the occipital bone (more inferiorly) are lateral.

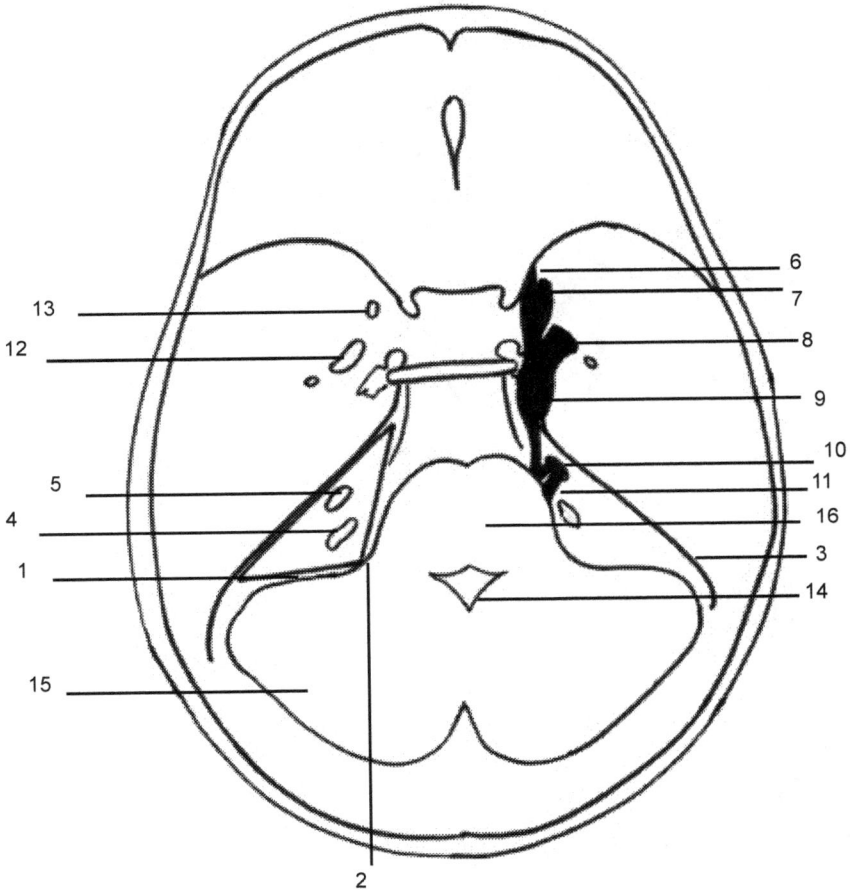

Figure 22. *The boundaries of the cerebellopontine angle. The course of the left trigeminal nerve is also shown. 1. Triangle representing the approximate boundary of the CPA in the axial plane 2. Triangle apex within the cerebellopontine fissure 3. Petrous ridge 4. Jugular foramen 5. Internal acoustic meatus (a.k.a. porus) 6. Ophthalmic nerve 7. Maxillary nerve 8. Mandibular nerve 9. Gasserian ganglion of trigeminal nerve 10. Facial nerve 11. Vestibulocochlear nerve 12. Foramen ovale 13. Foramen rotundum 14. Fourth ventricle 15. Left cerebellar hemisphere*

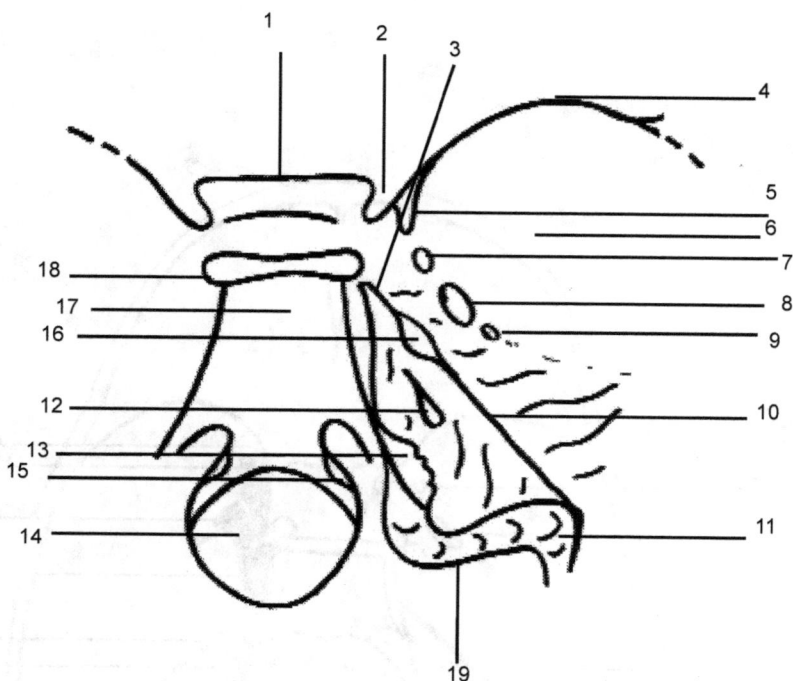

Figure 23. *The bony relations of the cerebellopontine angle. Viewed from behind. 1. Dorsum sellae 2. Anterior clinoid process 3. Petrous apex 4. Sphenoid wing 5. Superior orbital fissure 6. Floor of middle cranial fossa 7. Foramen rotundum 8. Foramen ovale 9. Foramen spinosum 10. Petrous ridge 11. Bony sulcus containing the junction of the superior petrosal and transverse sinuses as well as the origin if the sigmoid sinus 12. Internal acoustic meatus 13. Jugular foramen 14. Foramen magnum 15. Hypoglossal canal 16. Meckel's cave 17. Clivus 18. Posterior clinoid process 19. Sigmoid sinus*

The general relationship of the posterior circulation to the ventral brainstem.

The posterior circulation is supplied by the two *vertebral arteries*. These vessels enter the cerebral vault via the foramen magnum and run in the subarachnoid space of the premedullary cistern, overlying the medullary pyramids and the olive. The two *vertebral arteries* generally come together anterior to the pontomedullary junction to form the *basilar artery* although there is considerable variation as to the point at which this occurs.

The *vertebral arteries* give rise to the *posterior inferior cerebellar arteries (PICA)*. This occurs at the inferior aspect of the olive, although they may be absent entirely. The *PICA* then runs inferiorly along the medulla before passing into the cerebellar vallecula and dividing into *medial and lateral branches*. The *medial branch of PICA* supplies the cerebellar hemisphere and inferior vermis. The *lateral branch* supplies the inferior border of the cerebellum, the lateral aspect of the medulla and the choroid plexus of the forth ventricle. Occlusion of the *PICA* therefore leads to the 'lateral medullary syndrome'.

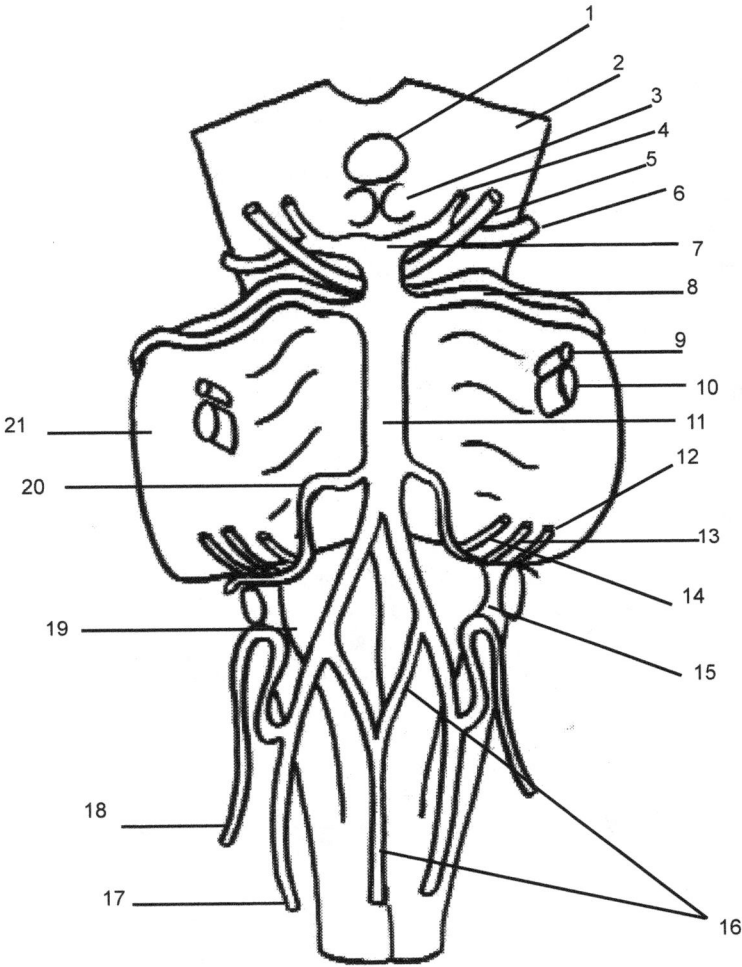

Figure 24. *The relationship of the posterior circulation and the brainstem. 1. Tuber cinereum 2. Cerebral peduncle 3. Mamillary body 4. Posterior communicating artery 5. Oculomotor nerve 6. Posterior cerebral artery 7. Basilar tip 8. Superior cerebellar artery 9. Motor root of trigeminal nerve 10. Sensory root of trigeminal nerve 11. Basilar artery 12. Vestibulocochlear nerve 13. Facial nerve 14. Abducens nerve 15. Post-olivary sulcus 16. Anterior spinal artery 17. Vertebral artery 18. Posterior inferior cerebellar artery 19. Olive 20. Anterior inferior cerebellar artery 21. Pons*

The *anterior spinal arteries* arise near the end of the *vertebral arteries* and pass inferiorly, joining in the midline (over the medulla) to supply the anterior areas of the spinal cord. The *anterior spinal artery* supplies the medial medulla and therefore occlusion will lead to the 'medial medullary syndrome'. The *posterior spinal artery* may also arise from the *vertebral artery* but more commonly it is a branch of PICA. The *vertebral arteries* also give off multiple tiny medullary vessels.

77

The *basilar artery* continues superiorly along the ventral surface of the pons in the midline. It terminates in the interpeduncular fossa (between the crus cerebri of the midbrain) by dividing into the two *posterior cerebral arteries*. The site of this bifucation is again variable and may be over the pons or as far up as the mamillary bodies. The most superior point of the *basilar artery* is called the basilar tip.

The *anterior inferior cerebellar arteries (AICA)* arise from the lower end of the *basilar artery* and run laterally around the pontomedullary junction, usually ventral to the *abducens, facial and vestibulocochlear nerves. AICA* may give rise to a loop that passes into the internal acoustic meatus below the *facial and vestibulocochlear nerves*. This loop often gives rise to the *labyrinthine (internal auditory) artery*, which supplies the inner ear.

The next major branch of the basilar is the *superior cerebellar artery*. This arises near the basilar termination and passes laterally, inferior to both the *oculomotor and trochlear nerves*. It divides into rostral and caudal trunks and supplies the superior cerebellar surface, the pons, pineal body and tela choroidea of the third ventricle.

The *posterior cerebral arteries* are the terminal branches of the *basilar artery* (see above).

The cerebellopontine angle is considered to contain three separate neurovascular complexes:

1. The upper neurovascular complex - the *superior cerebellar artery* and its relations.
2. The middle neurovascular complex - the *anterior inferior cerebellar artery* and its relations.
3. The lower neurovascular complex - the *posterior inferior cerebellar artery* and its relations.

The upper neurovascular complex.

The *trigeminal nerve* (V) joins the brainstem midway between the rostral and caudal borders of the pons on the lateral aspect. It then runs laterally and superiorly towards the petrous apex. On reaching the apex it passes underneath the tent and forms the *trigeminal (or gasserian) ganglion*, which sits in an indentation of the petrous apex called Meckel's cave. The nerve splits into its three major branches at the *gasserian ganglion*. These pass across the middle cranial fossa to exit via their separate foramina. The *mandibular nerve (V3)* is most lateral. It exits via the foramen ovale to pass into the infratemporal fossa. The *maxillary (V2) and ophthalmic (V1) nerves* pass through the *cavernous sinus* and exit the cranial vault via the foramen rotundum and superior orbital fissure respectively. Percutaneous treatment of trigeminal neuralgia is achieved via the foramen ovale.

In cross section, the *trigeminal root* is elliptical. The relative position of the fibres relating to the three division of the trigeminal nerve is consistent. *Ophthalmic (V1)* fibres are rostromedial and *mandibular (V3) fibres* are more caudolateral. The *maxillary fibres* are in between. However, caution should be taken when performing partial section of the trigeminal nerve as the long axis of the ellipse is variable it its orientation. It is therefore not reliable to assume that the most inferior part of the nerve root will contain *mandibular fibres*.

Motor input to the nerve initially comprises of motor rootlets, separate from this main sensory root. These are variable in number and tend to be clustered around the superior aspect of the sensory nerve root. Both the *ophthalmic* and the *mandibular nerves* are purely sensory. All trigeminal motor flow passes via the *mandibular nerve*. The motor root does not pass through the *trigeminal ganglion* but passes separately through the *foramen ovale* to join the *mandibular nerve* soon after leaving the foramen. This works in favour of the surgeon treating trigeminal neuralgia as partial section of the main sensory nerve root should not cause a motor palsy.

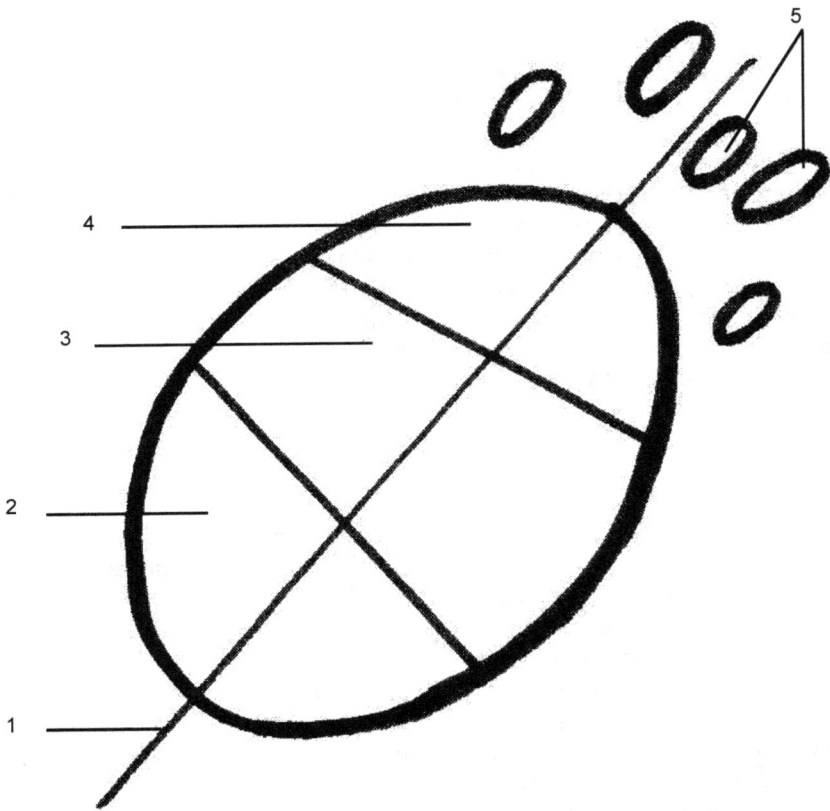

Figure 25. *The trigeminal nerve in cross section. 1. Longitudinal axis 2. Mandibular portion of the sensory root 3. Maxillary portion of the sensory root 4. Ophthalmic portion of the sensory root 5. Motor rootlets*

Vascular relations of the trigeminal nerve.
The *superior cerebellar artery (SCA)* runs around the brainstem above the *trigeminal nerve*. It often, however, takes a caudal deviation, running inferiorly along the lateral aspect of the pons. If this is marked, contact with the *trigeminal nerve* may arise. Generally this contact will be on the superior or superio-medial aspect of the nerve. During its journey across the pons the *SCA* bifurcates into rostral and caudal trunks and it is the bifurcation which most often compresses the nerve. The *SCA* then continues on its way to the cerebellomesencephalic fissure.

The *anterior inferior cerebellar artery* passes around the pons inferior to the *trigeminal nerve*, more closely associated with the *facial and vestibulocochlear nerves*. The *AICA* can form a superior loop sufficient to cause compression of the inferior aspect of the *trigeminal nerve*.

Other local vessels may also be adherent to the trigeminal root. A tortuous *basilar artery* can compress the medial aspect. Infrequently, the *posterior inferior cerebellar artery* can rise superiorly enough to touch the root. The *pontine arteries* arising from the *basilar trunk* generally enter the pons medial to the origin of the *trigeminal nerve* but a large *pontine artery* can pass either rostrally or caudally to insert laterally, passing above or below the nerve.

The *superior petrosal veins*, which drain into the *superior petrosal sinus,* are formed from the *transverse pontine veins, pontotrigeminal veins* and *veins of the cerebellopontine fissure and middle cerebellar peduncle* as well as *veins draining the lateral aspect of the cerebellum.* The *transverse pontine veins* are most likely to come into contact with the *trigeminal nerve* but any may do so (except the *lateral cerebellar veins*). The veins coalesce to from a single trunk before entering the *superior petrosal sinus*. This is usually lateral to the *trigeminal nerve* but may be medial, passing around the nerve to get to the sinus. Section of this vessel at surgery can lead to post operative swelling of the cerebellum.

The middle neurovascular complex.

The *facial nerve* exits from the lateral end of the pontomedullary sulcus very slightly anterior to the insertion of the *vestibulocochlear nerve* at the lateral end of the sulcus. The first of the roots contributing to the *glossopharngeal, vagus and spinal accessory nerves* are 2-3mm inferior to the facial nerve origin. The roots of *IX, X and XI* provide a reliable landmark for identification of the facial nerve at its origin. The foramen of Luschka is found at the lateral margin of the pontomedullary sulcus. It is therefore posterior to the junction of the *facial and vestibulocochlear nerves* with the brainstem. Although the foramen itself is not often seen on dissection, strands of choroid plexus (the only choroid plexus in the cerebellopontine angle) protrude from it and are readily identifiable. The flocculus of the cerebellum is seen at the margin of the lateral recess, posterior to the junction of the facial and vestibulocochlear nerves with the pontomedullary sulcus. Both the flocculus and the choroid aid identification of the *facial nerve.*

The *facial and vestibulocochlear nerves* pass directly across the cerebellopontine angle to the internal acoustic meatus. The *vestibulocochlear nerve* runs behind the *facial nerve* throughout their passage through the cerebellopontine angle. During its course, the *vestibulocochlear nerve* divides into three seperate parts: the *superior and inferior vestibular nerves* and the *cochlear (or auditory) nerve*. The three branches of the *vestibulocochlear nerve* and the *facial nerve* have a characteristic arrangement on entering the internal acoustic meatus.
The internal acoustic meatus contains bony landmarks, which aid the identification of the nerves at their lateral extent. These landmarks are within the meatus and are revealed by drilling away its posterior wall.
The lateral portion of the internal acoustic meatus is divided into superior and inferior sections by the transverse (or falciform) crest. The superior section contains the *superior vestibular nerve* (posteriorly) and the *facial nerve* (anteriorly). Also in the superior section is 'Bill's bar' (also called the vertical crest), which is a vertical ridge of bone separating the *facial nerve* anteriorly and the *superior vestibular nerve* posteriorly. The inferior section con-

tains the *inferior vestibular nerve* (posteriorly) and the *cochlear nerve* (anteriorly).
The internal acoustic meatus also contains *nervus intermedius* and the *labyrinthine artery* (see above). *Nervus intermedius* is the sensory branch of the *facial nerve*. It leaves the *facial nerve* in the internal auditory meatus and passes in close approximation to the *vestibulocochlear nerve* to enter the brainstem and pass to the *nucleus solitarius*.

The anterior position of the *facial nerve*, relative to the *vestibulocochlear nerve*, in the cerebellopontine angle means that it is usually displaced anteriorly by an acoustic neuroma (vestibular schwannoma). Variations in the direction of growth of the tumour may push it anterosuperiorly or inferiorly. A large vestibular schwannoma may also push the *trigeminal nerve* superiorly and the *glossopharngeal and vagus nerves* inferiorly. The brainstem may be compressed also.

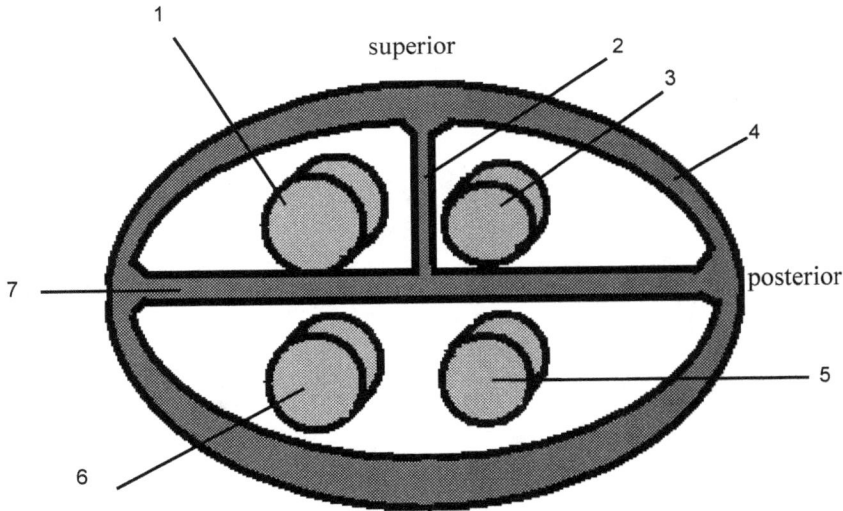

Figure 26. *Interior acoustic meatus. 1. Facial nerve 2. Vertical crest (Bill's bar) 3. Superior vestibular nerve 4. Border of internal acoustic meatus 5. Inferior vestibular nerve 6. Cochlear nerve 7. Transverse (or falciform) crest*

Vascular relations of the *facial and vestibulocochlear nerves*.
The *anterior inferior cerebellar artery (AICA)* arises bilaterally from the *basilar trunk* and passes around the brainstem below the *facial and vestibular nerves*. Less commonly the *AICA* passes over or between the facial and vestibulocochlear nerves. The *anterior inferior cerebellar artery* often loops into the porus. Preservation of the *AICA* during removal of an acoustic neuroma is vital. Occlusion may lead to infarction of the lateral pons, tegmentum and medulla, resulting in death.

The premorbid relationship of *AICA* to the *VIII* nerve determines its eventual position relative to an acoustic neuroma. Most commonly it runs inferior to the *vestibulocochlear nerve* and therefore will be pushed inferiorly. If the *AICA* runs over or between the nerves it will be pushed superiorly or anteriorly. Branches of *AICA* such as the subarcuate artery or the *labyrinthine artery* may also be draped over the tumour.

Vascular compression of the *facial nerve* may cause hemifacial spasm. *AICA* can impinge on the *facial nerve* exit should it become ectatic. In a minority of cases the *posterior inferior cerebellar artery* may come into approximation with the *facial nerve*. Compression by tortuous *vertebral or basilar arteries* is also reported.

The lower neurovascular complex.

The *posterior inferior cerebellar artery* is related to the lower four cranial nerves. It arises from the *vertebral artery* and passes around the medulla before entering the cerebellomedullary fissure near the inferior cerebellar peduncle. The anatomy of the lower four cranial nerve roots has been reviewed in the section on the surface anatomy of the brainstem.

3

PHYSIOLOGICAL ASPECTS

Matthew J Tait

Contents

Physiological spaces of the cranial vault
Blood and autoregulation
Extracellular fluid and the blood brain barrier
Cerebrospinal fluid and the choroid plexus
Intracellular fluid and the membrane potential

Intracranial pressure
Control of intracranial pressure
Raised intracranial pressure
The pathological sequelae of raised intracranial pressure

Pathophysiology of the intracranial spaces
Blood and acute haemorrhage
Intracellular and extracellular fluid and cerebral oedema
Cerebrospinal fluid and hydrocephalus

Pathophysiological response to common pathologies
Intracranial mass lesions
Brain injury
Subarachnoid haemorrhage

Much of the working of the various neural systems within the brain, such as the motor system and sensory systems is now understood, although this knowledge is far from complete. However, in relation to the daily practice of a neurosurgeon, knowledge of the physiological basis of the homeostasis of the brain (intracranial physiology) is of far greater importance. This branch of physiology is dominated by the rigid nature of the skull and the four physiological spaces that it contains.

Physiological spaces of the cranial vault

The cranial vault contains blood, CSF, intracellular fluid and extracellular fluid. These are the four physiological spaces. The intracellular and extracellular spaces are often referred to in combination as the brain parenchyma. Each of the spaces is regulated by different mechanisms, some of which are peculiar to the brain. The spaces show a high degree of physiological continuity.

The emergency cranial workload of a neurosurgeon is largely devoted to maintaining the integrity of these four spaces and controlling rises in intracranial pressure. Each will be considered in turn.

Typical values: 4% Blood (60ml)
9% CSF (140ml)
13% ECF (200ml)
74% ICF (1100ml)

Blood - Autoregulation of cerebral blood flow

Energy requirements of the brain
By weight, the brain is the heaviest user of oxygen in the body. Despite an average mass of about 1500g it receives 15-20% of cardiac output. It is the formation of the large quantity of ATP required to power the membrane pumps that maintain the electrical properties of the cells that consumes the majority of this oxygen. Oxygen consumption has been measured to be approximately 0.03mmol/100g/min.

Under normal circumstances, the brain exclusively uses glucose as the metabolic substrate and, in this sense, it is unique. In times of extreme starvation, the brain will, however, metabolise ketone bodies. Consumption of glucose is about 0.15-0.3mmol/100g/min. The brain has very little stored glycogen and it is not thought to be able to act as an effective glucose reserve.

Neurones are extremely sensitive to ischaemia. Both oxygen and glucose are delivered in far larger amounts than used by the cells. The proportion of delivered oxygen that is used by cells is termed the Oxygen Extraction Ratio (OER), the mean being 0.37. Glucose supply is, on average, 34mmol/100g/min (compared to the mean consumption of 0.15-0.3mmol/100g/min).

Increasing ischaemia has a graded effect on neurones. Initially, lack of oxygen leads to a breakdown in processes that have a high energy requirement. As a result, the resting potential cannot be maintained and the cell looses function. This situation is potentially reversible and is may form the basis of the ischaemic penumbra. Further falls in blood flow and oxygen delivery lead to irreversible cell damage or cell death.

Normal CBF	30-92 ml/100g/min
Minimum CBF for normal cellular function	15-23 ml/100g/min
Minimum CBF for membrane integrity	6ml/100g/min

Table 1. *The relationship between ischaemia and neuronal function. The probability of cell death if the CBF falls to a level between that required for normal function and that required for cell survival is related to both the severity and the duration of the fall in CBF.*

Cerebral blood flow

Cerebral blood flow (CBF) is the rate of blood flow through the cerebral capillary beds. It is not uniform throughout the brain. CBF to the grey matter is approximately 50ml/100g/min (30-92) although it declines throughout life after the third decade. White matter has a lower CBF of about 20-25ml/100g/min, which remains constant throughout life. The disparity in CBF between white and grey matter reflects the higher metabolic demand of the cell bodies of neurones compared to their axons. Local CBF is also adjusted to meet the immediate metabolic demands of groups of neurones. Increases in local activity lead to an increase in oxygen and glucose requirements. This is reflected in a local increase in blood flow. This process is known as flow-metabolism coupling.

Cerebral perfusion pressure

In most circulatory systems, the perfusion pressure is dependent on both arterial and venous pressures. The cerebral circulation differs due to the fixed volume of the cranial vault. This means that blood is pushed into a closed space with a pre-existing internal pressure. This intracranial pressure (ICP) is generally greater than the central venous pressure. As a result, cerebral perfusion pressure (CPP) is the difference between mean arterial pressure (MAP) and intracranial pressure. This is generally expressed as CPP = MAP - ICP.

Autoregulation

If unregulated, changes in MAP or ICP would alter the delivery of oxygen and glucose to neurones. Autoregulation is the process whereby CPP and CBF are dissociated. In health, a normal blood flow can be maintained over a CPP of about 50-150 mmHg (these values will increase in patients with chronic hypertension). Within the limits of CPP that can be autoregulated, the CBF is held steady by altering the vascular resistance. A rise in CPP leads to a decrease in the diameter of the cerebral vasculature. This increases vascular resistance and prevents a rise in CBF. Conversely, a fall in CPP is associated with an increase in vessel diameter to preserve CBF.

If CPP falls below the limits of autoregulation the oxygen supply can be maintained by increasing the oxygen extraction ratio (OER). Once the OER is maximal, a further fall in CPP will lead to ischaemia. Some brain areas appear to be more prone to ischaemia than others. The 'watershed' regions between the cortical territories of the major arteries are poor at autoregulation and therefore develop ischaemia at a higher CPP than other areas.

Mechanism of autoregulation

Any mechanism that maintains CBF by altering the diameter of the cerebral vessels must act by contraction or relaxation of vascular smooth muscle. This represents a final common pathway. In common with the vessels of other capillary beds, cerebral smooth muscle is under the control of both neural and humoral factors. Intrinsic properties of the vessel smooth muscle also play a role. It is thought that gross alterations of the CBF occurs in the larger vessels and smaller vessels are involved in fine tuning and the regional variations associated with flow-metabolism coupling.

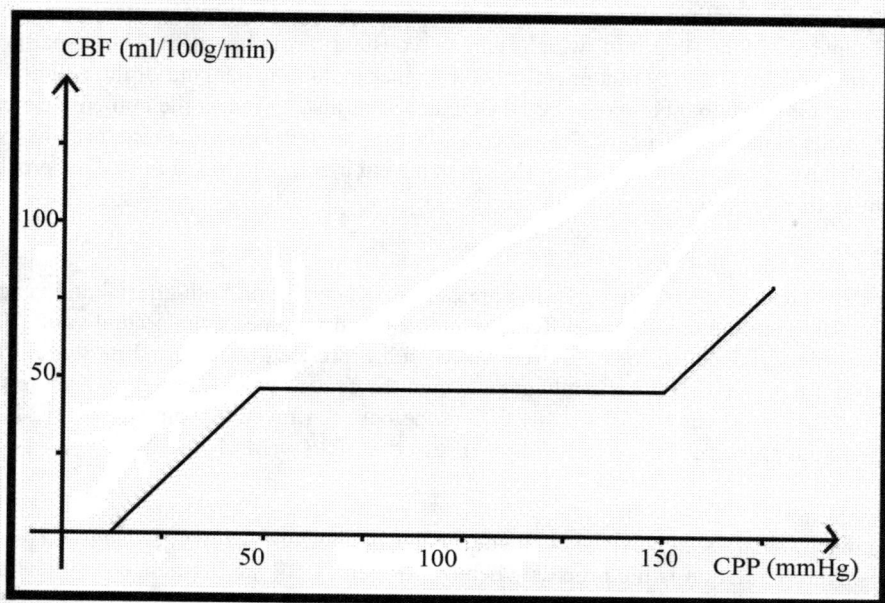

Graph 1. *Autoregulation. Increases in CPP between 50-150mmHg are compensated for by autoregulation to keep CBF constant.(Graph by S Bulled)*

Neurogenic control. The cerebral vessel walls express the various neurotransmitter receptors including adrenoceptors, muscarinic acetylcholine receptors, 5-HT1 and 5-HT2 receptors as well as receptors for vasoactive intestinal polypeptide, substance P, neuropeptide Y and neurokinin A. Of these systems, it is thought that the sympathetic drive exerts the strongest influence. Even so, this influence is weak and its exact physiological role is undetermined.

Humoral control. The blood brain barrier (see below) protects the cerebral vasculature from circulating systemic vasoactive substances. This allows autoregulation to remain independent of systemic changes in vascular tone. The principle humoral control is by locally produced metabolites. Rather than being involved in general autoregulation, it is thought that these factors are important for local control i.e. flow-metabolism coupling.

Rises in local arterial carbon dioxide tension ($PaCO_2$) cause marked vasodilatation. This is thought to be due to the associated fall in perivascular pH. Indeed, any factor that causes a local fall in perivascular pH (such as increased concentrations of lactic acid) will lead to vasodilatation. Despite this close correlation it has been found that increases in vessel diameter associated with increased local metabolism occur before there is a fall in local pH.

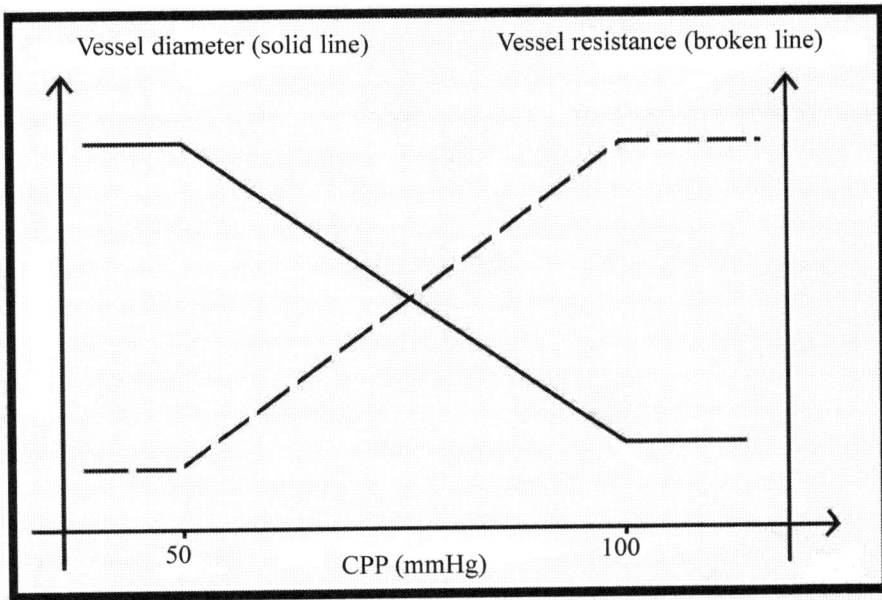

Graph 2. *Relationship of cerebral vessel diameter and resistance to CPP. Over the range of autoregulation increases in CPP lead to constriction of the cerebral vasculature and an increase in resistance. This maintains a consistent CBF. (Graph by S Bulled)*

As a result, CO_2 and pH are not thought to have a significant role in control of CBF under normal conditions. Lowering of systemic $PaCO_2$ by mechanical ventilation is used to help to control rises in ICP by reducing vasodilatation. It is important to note that this will be at the expense of CBF and therefore a careful balance is required. Furthermore, in circumstances of prolonged hypocapnia the CSF pH returns to normal and subsequent modulation of $PaCO_2$ is of questionable value.

Topical application of either K^+ or adenosine to pial vessels cause vasodilatation. Both show an increase in extracellular concentration when local neural activity is increased. They are thought to play an important role in flow-metabolism coupling. Additionally, perivascular adenosine concentrations rise in times of metabolic stress. Reduced oxygen delivery to cells caused by a fall in CPP will therefore trigger adenosine release and vasodilatation. Thus adenosine levels may play a role in general autoregulation although this is uncertain.

Myogenic control. The most likely mechanism of autoregulation relies on the intrinsic properties of the vessel smooth muscle. Cerebral smooth muscle contracts in response to distension of the vessel wall. This occurs to an appropriate extent to maintain a constant CBF. The timing of this process correlates well with the observed in vivo response to changes in CPP. Autoregulation may also exert an influence on the systemic circulation. Rises in ICP are associated with a rise in MAP. This is called Cushing's response. It is thought to be mediated by ischaemia of the medullary vasomotor nuclei.

CBF (ml/100g/min)

100

50

50   100   150

PaCO$_2$ (mmHg))

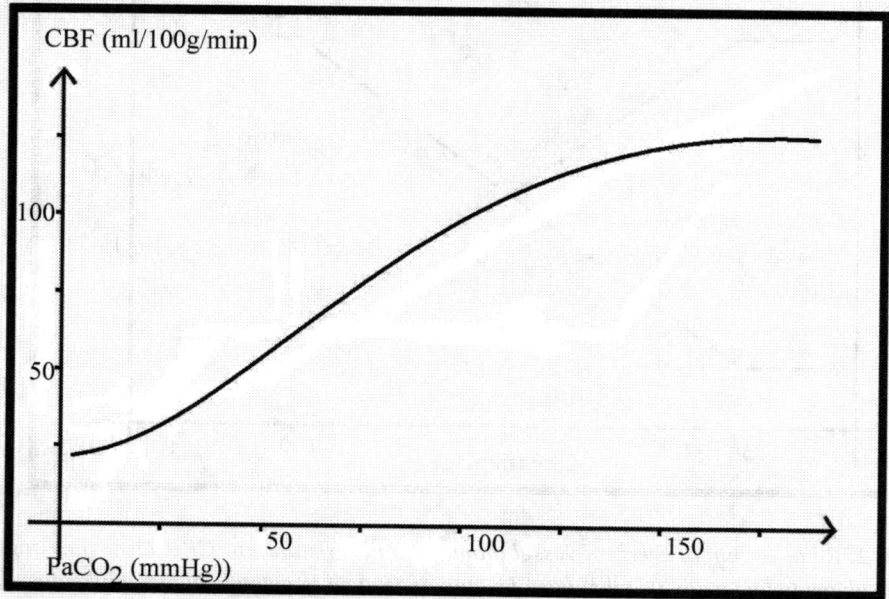

Graph 3. *The relationship of CO$_2$ tension and CBF. (Graph by S Bulled)*

Exracellular fluid - The blood brain barrier

Blood brain barrier

The term blood brain barrier refers to the prevention, by the cerebral endothelium, of extravasation of certain blood borne elements that are harmful to cerebral function and which pass through capillary walls elsewhere in the body. The endothelium thus plays an important and specific role in determining the composition of the extracellular environment of the brain. This role is not purely restrictive: other blood constituents, vital to neuronal function, are actively transported into the brain's internal milieu. The blood brain barrier is functionally active by, or shortly after, birth but continues to develop during early life.

The unique role of the cerebral capillaries is reflected in their structure. Blood is isolated from the brain at the endothelium by tight junctions that prevent the passage of plasma around the cells of the endothelium. There is also a lack of fenestrations and a reduction in the number of pinocytic vesicles compared with normal endothelium. Cerebral capillary endothelium also contains about 2-4 times as many mitochondria as normal epithelium, which may reflect increased active transport. Outside the basement membrane of the capillaries, astrocytes are found in close approximation to the endothelium and basement membrane. It is thought that these cells trigger the formation of the blood brain barrier.

The blood brain barrier contains some important anatomical gaps relating to brain structures that require an accurate picture of plasma constituents. These structures need access to specific blood elements or are involved in the production of CSF. Areas that lack a blood brain barrier are the choroid plexus, area postrema, median eminence, posterior pituitary gland, pineal body, subfornical and commissural organs and the supraoptic crest.

The physical nature of the blood brain barrier does not provide much of a hindrance to substances that are able to cross cell membranes, as these will bypass the tight junctions. Lipid soluble molecules, such as alcohol, therefore pass directly into the brain by simple diffusion. They freely cross the cell membranes, following their diffusion gradients. Both oxygen and carbon dioxide are also highly permeable. In the case of highly soluble molecules, the rate of diffusion is also related to the rate of supply of the substance to the blood brain barrier i.e. it is related to cerebral blood flow.

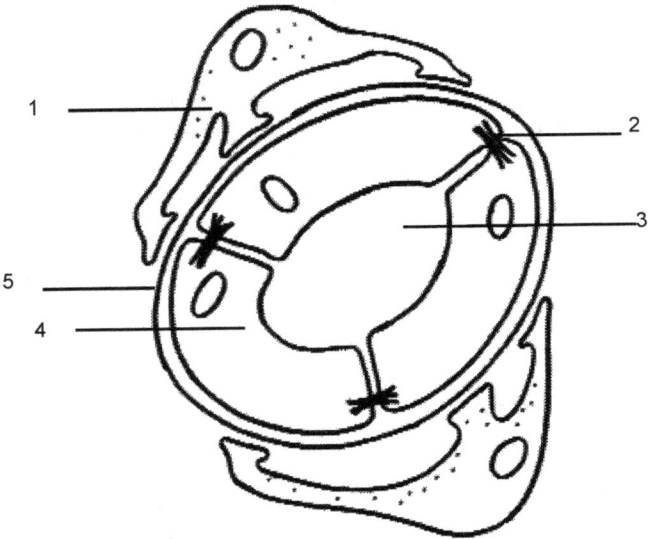

Figure 1. *The structure of the blood brain barrier. 1. Astrocyte 2. Tight junction 3. Intravascular space 4. Endothelial cell 5. Basement menbrane*

The passage of water across capillary beds is usually dependent on Starling's forces (hydrostatic and oncotic pressures). The tight junctions of the cerebral capillary bed reduce much of the impact of hydrostatic pressure and so oncotic pressure is the major determinant of water flow. Mannitol does not cross the blood brain barrier well so its administration will increase the intravascular osmolality and therefore cause water to enter capillaries. This requires an intact blood brain barrier, as mannitol within the cerebral milieu will have the opposite effect. Other methods of increasing the serum osmolality, such as infusion of hypertonic saline, have a similar effect to mannitol.

Polarised, non-lipid soluble compounds are, by contrast, efficiently excluded by the blood brain barrier. This is beneficial in the case of amino acids that are used as neurotransmitters, such as glycine. Other amino acids, such as tryptophan, which are essential precursors for neurotransmitter formation, are taken up by carrier mediated transport. Glucose is also taken up by carrier mediated transport, using the Glut-1 transporter. Neither of these carrier systems requires ATP and so they only serve to facilitate transport down the concentration gradient.

Other substances are transported against their concentration gradients. The $3Na^+/2K^+$ ATPase pump is found on the outside surface of the endothelial wall. This pump allows water and Na to be excreted into the brain extracellular fluid whilst removing K^+.

The blood brain barrier is not entirely under local control. The capillary walls contain a variety of receptors. Noradrenergic input from the locus ceruleus in the brain stem stimulates the $3Na^+/2K^+$ ATPase and is thought to influence active control of electrolyte balance. Other exogenous factors that influence the permeability of the blood brain barrier include steroids, such as dexamethasone, which tightens the tight junctions and atrial natriuretic peptide, which increases the permeability of the barrier to water.

Cerebrospinal fluid - Choroid plexus and the blood CSF barrier

Role of CSF

CSF is a colourless, viscous fluid, so much so that normal CSF is often described as being 'gin clear'. In anatomical terms, the CSF spaces are the ventricular system and the subarachnoid space (including the subarachnoid cisterns). The subarachnoid space of the spine is continuous with that of the brain, the most inferior part being the lumbar cistern. The CSF therefore acts as a bath in which the brain and spinal cord are immersed. It is therefore able to act as a support for the delicate neural tissue. Other functions of the CSF include cushioning trauma, acting as a sink for transependymal flow of extracellular fluid and contributing to a suitable environment for neuronal function. CSF may also be involved in the removal of waste materials, as evidenced by the increasing concentrations of proteins and neurotransmitters found as it flows along its pathways.

Composition of CSF

CSF may be thought of as an ultrafiltrate of plasma, modified using active transport by the choroidal epithelium. The ventricular cavities are lined by a thin membranous layer called the ependyma. The ependyma does not contain tight junctions and thus is 'leaky'. As a result CSF is physiologically continuous with the extracellular fluid of the brain parenchyma. It therefore has a very similar make up; indeed transependymal flow of extracellular fluid into the ventricles makes an appreciable contribution to the CSF volume.

Glucose concentrations in the CSF are generally 60-80% of plasma glucose concentrations. This figure falls when plasma glucose is pathologically elevated as glucose transfer is receptor mediated and these receptors become saturated at high concentrations. CSF glucose concentration tends to lag about 2 hours behind large changes in plasma glucose concentrations, reflecting the slow nature of carrier mediated transport.

CSF protein concentrations are low compared with interstitial fluid in other body areas (c. 0.5%). This is thought to aid the electrical activity of cells by making the CSF a better insulator. It is mainly the result of the tight junctions of the blood CSF barrier. Up to three-quarters of CSF protein is albumin, which is derived from the plasma. The remainder consists mainly of globulin (predominantly IgG). CSF protein concentration varies by anatomical location. CSF from the ventricles has a lower protein concentration (6-12mg/dl) than that in the lumbar theca (20-50mg/dl). Increases in the CSF protein count, although non-specific, are usually a reliable indicator of disease. Pathologically raised CSF protein may cause communicating hydrocephalus by interfering with CSF reabsorption.

The osmolality of CSF is similar to that of plasma in health. This is reflected in the sodium concentration of CSF, which is also approximately equal to that of plasma. Potassium, by contrast, has a lower concentration in CSF than plasma (c.60%). This may serve to help maintain the resting potential of neurones and is the result of the action of the $3Na^+/2K^+$ ATPase on the cerebral aspect of both the blood brain barrier and the blood CSF barrier (see below).

The cellular content of CSF in a healthy subject is largely made up of leucocytes. In adults 5 leucocytes/mm^3 is the upper limit of normal and this is doubled in children. No more than 40% should be polymorphonuclear leucocytes. Erythrocytes are not present in normal CSF.

	CSF	Plasma
Glucose (mg/l)	4.5-8.0	5.0-10
Protein (mg/dl)	6-50 (site dependent)	c6000
Osmolality (mosm/kg H_2O)	275-295	275-295
Na^+ (mmol/l)	135-145	135-145
K^+ (mmol/l)	2.5-3.6	3.5-5.0

Table 2. *Composition of CSF and plasma.*

CSF production - Structure and function of the choroid plexus
The ventricles and subarachnoid spaces generally contain about 150ml of CSF. CSF formation is predominantly by the choroid plexus in the lateral, third and forth ventricles (80-90%). An important but secondary contribution to CSF formation is made by flow of extracellular fluid from the brain parenchyma into the ventricles, through the leaky ependyma, or into the subarachnoid space, through the pia mater. The extracellular fluid probably accounts for about 10-20% of CSF volume.

The choroid plexus has rich blood supply. This blood passes into a highly vascularised region of the pial surface of the ventricular walls. Capillaries there lack the tight junctions that form the blood brain barrier of the majority of cerebral capillaries. The ependyma is generally a semipermeable membrane lacking tight junctions. In the choroid plexus, however, it forms a specialised covering of choroidal epithelium. The cells of the choroidal epithelium have apical tight junctions, giving them a controlled intercellular space. They also have invaginations on the basal surface (that adjacent to the capillary basement membrane) as well as microvilli on the ventricular surface, both of which serve to increase the surface area available for membrane transport. Thus the site of active formation of CSF is the choroidal epithelium (specialised ependyma) rather than the capillary endothelium. This interface is called the blood-CSF barrier.

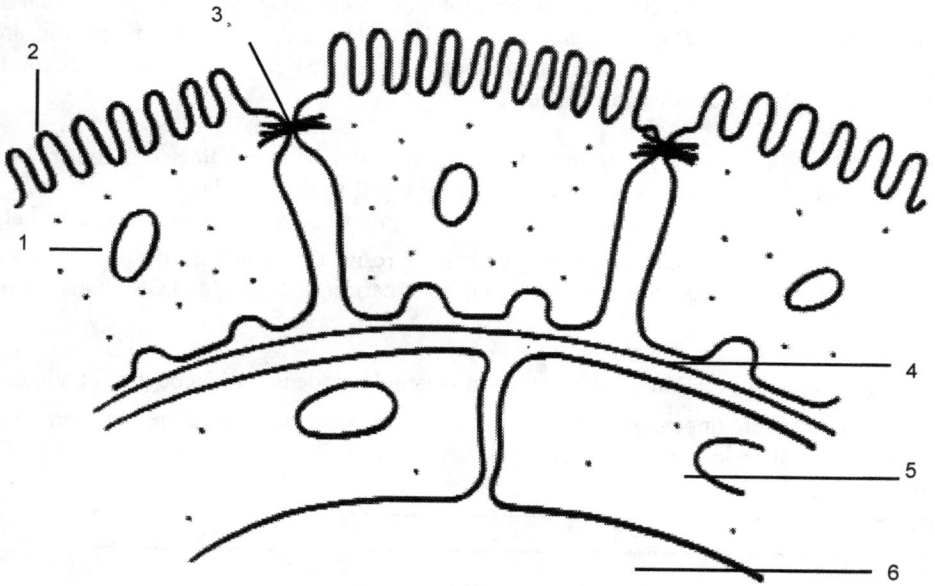

Figure 2. *The structure of the blood-CSF barrier. 1. Choroidal epithelial cell 2. Microvilli 3. Tight junctions between choroidal epithelium 4. Basement menbrane 5. Capillary endothelial cell (lacking tight junctions) 6. Intravascular space*

CSF is produced by a combination of ultrafiltration of plasma by the capillary endothelial wall and active transport of solutes by the choroidal epithelium. Despite the contrast in structure between the choroid plexus and the blood brain barrier the processing underlying the formation of both CSF and extracellular fluid are similar. The tight junctions of the choroidal epithelium play a very similar role to those of the endothelium of the blood brain barrier.

Much of the carrier mediated flow is the same: the $3Na^+/2K^+$ ATPase is again present (on the outside of the choroidal epithelium). Water flow is determined by osmotic gradients.

Control of CSF formation

CSF is formed at about 20ml/hour (0.35ml/min or 500ml/day). Factors influencing the rate of CSF formation are indicated in the box below

Increase	Low CSF osmolality
	Raised temperature
	Raised choroidal blood flow
Decrease	Raised CSF osmolality
	Low temperature
	Reduced choroidal blood flow
	Raised ventricular pressure
	Drugs such as steroids, diuretics and acetazolamide

Table 3. *Factors known to influence the rate of CSF production.*

CSF flow

Once in the ventricular system, the CSF flows caudally, towards the foramina of Magendie and Luschka by bulk flow. This movement is mediated by a pressure gradient between the sites of CSF production and its final absorption at the venous sinuses. CSF is also pushed through the ventricles by ependymal cilia and the arterial (and, to a lesser extent respiratory) pulsations. After exiting the ventricular system the CSF enters the subarachnoid space. It flows through the cisterns of the spinal cord and brain before ending its journey at the arachnoid granulations of the dural sinuses. The exact path or probably pathways of this flow remain to be elucidated.

The anatomy of the ventricular system is covered in the next chapter.

Absorption of CSF

CSF is predominantly reabsorbed via the arachnoid villi, into the venous sinuses. Other sites of reabsorption are the arachnoid villi of the spinal nerve roots, the cerebral capillaries and the choroid plexus (which is able to absorb as well as produce CSF).

The arachnoid villi have two mechanisms for absorption of CSF. Under normal conditions, absorption takes place by transcellular micropinocytosis. When ICP is raised, CSF reabsorption is increased by the opening of valve-like intercellular channels. Absorption of CSF by the cerebral veins and choroid plexus appears to be by diffusion or active transport of solutes. As a result of the valve mechanism, the reabsorption of CSF is greater when ICP is raised. In fact this relationship is proportional.

Intracellular fluid

The fluid contained within neurones is markedly different from that surrounding it. The most important distinction is in ionic concentrations. Intracellular potassium concentrations are far greater than in the extracellular space. The ubiquitous $3Na^+/2K^+$ ATPase membrane pump is found in high density on the neuronal cell membrane. It draws K+ ions into the cell accounting for much of this disparity. This effect is heightened by more $3Na^+/2K^+$ ATPase pumps on the cerebral aspect of the endothelium of the blood brain barrier which reduce extracellular K^+ concentration relative to plasma.

The reverse is seen for Na^+ concentrations. The neuronal cell membrane pumps expel sodium from the cell, keeping intracellular concentrations lower than both extracellular fluid and plasma. The water content of the cell is determined by its osmotic pressure. This pressure derives in part from a relatively stable content of intracellular proteins but predominantly from the ionic content of the cell.

It is the relative concentrations of intracellular and extracellular ions that account for the resting and action potentials of neurones, which form the basis of their function. Both Na^+ and K^+ form an equilibrium potential based on the potential difference required to balance the conflict of their electrical and chemical gradients when the cell is resting. The combination of these potentials (which can be calculated using the Nernst equation) gives the resting potential of the cell. Synaptic stimulation of the cell leads to changes in the membrane permeability, which trigger a stereotypical sequence of changes in membrane permeability to both Na^+ and K^+. The resultant ion currents, caused by flow down electrochemical gradients, cause local changes in cell membrane potential and trigger further local action potentials.

The volume regulation of the cells (and therefore the volume regulation of the intracellular space) is intimately related to their electrical function.

Intracranial pressure

ICP is measured relative to atmospheric pressure. It generally fluctuates between 5 and 10mmHg but values of less than 15mmHg are considered normal. Both cardiac and respiratory pressure waves are conducted to the CSF, becoming superimposed on one another.

High speed recordings of ICP demonstrate the transmission of the normal arterial wave form to the CSF: a sharp rise is seen as a result of contraction of the left cardiac ventricle (called the percussion wave), followed by a gradual fall due to relaxation of the great vessels. The dicrotic notch is a transient dip in pressure during the lag phase of the arterial pressure waveform caused by the small backflow that closes the aortic valve leaflets. This too is seen in the ICP waveform.

Fluctuations in ICP as a result of respiration are slower. They are caused both by the influence of the respiratory cycle on arterial blood pressure and venous drainage (via CVP). The respiratory influence is, however, less consistent than the arterial effect on ICP. In health, there is a fall in ICP during inspiration and a rise during expiration. This picture is complicated by mechanical respiration.

ICP is constant throughout the cranial vault. This is a result of pressure transmission by the CSF in accordance with physical principles described by Pascal's law. This law states that the pressure of a liquid in a confined spherical space, such as CSF within the cranial vault, is uniform. Thus, measurement of the ICP from one point within the vault gives a reading of the pressure throughout. Two factors complicate this picture. First is the presence of the falx and tentorium, which may shelter certain areas. The second is the columnar nature of the spinal extension of the subarachnoid space. The pressure of fluid in a column is greatest at its base. As a result ICP varies with posture, being reduced by making the neuraxis more vertical. Overall, this effect is secondary to Pascal's law.

Three clinical implications are that (1) subdural, intraparenchymal and intraventricular ICP recordings all give reliable indications of ICP throughout the vault, that (2) control of raised ICP requires the head to be raised and that (3) ICP readings done via lumbar puncture must be performed with the patient horisontal.

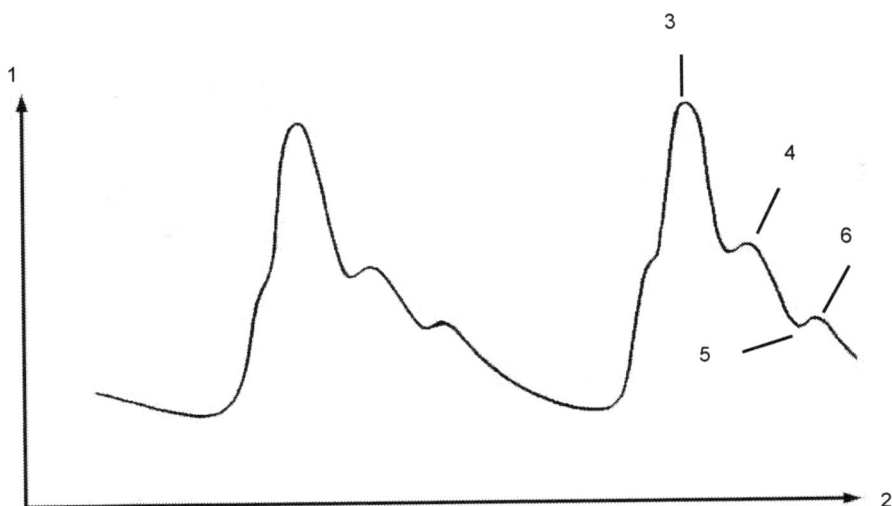

Figure 3. *Normal ICP trace. 1. ICP 2. Time 3. Percussion wave 4. Tidal wave 5. Dicrotic notch 6. Dicrotic wave*

Control of ICP

As is apparent from the previous discussion, the volume of each intracranial space is controlled separately. Fluid passes freely between the spaces, mainly controlled by osmotic pressures generated by the movements of ions (predominantly sodium). Thus there is no one mechanism for the control of ICP; rather it is the result of the sum of each separately controlled but interdependent process. Pathological processes that increase the content of a physiological space sufficiently to overcome buffering mechanisms will lead to a rise in ICP.

Raised intracranial pressure

Increases in ICP are either the result of failure to regulate the physiological spaces or a decrease in the effective volume of the cranial vault, caused by a mass lesion. In the early stages of volume change, a rise in ICP is deferred by buffering mechanisms.

The best known buffering mechanism is concomitant displacement of fluid from another physiological space. This effect is known as volume buffering and is the basis of the Monroe-Kelly doctrine. Both CSF and blood can be rapidly displaced from the cranial vault. Blood displacement occurs by compression of the venous system. CSF is displaced caudally to the lumbar theca. As abnormal volume changes occur, blood and CSF are squeezed from cranial vault so that the overall intracranial volume and thus the ICP remain constant. Clearly there is only a finite amount of either CSF or blood that can be displaced. Once this has been exhausted, further increases in volume lead rapidly to increases in ICP. Rises in ICP also lead to increased CSF absorption (see above)

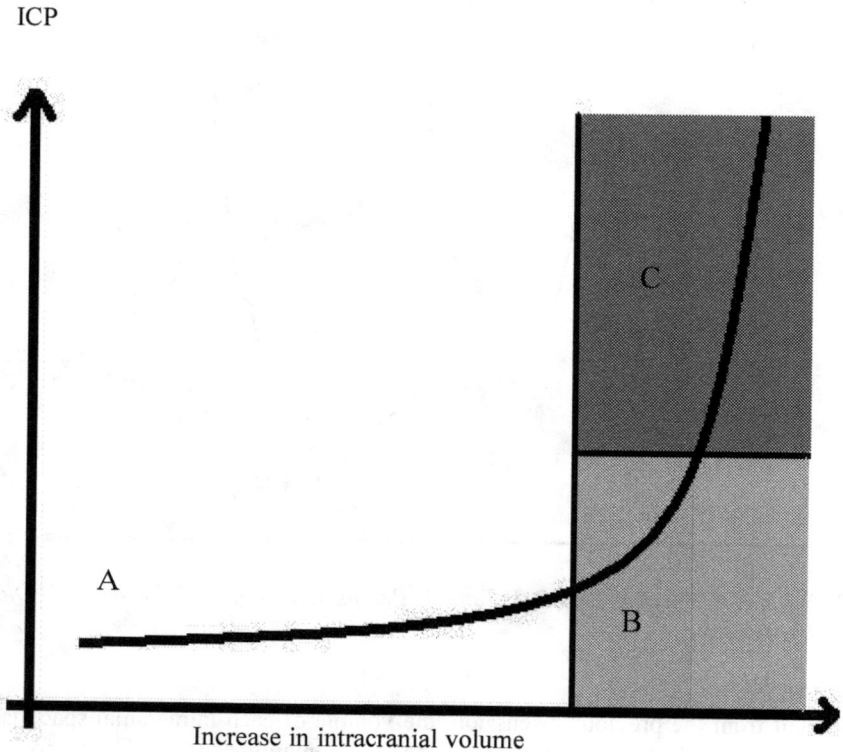

ICP

A

C

B

Increase in intracranial volume

Graph 4. *The relationship between intracranial volume and intracranial pressure. As additional volume is added to the intracranial space compliance is initially high due to the expulsion of blood and CSF (area A). As volume buffering begins to fail compliance falls and addition of further volume causes a greater increase in ICP (area B). Once the compensatory mechanisms have been exhausted compliance is very low and ICP rises rapidly.*

It is not only blood and CSF that can provide volume buffering. If volume changes are sufficiently gradual, large changes in both the intracellular and extracellular spaces can occur. The volume of brain parenchyma may reduce by as much as 50% allowing accommodation of chronic expansions of mass lesions or of the ventricular system in chronic hydrocephalus.

Once the ICP has begun to rise, the vascular autoregulatory mechanisms described above are initially able to preserve cerebral blood flow. Rises in ICP trigger both increases in systemic blood pressure (Cushing's response) and cerebral vasodilatation (increases in ICP lead to a fall in CPP and therefore vasodilatation by autoregulation).

Pathological Sequelae of raised intracranial pressure

Uncontrolled rises in intracranial pressure cause, reduced cerebral blood flow, displacement of cerebral tissue (brain herniation) and papilloedema

Vascular consequences of raised intracranial pressure:

As described above, the cerebral perfusion pressure is equal to the mean arterial blood pressure (MAP) minus the intracranial pressure (ICP).

$$CPP = MAP - ICP$$

Thus a rise in ICP will lead to a fall in CPP. If autoregulation is undamaged there will be a resultant increase in the diameter of the cerebral vessels to preserve CBF. This increases the volume of the intravascular space further contributing to the rise in ICP. If ICP rises to a point where the CPP is too low to allow maintenance of the CBF ischaemia will develop. Ischaemic brain tissue will generate oedema, which contributes further to raised ICP. If untreated, this downward spiral will result in death.

Brain herniation

Pascal's law ensures that CSF transmits rises in intracranial pressure throughout the cranial vault and also down into the spinal subarachnoid space and cisterns. If CSF is no longer able to pass freely throughout the subarachnoid spaces, pressure gradients will occur. The most common sites of blockage are the tentorial incisura (between the supratentorial and infratentorial spaces) and the foramen magnum (between the infratentorial space and the spinal subarachnoid space). Mass lesions such as haematomas or tumours may displace the brain parenchyma in such a way that CSF passage at the tentorial incisura or foramen magnum is blocked. There are five recognised patterns of herniation.

Subfalcine herniation

A large unilateral mass lesion in the supratentorial space will displace the brain parenchyma away from it. This pushes the ipsilateral cingulate gyrus under the free edge of the falx. The falx is not of uniform depth. Anteriorly it terminates nearer to the superior hemispheric border than posteriorly and therefore the herniation is more pronounced in the frontal part of the brain. Compression of the internal cerebral veins or ipsilateral anterior cerebral artery may occur. Subfalcine herniation is described as midline shift when seen on CT scans.

Bilateral transtentorial herniation (central herniation)

If both cerebral hemispheres swell equally, a downward displacement of the hemispheres pushes the diencephalon and midbrain through the tentorial incisura. Initially, the diencephalon is distorted. Then, as the pressure increases, the midbrain, pons and medulla are compressed in sequence. As each segment becomes compressed in turn it looses function giving an evolving clinical picture. Whilst a complete description of the examination findings at each stage is outside the scope of this chapter, the pupillary responses provide a good example. At the stage of diencephalic compression the pupils are small and reactive. Progression to the midbrain stage leads to midsize unreactive pupils. This persists throughout the pontine stage until, with compression of the medulla, they become bilaterally dilated. Further compression leads to brain death.

Unilateral transtentorial herniation (uncal herniation)

Large unilateral supratentorial mass lesions also displace the ipsilateral uncus of the temporal lobe. This causes the uncus to move medially into the anterior tentorial incisura, bringing it into contact with the contents of the suprasellar region. The resultant compression of the brainstem leads to reduced consciousness. Compression of the oculomotor nerve causes ipsilateral pupillary dilatation (a 'blown pupil'). Compression of the ipsilateral posterior cerebral artery may cause cortical blindness of the contralateral hemifield.

The third nerve palsy is a reasonably reliable indicator of the side of the lesion, however if the contralateral aspect of the brainstem is compressed against the contralateral free edge of the tentorium (Kernohan's notch) a misleading contralateral blown pupil may occur.

Further progression of uncal herniation leads to sequential brainstem compression in the same way as is seen in central herniation.

Upward tentorial herniation and transforaminal herniation

Mass lesions within the posterior fossa causing raised pressure within the infratentorial space can cause occlusion of and herniation through either the tentorial incisura (up into the supratentorial space) or the foramen magnum.

Papilloedema

Papilloedema is swelling of the optic discs caused by raised intracranial pressure. If chronic or severe and acute this may cause permanent loss of vision. It is most commonly associated with gradual rises in intracranial pressure such as that associated with chronic hydrocephalus or slow growing tumour masses.

The optic nerve has more in common with a tract of fibres within the brain than a peripheral nerve. It is surrounded by sheaths of both arachnoid and dura, both of which are attached to the sclera of the eyeball at the point where the nerve exits the back of the globe. The central retinal vein, which drains the retina, runs in the subarachnoid space of the optic nerve. The optic nerve sheath allows the transmission of raised intracranial pressure to the optic disc. This compresses the central retinal vein elevating the pressure within the capillary bed of the retina and therefore reducing retinal perfusion pressure. This decrease in perfusion pressure reduces the energy delivery to the cell bodies of the projection neurones of the retina (called ganglion cells). As a result, axonal transport is inhibited and the build up of untransported proteins causes swelling of the optic disc.

The symptoms of papilloedema consist of visual symptoms superimposed on a background of symptoms of raised intracranial pressure. Papilloedema may cause gradual loss of vision, usually beginning as blurring of the peripheries. Patients sometimes report flashing lights (photopsia) or horisontal diplopia (due to abducens nerve palsy). If present, transient obscurations of vision are pathognomonic. These are visual blackouts associated with changes in posture. If untreated, severe visual loss and, finally, blindness will ensue. Treatment is by either reducing intracranial pressure or decompression of the optic nerve sheath (to restore flow in the central retinal vein).

Pathophysiology of the intracranial spaces

Disorders of the intracellular and extracellular spaces: Brain oedema

Brain oedema has been defined as an increase in brain water content leading to an increase in tissue volume. Four types are recognised. Vasogenic oedema, cytotoxic oedema, hydrocephalic oedema and osmotic oedema.

Vasogenic oedema

This type of oedema is caused by dysfunction of the blood brain barrier. Leaky cerebral capillaries allow a protein rich exudate to escape into the cranial interstitium. Extravasation of plasma proteins, leads to an increase in the osmotic pressure within the extracellular fluid of the brain and fluid accumulation.

The manner of capillary disruption appears to influence the development of vasogenic oedema. Distension of the capillary wall by large increases in blood pressure or shrinkage of the endothelial cells by hyperosmotic extracellular fluid can both cause mechanical disruption of the tight intercellular junctions but neither are associated with significant development of oedema. It has therefore been suggested that vasoactive factors, released by damaged brain, must play an important role. Experimental models of vasogenic oedema involve freezing areas of brain to cause local damage. In this model, vasogenic oedema arises locally and its formation terminates with removal of the damaged focus.

Cytotoxic oedema

Cytotoxic oedema is characterised by swelling of the cellular components of the brain i.e. an increase in the intracellular fluid volume. There is a concomitant decrease in the extracellular space. This occurs in the presence of an intact blood brain barrier. Neuronal cell membranes are highly permeable to water. As a result, maintenance of cell volume is dependent on electrolyte loads, particularly sodium. An influx of sodium, down its concentration gradient will drag water with it resulting in an increase in cell volume. This alone will not increase overall volume. A fall in extracellular osmotic pressure causes increased sodium uptake from the capillaries. Formation of cytotoxic oedema therefore requires local perfusion.

Intracellular sodium influx is counterbalanced by the Na^+/K^+ ATPase. Thus, increases in the membrane permeability to sodium or failure of the Na^+/K^+ ATPase (either due to pump failure or lack of ATP) will to lead to intracellular accumulation of sodium and thus oedema. As well as swelling, the cell will also lose its depolarisation and thus its ability to function.

The underlying mechanism is thought to be related to high extracellular concentrations of toxins released by cell injury due to the underlying pathology (e.g. ischaemia). Glutamate, for example, binds to specific membrane receptors leading to an increase in membrane permeability to sodium. Attempts by the Na^+/K^+ ATPase to counteract this imbalance lead to exhaustion of the cell's ATP reserves and therefore pump dysfunction.

Hydrocephalic oedema.

A rise in CSF pressure e.g. that due to obstructive hydrocephalus causes CSF to be pushed across the ependyma of the ventricular system into the interstitial space. This is seen as periventricular lucency (also known as transependymal oedema) on radiological imaging. The resulting increase in interstitial hydrostatic pressure prevents drainage of interstitial fluid in the usual manner.

Osmotic oedema

The tight junctions of the blood brain barrier ensure that oncotic pressures are the major determinant of water flow across cerebral capillary walls. As a result, the brain is particularly sensitive to hypo-osmolar states. This is why infusion of large amounts of hypotonic solutions causes cerebral oedema and dysfunction in preference to other organ systems. Low plasma osmolality can also occur as a result of the syndrome of inappropriate antidiuretic hormone release (SIADH) or cerebral salt wasting, either of which may cause cerebral oedema and coma.

99

Disorders of the intravascular compartment: Acute haemorrhage

Strictly speaking, an increase in the volume of the intravascular space is associated with unruptured vascular abnormalities such as arterio-venous malformations or giant aneurysms. These increases are not great and are easily buffered without causing changes in ICP. Of far greater relevance to intracranial physiology is the effect of blood escaping from the intravascular compartment into the other physiological spaces.

Intracranial haemorrhage may be the spontaneous or traumatic. Spontaneous bleeding is the result of inherent weaknesses of the vasculature, such as an aneurysm or AVM. Haemorrhages are classified according to their anatomical location. They may be extradural, subdural, subarachnoid, intraparenchymal or intraventricular. Many bleeds are a combination of the above. Most intracranial bleeding is arterial in origin and thus blood escapes into the cranial vault at pressures way in excess of normal ICP. This results in a rapid rise in ICP, often associated with brain herniation.

The development of loss of consciousness caused by an extradural haemorrhage following vascular trauma gives a good illustration of the buffering of ICP by the Monroe-Kelly doctrine. In the initial stages following the injury the volume of the expanding extradural blood can be accommodated by the displacement of CSF and intravascular blood. This period is called the 'lucid interval', during which the patient remains conscious. If the clot continues to expand the buffering mechanism will be overcome and ICP rises rapidly, resulting in brain herniation, loss of consciousness and ultimately death by coning. The lucid interval is less often seen in acute subdural haemorrhage as loss of consciousness due to the underlying brain injury may supervene.

Haemorrhage into the subarachnoid space may lead to a sudden massive rise in ICP to that of arterial pressure. This is mediated by Pascal's law (the CSF space becomes suddenly continuous with the intravascular space). These radical changes in ICP may account for the high incidence of sudden death with subarachnoid haemorrhage.

Haemorrhage into the intraventricular spaces may lead to either acute non-communicating hydrocephalus or more chronic communicating hydrocephalus. Acute hydrocephalus arises as a result of physical blockage of the CSF pathways, particularly the forth ventricle and aqueduct of Sylvius. Chronic hydrocephalus is thought to be due to dysfunction of CSF reabsorption at the arachnoid granulations. This is perhaps due to inflammatory damage brought about by accumulation of blood products at the granulations at the time of the intraventricular bleed.

Disorders of the CSF space: Hydrocephalus

Increases in the volume of the CSF space mainly alter the volume of the ventricular system, rather than the subarachnoid cisterns. This increase in CSF volume is referred to as hydrocephalus. Hydrocephalus is either the result of an imbalance between CSF production and absorption or due to obstruction of the ventricular flow channels. CSF overproduction causing hydrocephalus is rare, being largely restricted to children with choroid plexus papillomas. Thus the most common causes of hydrocephalus are failure of CSF absorption at the arachnoid villi and obstruction of CSF flow. These patterns of hydrocephalus are referred to as communicating and non-communicating hydrocephalus respectively. Non-communicating hydrocephalus is also known as obstructive hydrocephalus. This may be confusing as communicating hydrocephalus may be caused by obstruction of the arachnoid villi.

Communicating hydrocephalus is associated with high protein or cell loads within the CSF. This may occur with subarachnoid haemorrhage or with protein shedding tumours, such as an acoustic neuroma.
Non-communicating hydrocephalus may be caused by obstruction of the ventricular channels at any point. Occlusion of the forth ventricle or Sylvian aqueduct by mass lesions within the posterior fossa is a well appreciated cause.

A further important distinction is the duration over which hydrocephalus occurs. The brain is far better able to withstand gradual increases in CSF volume than sudden changes. As a result, relatively small changes in CSF volume in an acute process (e.g. sudden blockage of both foramina of Monroe by a colloid cyst) may prove rapidly fatal. This may be due to the compensatory reduction in the volume of the brain parenchyma which is possible over time. Hydrocephalus ex vacuo is a dilation of the ventricles which is independent of CSF physiology for its aetiology. Brain atrophy leads to a loss of parenchymal volume and therefore the CSF space (including the ventricles enlarges).

Increases in the intracranial volume of CSF have several effects. Chronic hydrocephalus causes hydrocephalic oedema, ventricular dilatation and papilloedema. It may also lead to loss of volume of the brain parenchyma. Acute hydrocephalus causes ventricular dilatation, loss of consciousness, cerebral herniation and death.
The degree of ventricular dilatation caused by hydrocephalus is related to the increased pressure within the ventricles but there is much variation between individuals as to how much dilation is produced by a given pressure increment. Patients with 'stiff' ventricles may show very little ventricular dilatation thus a lack of ventriculomegaly on a CT scan does not exclude a high CSF pressure.

Ventricular dilatation leads to tearing of the subependymal lining and septum pellucidum. The ependymal lining often remains intact. The raised pressure within the ventricular system prevents drainage of the extracellular fluid of the brain into the CSF. This results in periventricular hydrocephalic oedema.

Ventricular dilatation is responsible for the neurological signs associated with hydrocephalus. Long tract weakness is caused by elongation of the corticospinal tracts as they pass laterally around the enlarged lateral ventricles. The lower limb fibres are preferentially affected as they arise from the medial aspect of the motor strip and thus have a longer course around the lateral ventricle. Weakness is therefore more pronounced in the lower limbs. Downward displacement of the brainstem due to ventriculomegaly causes the abducens nerves to become stretched over the petrous apices. This leads to abducens nerve palsy and diplopia - the classical 'false localising' sign of hydrocephalus.

Pathophysiology

Thus far diseases which predominantly effect individual physiological spaces have been considered (although these will have 'knock on' effects). Other common pathologies have concurrent effects on more than one space. They are considered below. I have restricted the discussion to issues relating to the fluid spaces.

The response to intrinsic tumour formation. The slow growth of a tumour within the cranial vault gives rise to a 'mass lesion'. Although both take up space, the effects of tumours are not the same as those of acute haematomas (described above). As the tumour increases in size it will exert 'mass effect'. This is the compression of adjacent neurological structures. Mass effect may lead to brain herniation, particularly subfalcine herniation and midline shift. Larger space occupying lesions can be tolerated if growth is slow. This is because reduction in extracellular and intracellular fluid volumes are possible.

Compression or occlusion of the ventricular system will cause obstructive hydrocephalus. This is particularly common with tumours of the posterior fossa, which may compress the fourth ventricle.

Tumours also tend to give rise to cytotoxic oedema via the mechanism described above.

All these effects contribute to a rise in ICP. This may be sufficient to cause the patient to become obtunded. Further rises in ICP lead to brain herniation and death.

The response to physical injury. Although there are many patterns of head injury, this section will deal with severe closed head injuries.

1. Loss of autoregulation. Maintenance of the CBF by both response to metabolites and the intrinsic smooth muscle mechanisms may fail after severe head injury. The mechanism for this or even which patterns of injury are most likely to cause it are unknown. Once autoregulation is lost, CBF passively follows MAP. Without autoregulation, the MAP below which CBF is inadequate will be greater and the MAP above which vascular damage and oedema occur will be lower. The extent to which MAP alters CBF is dependent on the residual resistance of the cerebral vasculature.

2. Damage to the blood brain barrier. The BBB may be physically disrupted by diffuse physical injury. This may be sufficiently widespread to cause formation of vasogenic oedema. Once again, the mechanism of diffuse opening of the BBB is poorly understood. It is important to note that osmotic diuretics depend on the BBB for maximal effect.

3. Formation of cerebral oedema. As well as vasogenic oedema caused by BBB dysfunction, cell damage due to physical injury or infarction (due to impaired CBF) will lead to cytotoxic oedema

4. Cerebral metabolism. Severe head injury is followed by hyperglycolysis, the extent of which has been shown to relate to severity of functional impairment in survivors. The mechanism for this is unclear but it is probably triggered by the mechanical injury. This raised metabolic demand makes cells more vulnerable to hypoxia, resulting in increased risk of cytotoxic oedema or cell death.

5. Excitatory amino acids. Significant head injuries are associated with a rise in the extracellular concentration of excitatory amino acids (EAA), particularly glutamate. High concentrations of EAA lead to cell swelling in the acute phase, followed by cell death.

The cumulative effect of each of these processes, each of with is triggered by the injury itself is to engender tissue swelling and a rise in ICP. In a brain lacking autoregulation, a rise in

ICP will reduce CPP and therefore CBF. The resultant ischaemia and tissue damage will a cause further rise in ICP and a vicious circle is formed. This leads to higher and higher intracranial pressures culminating in death due to cerebral herniation or diffuse ischaemia.

If autoregulation is intact then there will still be swelling as a result of the physical injury. As long as the rise in ICP is less than that required to reduce the CPP to below the limits of autoregulation, the vicious cycle should be avoided.

The treatment of severe closed head injuries hinges around control of ICP and CPP. This is covered in the chapter on ITU management.

4

HISTORY AND EXAMINATION

W Adriaan Liebenberg

Contents

Taking a neurosurgical history
Introduction
Where to start
Presenting complaint
History of the presenting complaint
The rest of the history

Examination of the neurosurgical patient
Alertness and mental function
Cranial nerves
Gait
Romberg
Examination of the motor system
Examination of the sensory system
Examination of the comatose patient

Taking a neurosurgical history

Introduction

I have seen patients mismanaged because they were not properly examined or their history not adequately taken. For instance, a patient who presents with walking difficulties and weakness in his lower limbs (paraparesis) can have pathology localised to his lumbar spine, his thoracic spine, his cervical spine, his brain or a combination of these. Decompressing a patient's spinal stenosis to alleviate walking problems will be unsuccessful if the walking problems are due to an intracranial parafalcine meningioma. It is important to understand the pathology and important to learn to ask those questions that will distinguish the different types of pathology from each other. The neurological examination in neurosurgical practice is frequently different from that employed by neurologists and other physicians. There are many ways to go about this and I have outlined what I have found to be an effective approach below.

Where to start

A neurosurgical history should focus on the presenting complaint and the history of the presenting complaint but great attention should also be paid to the whole patient and to the patient's pre-existing level of function. For instance, a mathematician who has trouble doing basic sums is clearly not normal whereas someone who never finished formal schooling who has problems doing basic sums might not be abnormal. It is also important to note whether the patient is right - or left-handed as this indicates which cerebral hemisphere is the dominant hemisphere containing speech and language centres. All right handed people have a left dominant hemisphere. Most left-handed people also have left dominant hemisphere but there is a small proportion who have a right dominant hemisphere. The history has to be structured and has to start off with the demographics of the patient and the presenting complaint.

Presenting complaint

When presenting the history to colleagues we might say something like: *"Mr A is a 68-year old, right-handed, bank manager who presents with seven days of progressive headache and confusion..."*

History of the presenting complaint

Having stated the basic problem, the history of the presenting complaint is then described. We would, for example, say: *"The headache was slowly progressive in nature, was occipital and spread frontally, was exacerbated by coughing, was worse in the morning and improved by walking around and taking simple analgesics. Towards the end of the week even very strong painkillers had no effect on the headache. The patient experienced associated nausea, vomiting and photophobia."*

The rest of the history

Now we go on to describe the patient more in total including looking at his previous medical history, habits and the usual family and social history is also obtained as with any patient: *"This gentleman had prostatic cancer ten years ago. This was treated with a radical prostatectomy, orchidectomy and radiation therapy. He has had a clear follow up for his disease since then, with a prostate specific antigen within normal limits. He suffers from mild asthma and is allergic to Penicillin but otherwise very fit and still walks 3 miles daily. He is a smoker and takes approximately four units of alcohol a week, is married and lives independently with his wife in a single story house which they own."* Now everybody has a mental picture of the total patient and his problem. More information will be revealed by reporting his physical examination and finally by reviewing the patient's imaging.

Examination of the neurosurgical patient

The full and thorough examination of a neurosurgical patient should be a seamless, fast process and comes only with practice. Following the detailed history you will already have a very good idea of what it is that you are dealing with and you can tailor your examination to this. When there is a good understanding of the pathology it becomes quite easy to focus on certain aspects.

Alertness and mental function

Patients with neurological disease frequently have differing levels of consciousness and examination of unconscious patients obviously differs markedly from that of the patient who is conscious, awake and alert. In the patient who is awake the first thing to assess is their mental function and orientation in time, place and person. Two bedside tests are the abbreviated mental test score and the mini mental state examination. See tables 1 and 2

Task	Instructions	Scoring	
Orientation (Date)	"Tell me the date?" Ask for omitted items	One point each for year, season, date, day of week, and month	5
Orientation (Place)	"Where are you?" Ask for omitted items	One point each for state, county, town, building, and floor or room	5
Register 3 objects	Name three objects slowly and clearly. Ask the patient to repeat them	One point for each item correctly repeated	3
Serial sevens	Ask the patient to count backwards from 100 by 7. Stop after five answers. (Or ask them to spell "world" backwards)	One point for each correct answer (or letter)	5
Recall 3 objects	Ask the patient to recall the objects mentioned above	One point for each item correctly remembered	3
Naming	Point to your watch and ask the patient "what is this?" Repeat with a pencil.	One point for each correct answer	2
Repeating a phrase	Ask the patient to say "no ifs, ands, or buts"	One point if successful on first try	1
Verbal commands	Give the patient a plain piece of paper and say "Take this paper in your right hand, fold it in half, and put it on the floor"	One point for each correct action	3
Written commands	Show the patient a piece of paper with "CLOSE YOUR EYES" printed on it	One point if the patient closes their eyes	1
Writing	Ask the patient to write a sentence	One point if sentence has a subject, a verb, and makes sense	1
Drawing	Ask the patient to copy a pair of intersecting pentagons onto a piece of paper	One point if the figure has ten corners and two intersecting lines	1
	A score of 24 or above is considered normal		30

Table 1. *Folstein's Mini Mental Status Examination*

Age	Must be correct
Time	Without looking at watch/clock; correct to nearest hour
42 East Street	Give this address. Check registration. Check memory at end of test.
Month	Exact
Year	Exact, except in Jan/Feb when previous year OK
Name of place	If not in hospital ask type of place or area of town
Date of birth	Exact
Start of WW1	Exact
Name of present monarch/president	Exact
Count backwards from 20 to 1	Can prompt with the first few numbers, but no further prompts, patient can hesitate and self correct but no other errors
Score 8-10	Normal
Score 7	Probably abnormal
Score < 6	Abnormal

Table 2. *Abbreviated Mental Test score. One point for each correct answer.*

These are quite rough tools which will not pick up subtle deficiencies, so if these are suspected then assessment by a neuropsychologist is indicated. This is especially true in those patients who are recuperating from an insult to the nervous system such as subarachnoid haemorrhage or traumatic brain injury. It is always good to quantify a baseline in these patients so that progression and improvement can be seen. Following the testing of mental function and orientation of the patient it should be recorded as follows: AMT (score)/10 and MMSE (score)/30 with the orientation noted as "orientated in time, place and person."

Cranial nerves
CN I
The first cranial nerve is frequently involved in tumours of the anterior skull base or in trauma of the anterior skull base and can be tested with different substances. Oil of cloves or coffee is frequently used. The olfactory nerves can be tested independently by pinching the opposite nostril shut and testing one side at a time.

CN II
Visual fields. The second cranial nerve carries visual signals from the retina to the occipital cortex. Compression of the optic nerve or the optic tract and its radiations will lead to deficiencies in the visual field. There will be different clinical manifestations depending on where the compression is. See figure 1. Deficiencies are diagnosed with confrontation testing. See figure 2.

Visual acuity. Visual acuity is tested with a Snellen chart over a set distance of 20 feet and noted as a value which is a fraction of one. Therefore, if the set distance is 20 feet and the patient can see the letters that the chart indicates you should be able to see over a distance of 20 foot and therefore has 20/20 vision, it indicates a value of one, which is normal. If the patient can only see the large letters which you should be able to read at 200 feet then the vision is recorded as 20/200 or 1/10 of normal vision. Countries with the metric system use a Snellen chart that is measured at 6 metres and normal vision is 6/6 vision.

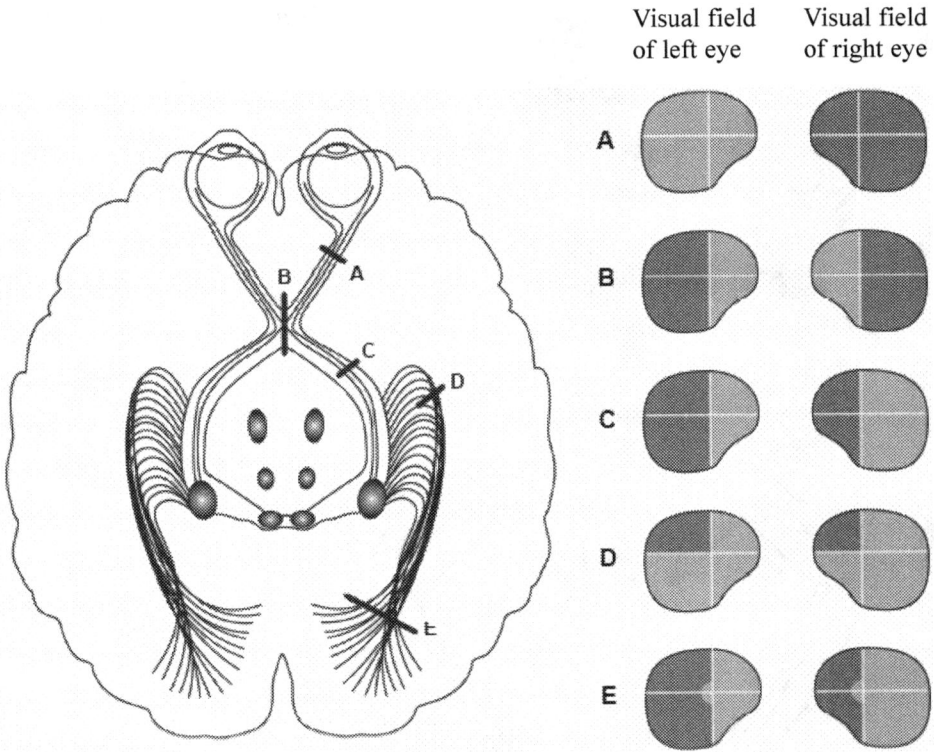

Visual field of left eye   Visual field of right eye

A
B
C
D
E

Figure 1. *Visual field deficits according to the site of the compression - A. complete vision loss in right eye, B. bitemporal hemianopia, C. left homonomous hemianopia, D. left upper quadrant hemianopia, E. macular sparing in left homonomous hemianopia. It is important to note that the images transmitted in the nasal fibers of the optic nerve cross over in the chiasm and that the temporal fibers continue straight backwards. It is also important to note that the lower retinal fibers cross anteriorly and the upper retinal fibers cross posteriorly in the chiasm. The lower retinal fibers carry the upper temporal visual field and the upper retinal fibers carry the lower temporal field. Beyond the lateral geniculate body, the fibers fan out into the optic radiation and the fibers serving the lower nasal retina (the upper temporal field) dip into the temporal lobe. These fibers are called Meyer's loop. Compression of these fibers leads to a contralateral upper quadrantanopia. It will be a homonomous hemianopia since the nasal fibers from the contralateral eye would have crossed over in the chiasm. Visual fields can be assessed by visual confrontation testing. See figure 2. The most sensitive way to do this is to use a red pin because red is the first colour that we experience inability to see when there is compression of the optic nerve.*

It is important to remember that patients can have near normal visual acuity with large deficits in their visual fields. Having tested both visual fields and visual acuity it is now important to perform fundoscopy.

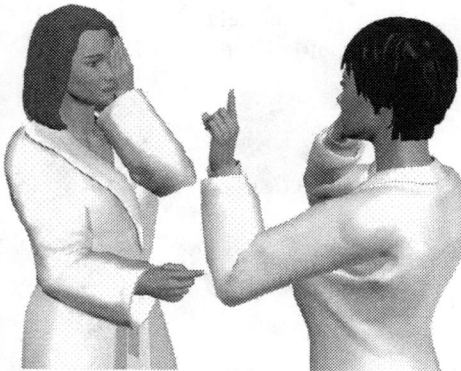

Figure 2. *Visual confrontation testing. Whilst sitting opposite the patient you ask them to occlude their left eye while you occlude your right eye and, using the limits of your own visual field, you test whether the patient has the same extent of visual field. Repeat this with the other eye. Visual fields are recorded as the patient sees them. There fore the left temporal field will be recorded on the left and the right temporal field on the right.*

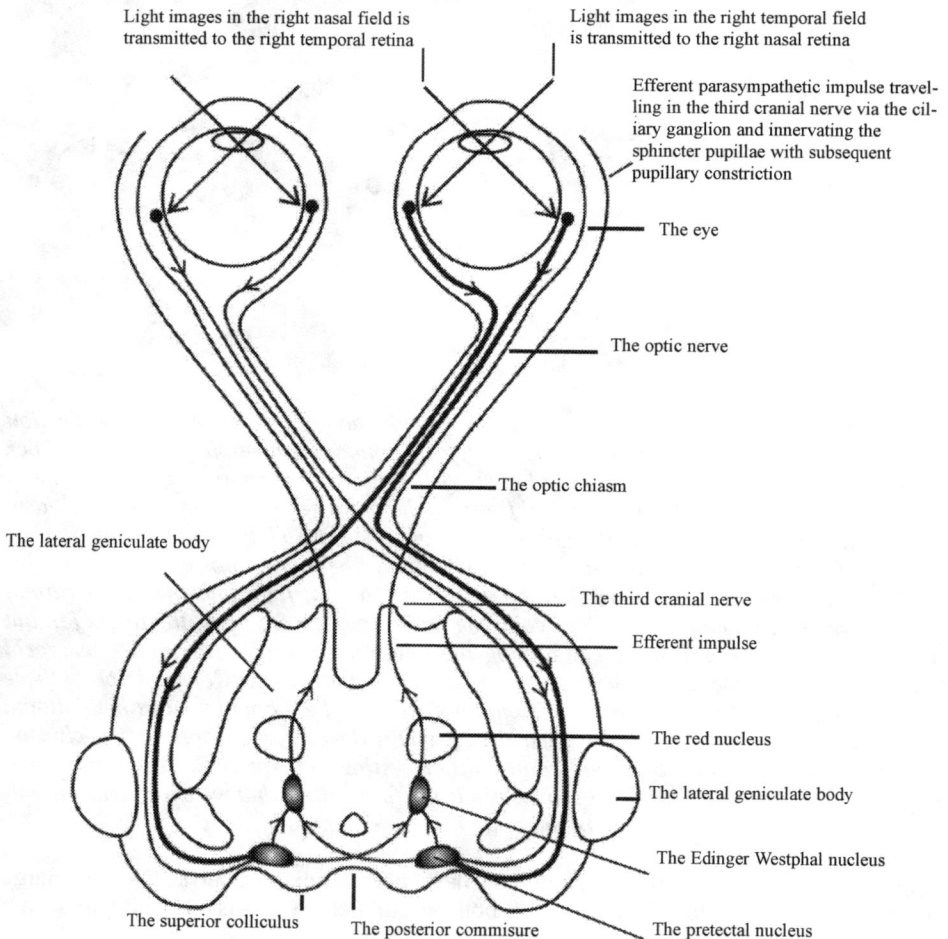

Light images in the right nasal field is transmitted to the right temporal retina

Light images in the right temporal field is transmitted to the right nasal retina

Efferent parasympathetic impulse travelling in the third cranial nerve via the ciliary ganglion and innervating the sphincter pupillae with subsequent pupillary constriction

The eye

The optic nerve

The optic chiasm

The lateral geniculate body

The third cranial nerve

Efferent impulse

The red nucleus

The lateral geniculate body

The Edinger Westphal nucleus

The superior colliculus

The posterior commisure

The pretectal nucleus

Figure 3. *Pupillary light reflex - pupillary constriction is a parasympathetic function and is mediated by the Edinger-Westphal nuclei. Light impulses travel back in the second cranial nerve and in the brain stem at the level of superior colliculus bilaterally innervates the Edinger-Westphal nuclei. Efferent impulses then travel forwards in both third cranial nerves and therefore light shone into one eye activates constriction in both eyes.*

Fundoscopy
This is a skill that is learnt only with a lot of practice and it is frequently reported incorrectly. It is important to note that papilloedema (bilateral optic disc swelling) takes 10-14 days to develop and is not present in the patient with acute head injury. It is rather a hallmark of chronic raised intracranial pressure or chronic optic disc pathology. It is frequently said that patients who have no papilloedema are safe to undergo a lumbar puncture without resorting to any cranial imaging. This is incorrect, as a patient who has a large acute subdural haematoma or intracerebral haematoma will not have papilloedema and performing a lumbar puncture on these patients can lead to coning and death.
Papilloedema has four stages. See table 3.

Stage one	There is decreased drainage of the veins of the optic nerve and this leads to the veins swelling and becoming tortuous. An experienced observer will also be able to see decreased venous pulsation
Stage two	The optic discs swell and, where the vessels of the optic disc in the normal situation have an acute posterior kink plunging into the optic discs, they now stop at the margin of the disc. The discs frequently changes colour from a pale yellow to pink as this occurs
Stage three	The disc margins swell more and become increasingly indistinct and blurred
Stage four	There is even more swelling of the discs with obvious elevation and scattered haemorrhages frequently seen

Table 3. *Grades of papilloedema*

CN III, IV, VI
These three nerves work together to move the eyeball around in its socket. The third cranial nerve has the added function of pupil constriction and carries sympathetic fibres that mediate eyelid elevation. Most of the muscles of the eyeball are supplied by the third cranial nerve, but the *lateral rectus* is supplied by the sixth cranial nerve and the *superior oblique* by the fourth cranial nerve. This causes a patient with a third nerve palsy to have an eyeball which looks downwards and outwards because of the unopposed pull of the *lateral rectus* and *superior oblique muscles*. In cases of *lateral rectus* palsy, the eyeball loses the ability to look laterally. In an isolated fourth nerve palsy, the patient develops diplopia on looking outwards and downwards. The *superior oblique* pulls the eye downwards and medially as it acts by hooking around the trochlea and the *inferior rectus* pulls the eye down and laterally. In a patient with fourth cranial nerve palsy, downward gaze results in unopposed action of the *inferior rectus* pulling the affected eye downwards and outwards. Downward gaze therefore precipitates or worsens diplopia. Pupillary constriction is a parasympathetic function and is mediated by the Edinger-Westphal nuclei. Light impulses travel back in the second cranial nerve and in the brain stem at the level of superior colliculus bilaterally innervates the Edinger-Westphal nuclei. Efferent impulses then travel forwards in both third cranial nerves and therefore light shone into one eye activates constriction in both eyes, see figure 3.

If there is compression or dysfunction of the afferent pathway of the pupillary reflex (second cranial nerve) this will lead to a Marcus Gunn pupil: light falling on the affected pupil will lead to a larger pupil than when light falls on the unaffected pupil. This is due to the ipsilateral input to the Edinger-Westphal nucleus being weaker (because of the damage to the afferent pathway) than when light is shone into the contralateral eye with the unaffected optic nerve (consensual light reflex). This is demonstrated by swinging a flashlight between the two eyes and seeing a slight dilatation when the light falls directly on the affected eye.

Compression of the efferent pathway (third cranial nerve), causes dysfunction of pupil constriction and that leads to a persistently dilated pupil. The pupillary constrictor fibres lie quite superficially in the third nerve and a hallmark of external compression is that of pupillary dilatation. The third nerve also carries sympathetic fibres which innervate the superior tarsal muscles and assist eye opening. Thus a patient with an external compressive third nerve lesion will have a dilated pupil, ptosis and a downward and outward deviated eye (ophthalmoplegia). Pupillary dilatation is a sympathetic activity and is initiated in the hypothalamus with the signals descending in the spinal cord to the level of T1. At the level of T1, the white rami of the nerve roots of C8 and T1 pass through the cervical sympathetic ganglion. Impulses travel from there in sympathetic nerves into the cranial cavity on the surface of the carotid artery and arrive at the pupil via a branch of the ophthalmic artery. When there is dysfunction of the sympathetic system it leads to ptosis because of the decreased innervation of the tarsal muscles, pupillary constriction due to a loss of pupillary dilatation and loss of facial sweating due to autonomic dysfunction. This is called Horner's syndrome and is easily remembered by the rhyme "ptosis, myosis and anhydrosis." The pupillary abnormality is best demonstrated by taking the patient into a darkened room. In normal circumstances, both pupils will dilate in a darkened room but in a patient with Horner's syndrome, the affected pupil will remain constricted.

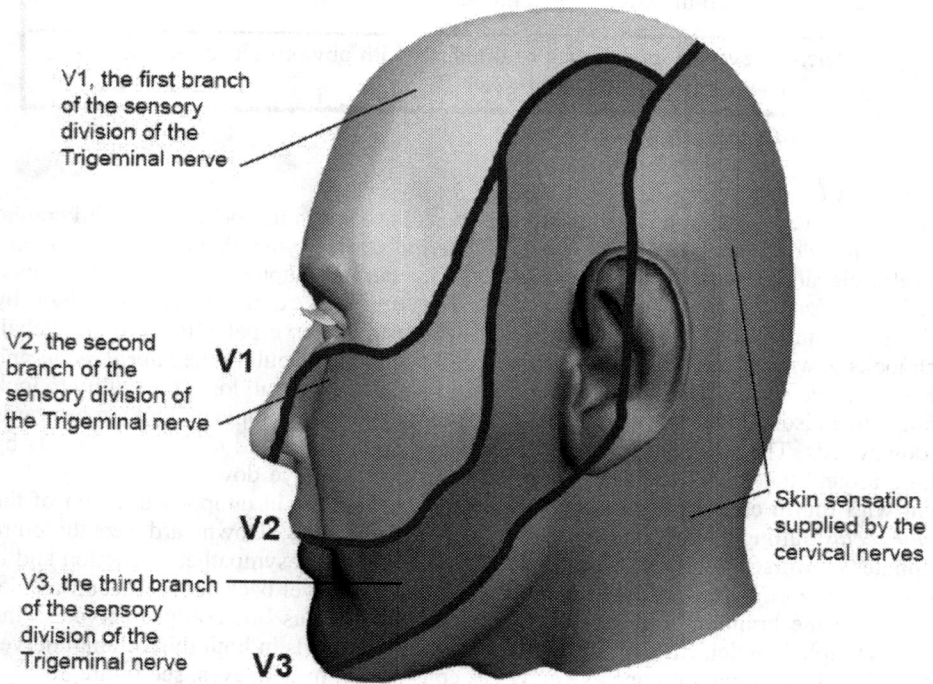

Figure 4. *Distribution of the Trigeminal nerve's sensory divisions. Note that the sensation in front of the tragus is supplied by the 7th and 9th cranial nerves (not demonstrated)*

CN V

The first division of the fifth cranial nerve accompanies the third, fourth and sixth cranial nerves through the cavernous sinus and these four nerves are frequently compromised together by lesions in the cavernous sinus. The fifth cranial nerve's largest component is the sensory division but it also has a motor division that serves mastication. It is assessed by testing sensation over the face and by testing corneal sensation (first division) and the jaw jerk. It is important to realise that the first division of the fifth cranial nerve actually supplies sensation as far back as the coronal suture, but does not supply the jaw line. See figure 4.

CN VII

The seventh cranial nerve is almost purely made up of motor fibers and supplies the muscles of the face. The facial nerve has a supranuclear input which supplies the ipsilateral side of the face and also a reflex component that is primarily concerned with reflex eye closure and has no cortical component. Both eyes will shut if there is danger to either individual eye and therefore there is dual innervation of both sides of the forehead. If there is dysfunction of the cortical innervation (supranuclear innervation) this leads to deficient lower face muscle function and intact upper face function. The seventh cranial nerve also has a small sensory function and carries sensation from the external auditory canal and taste sensation from the anterior two-thirds of the tongue via the chorda tympani.

CN VIII

The vestibulocochlear nerve consists of the vestibular nerve and the cochlear nerve. The vestibular nerve serves balance and the cochlear nerve hearing. Hearing can be tested by rubbing your fingers next to the patient's ears and determining whether they can hear that or, alternatively, whispering numbers in their ears and asking the patient to relay which numbers have been whispered. Weber and Rinne's tests are useful in distinguishing between conductive and sensory neural deafness. Weber's test consists of placing a vibrating tuning fork on the patient's vertex and asking if the patient feels or hears it best on one side or the other. A patient with no abnormalities will experience no difference. In cases with unilateral neurosensory hearing loss, the hearing will be best in the normal ear, while in cases of a unilateral conductive hearing loss, it is best heard in the abnormal ear. In Rinne's test, bone conduction (placing the tuning fork on the mastoid process) is compared to air conduction (placing the tuning fork in front of but not touching the pinna). Normally, air conduction is greater than bone conduction. In cases of partial neurosensory hearing loss, air conduction is still greater than bone conduction but in cases of conduction hearing loss bone conduction will be greater than air conduction. It is sometimes difficult to remember which test does what but I remember Weber's test as being the one where you put the tuning fork on top of somebody's head by the fact that a 'W' looks a bit like a crown.

CN IX, X, XI

These nerves share the same motor nucleus (nucleus ambiguus) and all exit the skull through the jugular foramen. The **glossopharyngeal nerve (IX)** is the main afferent pathway of the gag reflex and also, along with the seventh cranial nerve, supplies some sensation in the external auditory canal and conveys taste, in this case, from the posterior third of the tongue. The only function that we routinely test is the gag reflex and the efferent pathway of the gag reflex is the tenth cranial nerve **(vagus)**. The tenth cranial nerve also supplies motor fibres to the muscles of the palate. Testing the ninth and tenth nerves together then consists of testing the gag reflex and also testing the patient's palatal muscles by asking them to open their mouth widely and saying "aaaahh" whilst using a light to illuminate the back of the mouth. If there is a palsy of the vagus, there will be asymmetry of the palate and a left-sided nerve palsy will cause the intact muscles on the right-hand side to pull the palate over to the right and vice-versa. Having a depressed gag reflex can either be because of dysfunction in the ninth or tenth cranial nerve. Patients with a ninth nerve palsy will usually have normal

113

palatal function. The gag is tested by stimulating the uvula and posterior pharynx with a tongue depressor. The tenth cranial nerve also supplies the larynx and a vagal or recurrent laryngeal nerve palsy causes ipsilateral vocal cord paralysis and a hoarse voice.

The **spinal accessory nerve (XI)** originates in a nucleus in the spinal cord and leaves the spinal cord through the cervical branches supplying the *sternocleidomastoid and trapezius muscles* on the same side. The unusual feature of this nerve is that the higher control is not crossed and a right-sided lesion will therefore lead to a right-sided nerve dysfunction. The *sternocleidomastoid muscle* pulls the patient's head towards the opposite side and right *sternocleidomastoid muscle* (right eleventh nerve) function is therefore tested by asking the patient to look towards the left against resistance and simultaneously palpating the muscles on the right-hand side. A patient with a right hemisphere lesion will not be able to look towards the left-hand side and if we remember the anatomy of the second cranial nerve, they will have inattention of the left visual field. Therefore patients with extensive right hemisphere damage will not be aware of the left-hand side and will not be able to look towards the left-hand side.

CN XII

The twelfth cranial nerve supplies the motor function of the tongue and is tested by both observation and active movement. Observing the tongue lying in the floor of the mouth with the patient's mouth open will demonstrate any fasciculation if present. The patient is then asked to push the tongue out of their mouth and move it from side to side. If there is a palsy, the stronger intact muscles will push the tongue towards the affected weaker side and therefore the tongue will deviate towards the affected side (whereas in the case of a tenth nerve palsy, the palate will pull away from the affected side). This can be remembered by the fact that the tongue muscles push out and the palatal muscles pull up. See table 4 for a summary of the cranial nerve examination.

CN I	Usually reserved for cases where the patient reports a decrease in olfaction
CN II	Visual confrontation, acuity and fundoscopy
CN III, IV, VI	Eye movements
CN V	Facial sensation
CN VII	Facial movements
CN VIII	Rubbing your fingers next to the ear (Rinne, Weber)
CN IX - XII	Gag reflex, palatal function, shoulder and neck movements and looking at tongue movements

Table 4. *Examination of the cranial nerves*

Examination of the motor system

The left hemisphere controls the right-hand side of the body and vice versa. The motor system is made up of two parts: the main controlling pyramidal system (named after the pyramids in the medulla oblongata) and the extrapyramidal system which modulates the pyramidal system and does not cross over. Motor signals are generated in the cortex and then travel via the corona radiata and the internal capsule down to the brainstem. They cross over in the medulla oblongata to the opposite side to control motor movement. The extrapyramidal system modulates the actions of the pyramidal system based on proprioception and feedback via the cerebellum. In a hemispheric deficit there is dysfunction of the motor system on the whole of the contralateral side. A large left hemispheric infarct will produce a paralysis of the right side of the face, the right arm and the right leg. Because the reflex arc of the spinal cord is independent of cerebral input, patients who are completely paralysed will still have intact reflexes. Reflexes are however modulated by higher input and if there is dysfunction anywhere in the brain or the spinal cord the effect downstream of that will be a decrease in modulation of the reflex activity. Therefore patients who have a left hemisphere infarct will have spastic right arm and leg reflexes due to non-modulated reflex arc activity. This is also true if the cause of the paralysis is in the spinal cord which will lead to decreased muscle power below the level of the lesion and increase in the reflexes (hyperreflexia). This is extremely useful in delineating the level of the pathology. Somebody who has damage to the spinal cord at C6 level will have increased reflexes below the level of C6 as well as weakness below that level with normal power and reflexes above that level. The rule for establishing the level of spinal pathology is that at the level of injury there will be decreased reflexes and weakness (lower motor neurone signs) and below the level there will be weakness and increased reflexes (upper motor neurone signs). Lesions distal to the anterior horn cells in the spinal cord lead to lower motor neurone signs (decreased or absent reflexes and weakness). Patients who have only dysfunction of a nerve root might have a radiculopathy and the myotome as well as the dermatome served by this nerve will show dysfunction. For instance somebody with a centrally herniated intervertebral disc (slipped disc) at the L4/5 lumbar level might have a L5 radiculopathy which, if it only involves the sensory component will produce numbness on the dorsum of the foot. If it is severe and also involves the motor component, they will have difficulty with extension (dorsiflexion) of their ankle. When examining the motor system you have to test the tone of the muscles, the muscle power (table 6) and reflexes (table 5).

Description	Score
Absent	-4
Just elicitable	-3
Low	-2
Moderately low	-1
Normal	0
Brisk	1
Very brisk	2
Exhaustible clonus	3
Continuous clonus	4

Table 5. *Mayo Clinic scale for tendon reflex assessment*

Extrapyramidal system (cerebellar function)
Pathology in the cerebellum causes ipsilateral deficits so that an infarct of the left cerebellum will lead to left-sided weakness and hypotonia. It is important to note that extrapyramidal weakness is not associated with hyperreflexia. Pathology causes a dysfunctional proprioception feedback system and will cause the limbs on the ipsilateral side to be ataxic. Lesions of the vermis, on the other hand, will lead to truncal ataxia. Limb ataxia can be tested by checking the patient for past pointing with the ability to do the finger-nose test and testing for the

presence of dysdiadocokinesia. In the lower limbs ataxia can be tested by asking the patient to tap his foot on the floor or to do the heel-to-shin test. Another marker of possible cerebellar pathology is nystagmus.

Score	Muscle Response
0	No Movement
1	Muscle belly moves but the joint does not move
2	Joint moves with gravity eliminated
3	Joint moves against gravity
4	Joint moves against gravity and some resistance
5	Full strength

Table 6. *MRC Scale for Grading Muscle Strength*

Muscles	Root Levels	Clinical
Trapezius	C3-C4	Shrug shoulders
Deltoid	C5-C6	Abduct shoulder
Biceps	C5-C6	Flex elbow
Triceps	C6-C8	Extend elbow
Wrist extensors	C6-C7	Extend wrist
Wrist flexors	C6-T1	Flex wrist
Hand intrinsic muscles	C8-T1	Spread fingers
Opponens pollicis and digiti minimi	C8-T1	Make "o" with thumb and 5th finger
Iliopsoas	L2-L3	Flex hip
Quadriceps	L3-L4	Extend knee
Hamstrings	L5-S1	Flex knee
Gluteus maximus	S1-S2	Extend hip
Tibialis anterior	L4-L5	Dorsiflex foot
Tibialis posterior	L4-5	Invert foot
Peroneii	L5-S1	Evert foot
Extensor hallucis longus	L5	Extend (dorsiflex) great toe
Gastrocnemius	S1-S2	Plantar flexion

Table 7. *Myotomes*

Tendon	Root
Bicep reflex	C5/6
Brachioradialis reflex	C6
Triceps	C7
Patella (knee) reflex	L4
Achilles (ankle) reflex	S1

Table 8.

Deep tendon reflexes

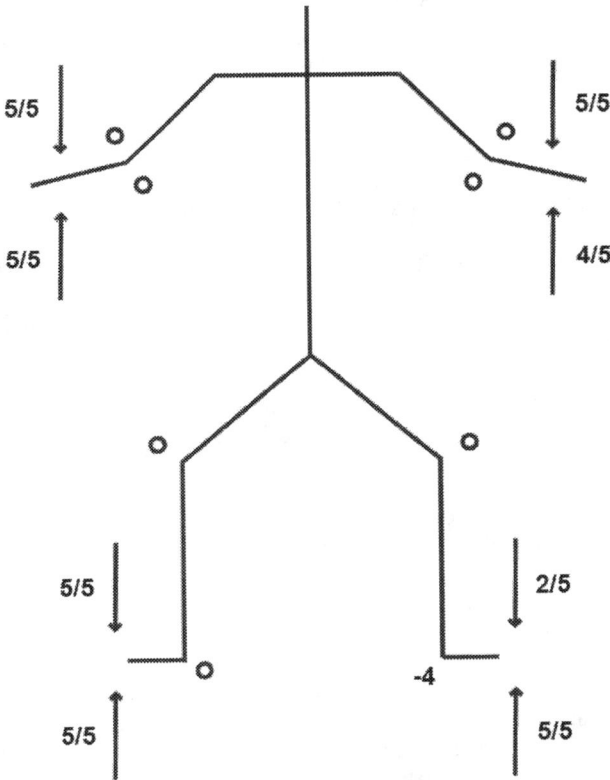

Figure 6. *Notation of the motor system examination. The motor strength (Table 6) and reflexes (Table 5) should be noted on a visual chart as above.*

Gait

The last part of evaluation of the motor system is to test the patient's gait. A lot can be learned from a patient's gait. Patients with severe lower back pain and radicular pain will have a type of gait where they put less pressure on the affected side and walk with a limp. This is called an antalgic type of gait. Patients who have suffered cerebrovascular accidents, often have a fixed flexion of their upper limb and a straight, outstretched leg with a plantar-flexed foot which causes them to walk by circumducting the affected leg. They do this by swinging the stiff leg out and around before putting it down. Where there is cerebellar pathology the patient may have a general unsteadiness due to limb ataxia. Patients who are myelopathic have a stiff, spastic gait and frequently shuffle along.

Romberg

Following assessment of gait you may want to do a Romberg's test. Romberg's test is based on the fact that we need at least 2 out of 3 senses to be able to stand unaided (proprioception, vestibular function, vision). If patients close their eyes and they have a deficit in either their vestibular function or proprioception, they will fall over. This is, however, not a very specific test.

Overview of the motor examination

The suggested sequence for examining the motor system is as follows:
Ask the patient to hold their arms stretched out in front of them with palms upward facing. Ask them to close their eyes. Any subtle weakness will result in a drift of the arm on the weak side. Now ask the patient to open their eyes, turn their palms downwards towards the floor and to make piano playing movements with their fingers. If they can do this, you have successfully screened for subtle motor weakness. You have also tested proprioception and fine motor movements and therefore have tested both pyramidal and extrapyramidal systems. This can be followed up by testing tone in all 4 limbs, one at a time and then testing motor function in all the myotomes. The last step is to test the reflexes. Examination for the motor system should be noted down as demonstrated in figure 6.

Examination of the sensory system

When testing the sensory system it is always very important to ask the patient whether they are aware of any abnormal sensation. If they are not then it is unlikely that you will find any deficit. In testing for sensation it is important to test the different sensory modalities (light touch, temperature, pain and joint position sense).

If you are testing for pain it usually negates the necessity to test for temperature sensation as well, except in patients where we have reason to suspect hydromyelia or syringomyelia where the loss of temperature sensation is quite typical. We therefore effectively have 3 modalities that we test for – proprioception, the fibres of which are located in the posterior part of the spinal cord, light touch, the fibres of which are located in the anterior part of the spinal cord and pain, the fibres of which are located in the lateral part of the spinal cord. Light touch can be tested by running your fingertips or cotton wool lightly along the patient's skin. Pain sensation is tested with a pinprick. Proprioception and joint position sense is tested by moving the patient's toes, feet, fingers or hands with their eyes closed. When testing pain sensation it is important to realise that the pain fibres cross over in the spinal cord and not at the brain stem unlike the other fibres. Therefore a lesion that is restricted to only one half of the spinal cord will lead to ipsilateral proprioceptive and light touch abnormalities, and contralateral pain sensation abnormalities below the affected spinal level (dermatome). This is the basis for the Brown-Séquard syndrome.

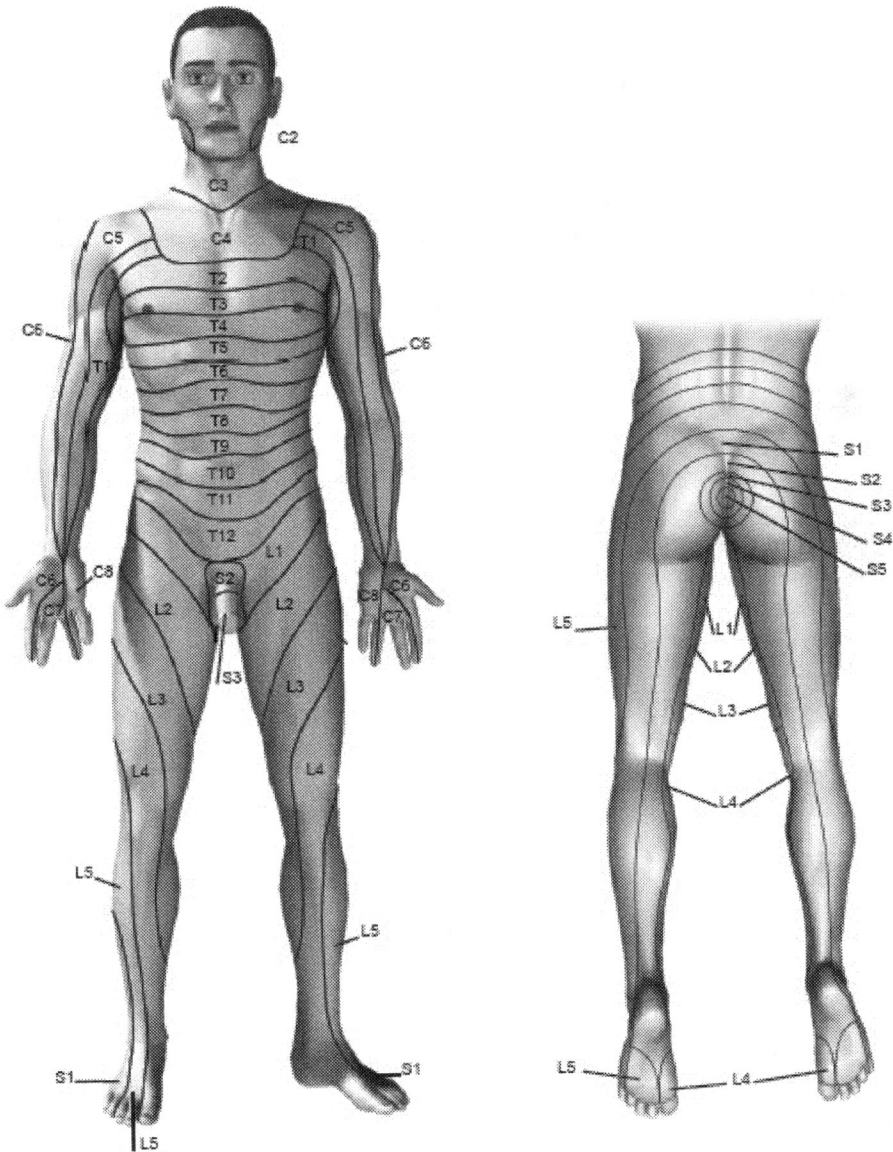

Figure 7. *Human dermatomes*

It is important not to fall in the C4/T2 trap and to realise that the dermatomes on the chest for C4 and T2 are close to each other and therefore a C4 lesion can be mistaken for a thoracic lesion if the sensation in the arms is not tested. Somebody who is numb from just above the level of their nipples downwards and therefore has a sensory level just above their nipples might have a T3/4 lesion but, if you were to examine their arms that contain the cervical dermatomes and find that they were numb as well, you would have to conclude that this was actually a cervical rather than a thoracic lesion. See figure 7 for the anatomical pattern of dermatomes. Another type of sensory deficit is a cortical sensory deficit and patients with lesions in their parietal lobe might have a deficiency in two point discrimination and discrimination of objects.

Examination of the comatose patient

Examination of the comatose patient is restricted to testing the pupillary reactivity, the Glasgow Coma Scale, the presence of a paresis or paralysis and the patient's reflexes including pathological reflexes (Babinski). The Glasgow Coma Scale is made up of the motor response, the verbal response and eye opening.

The motor response comprises 6 points. See table 8. The notation for a patient's GCS is as follows: GCS (total score)/15, M (score), V (score), E (score). Patients who are intubated have an annotated T added to indicate intubation (GCS 7/15 T). Following notation of the GCS, the pupillary activity is then noted and the term "PEARL" can be used which stands for pupils equal and reactive to light. Following notation of the GCS and the pupillary activity, the focal deficit must be noted down for paresis or paralysis of any of the limbs. Verbal response is scored out of 5. It needs to be remembered that someone who has a lesion focally in Broca's area will not be able to speak properly and will therefore drop several points on the Glasgow Coma Scale. Therefore somebody with a Glasgow Coma Scale of 11/15 may be completely awake and orientated,but completely aphasic, see table 9 for a summary of the verbal response. Eye opening response is scored out of 4. See table 10 for a summary of the eye opening response.

6/6	Ability to follow commands which requires a rather sophisticated train of events to occur in the nervous system
5/6	The awareness and localisation of painful stimuli. Painful stimulus on the chest wall will therefore lead to the patient grasping your hand and even trying to pull it away
4/6	The patient is aware of the pain or threat and attempts to localise it but cannot. Patients who flex their limbs but are unable to localise the painful stimulus.
3/6	The patient's arms are spasmodically fully flexed next to the body. This is an action that has no reliance on cognition of the cortex and is therefore called decorticate posturing
2/6	The arms are spasmodically extended on either side of the body; the legs are also spastic and extended. This is a final reflex stage that does not rely on the cerebrum at all and so it is called decerebrate posturing. Posturing, both decorticate and decerebrate carry a poor prognosis
1/6	No motor response. Therefore somebody who has even a flicker of movement will get a score of 2/6

Table 8. *Motor response (GCS)*

5/5	Patient is fully orientated to person, time and place
4/5	Confused speech
3/5	Words only
2/5	Sounds only
1/5	No sound whatsoever

Table 9. *Verbal response (GCS)*

4/4	The patient spontaneously opens the eyes
3/4	The patient opens the eyes to verbal stimuli
2/4	The patient opens the eyes to painful stimuli
1/4	The patient does not open the eyes at all

Table 10. *Eye opening response*

5

INTERPRETATION OF CRANIAL CT AND MRI SCANS

W Adriaan Liebenberg

Contents

Introduction
CT scans
Tissue densities
MRI scans
Physics
Sequences
Tissue intensities
Blood changes with time on MR scans
An approach to reading scans and radiological anatomy
Hydrocephalus and ventriculomegaly

Trauma
Skull fractures
Diffuse Brain Injury
Intracerebral haemorrhage
Extra axial collections

Brain Tumours
Primary brain tumours
(Low grade) astrocytoma
Anaplastic astrocytoma
Glioblastoma Multiforme
Pilocytic astrocytoma
Oligodendroglioma
Ependymoma
Meningioma
Primary central nervous system lymphoma

Intracranial cyst-like lesions
Dermoid cyst
Epidermoid cyst
Colloid cyst of the third ventricle
Arachnoid cyst

Pituitary region tumours
Microadenomas
Macroadenomas
Craniopharyngiomas

Neuronal tumours
Central neurocytomas

Pineal region tumours
Germinoma
Pineal parenchymal tumours

Tumours of the posterior fossa
Hemangioblastoma
Medulloblastoma
Astrocytoma

Skull base tumours
Chordoma
Vestibular schwannoma

Metastatic tumours

Vascular Pathology
Arterial infarct
Venous infarct
Spontaneous haemorrhage
Subarachnoid haemorrhage (aneurysmal)
Parenchymal hypertensive haemorrhage
Vascular anomalies
Arteriovenous Malformation
Cavernous malformation
Venous angioma

Infection
Empyema
Cerebritis
Abscess

Introduction

I remember being amazed at the skill of the neurosurgical registrars in reading CT and MRI scans when I was a trauma doctor. A scan was quite a frightening investigation to me and I was unsure how to evaluate them. I think this is probably true for many doctors. The scan can however be an exceedingly straightforward test to read since the brain is a relatively symmetrical structure and it is therefore quite easy to pick up asymmetry denoting underlying abnormalities. Once you can identify the normal anatomy, there are a few simple rules to follow to lead you to a differential diagnosis. Even the most experienced physicians and radiologists can only take a diagnosis up to a certain level and will mostly end up saying that "this is most probably lesion x but it could also be lesion y or z". For me, the cranial scan is a clinical test in the sense that it has much less relevance if not interpreted in the context of the clinical setting. The patient's history and examination should really have brought you quite close to a diagnosis in the first place and should have set a differential diagnosis in your mind already. If you combine the history and examination with a few simple rules in this chapter then you should be able to narrow down the diagnosis quite efficiently without needing a great deal of knowledge about neurosurgery.

CT scans

A Computed Tomography scan is a process where ordinary X-rays (tomograms) are fed through a computer (computed - therefore the term computed tomography) to form a 2D or 3D picture. Different tissues have different densities to X-ray penetration and are reported as hypo, iso and hyperdense. Iodine based contrast is used to enhance areas of increased blood flow or capillary leakage which show up as more dense areas on CT scans since these areas have a higher load of radiodense contrast material.

Tissue densities:
There are four shades of grayscale that tissues can have on a CT scan: white, grey, dark grey and black.
White (hyperdense)
Bone
Calcium deposits
Blood (fresh)
Melanin
Contrast enhancement
Grey (isodense)
Brain
Glial tumours
Blood (subacute)
Dark grey (hypodense)
Most fluid is seen as dark grey, quite close to pure black and if there are different densities, it usually indicates deposits within the fluid.
CSF (ventricles, subarachnoid spaces)
Brain oedema
Fat
Dermoid tumours are black due to fatty deposits
Blood (chronic)
Black (hypodense)
Air

Hounsfield units
The pixels that make up a CT scan image are assigned a numerical value and these values can be used to identify the type of tissue shown on the image. These values range between - 1000 for air and + 1000 for bone and water is designated as 0. Fat generally has a value of - 50 and soft tissues a value of + 40.

MRI scans

Physics
Magnetic Resonance Imaging is a process where the body's hydrogen atoms are aligned by a strong magnet (the magnetic part) and is then subjected to powerful radio wave frequencies that are used to push them out of alignment. The hydrogen atoms alternately absorb and emit radio wave energy, vibrating backwards and forwards between their magnetised resting state and their agitated state caused by the radio pulses (the "resonance" part of MRI). Depending on how quickly these atoms return to their original state, the computer can deduce what kind of tissue is represented by the signals returned. This is based on the intensities of the returned signal and therefore the tissues are reported as being hypo, iso and hyperintense (compared to *densities* in CT scans). A paramagnetic contrast medium, Gadolinium is used in a similar fashion as iodine-based contrast is used in CT scans.

Sequences

The different imaging techniques generated by the radio frequency pulses are called pulse sequences. They include amongst other, spin-echo, inversion recovery, gradient echo and FLAIR (fluid attenuation inversion recovery) sequences. By changing the scan repetition time (TR - the time between RF pulses) and the echo time (TE - the time between the RF pulse and recording the MR signal), it is possible to change the sequence. The two main types of MRI sequences that are used are T1 and T2 weighted images. The terms T1 and T2 refer to the relaxation of the excited nuclei to their original alignment after being excited by the radio waves (relaxation times).

A variant T1-weighted image (T1 WI) is the **STIR** (short tau inversion recovery) sequence which removes bright fat that obscures the signal of interest in orbital or spine images, with pathology being conspicuously bright.

Proton density is neither a T1 nor a T2-weighted image (T2 WI) and is designedto minimise the effects of T1 and T2 WI. Proton density is the concentration of protons in the tissue in the form of water and macromolecules.

FLAIR (fluid attenuation inversion recovery) sequences are a variant of T2 WI where normal body water is suppressed to show pathological oedematous tissue, which is conspicuously bright.

T1 WI are useful in delineating anatomy and return high intensity signals in the following tissues:

Fat
Melanin
Subacute blood
Fluids with high protein content
Paramagnetic contrast agents

T2 WI are very sensitive to most types of pathology and tissues that return high intensity signals are:

Fluid collections (CSF, tissue oedema)
Infarcted brain
Demyelination
Infection
Neoplasms (most)

T1 WI and T2 WI

Flowing blood moves through the plane of the imaging and does not remain present long enough for the spinning hydrogen atoms to return their signal and therefore return little or no signal. Flowing blood is therefore dark on both T1 WI and T2 WI and the signal returned is referred to as a flow void. Air, calcification (bone) and fibrous tissue also return little or no signal due to a paucity of mobile protons and appear dark on both sequences.

Tissue intensities

White matter, because of its high lipid and low water content, is hypointense (relative to grey matter) on T2 WI and hyperintense on T1 WI. On the other hand, grey matter has higher water content than white matter and will therefore be less intense on T1 WI and more intense on T2 WI. CSF therefore appears dark on T1 WI and has a very high signal on T2 WI. The pituitary gland and infundibulum appear grey on T1 WI and T2 WI. When disease processes infiltrate the white matter and displace the hydrophobic tissue with more hydrophilic tissue, the intensities decrease on T1 WI and increase on T2 WI. Most brain tumours return decreased signal intensity on T1 WI and increased signal intensity on T2 WI. In general, pathological processes increase the water content of tissues and appear bright on T2 WI and have decreased signal on T1 WI but there are a few important exceptions to this rule:

Blood (subacute) and melanin is intrinsically bright (white) on T1 WI.

Tumours with a high nuclear to cytoplasmic ration such as lymphomas and primitive neuroectodermal tumours (PNET) are also iso/ hyperintense on T1 WI.

Multiple areas of increased signal intensity on T2 WI raise the suspicion of secondary metastatic disease, demyelination or vascular disease.

Blood changes with time on MR scans
Depends on age of clot
In T1 WI – remember 'Big Great White Bear!'
Hyperacute, within hours - Black (hypointense)
Acute stage, less than 3 days - Grey (isointense),
Subacute stage, 3 to 14 days - White (hyperintense),
Chronic stage, more than 14 days - Black (hypointense)

In T2 WI – remember 'Bear, What Bear?'
Acute stage – Black (hypointense)
Subacute – White (hyperintense)
Subacute stage and chronic stages – Black (hypointense)

An approach to reading scans and radiological anatomy

Both MRI and CT scan images are presented as slices through different parts of the skull and brain. On the scan there is usually a scout or survey image that shows a lateral view of the head and neck with lines that have corresponding numbers on them. This is a road map to the slices that can be seen in the rest of the scan. Following the road map indicates which of the axial slices go where in the 3-dimensional anatomic model, see figure 1. About a quarter of the way down through the cranium the ventricles start to appear. They can be discerned from the brain, which is grey, by the fact that they are darker in colour, and nearly pitch black on CT scans and T1 WI and hyperintense on T2 WI. The ventricular system consists of a pair of lateral ventricles, the third ventricle and a fourth ventricle. The third and fourth ventricles are connected by the aqueduct of Sylvius, which we can see on a MRI scan, but not a CT scan. The lateral ventricles have frontal and occipital horns and, in cases of hydrocephalus, we can see the temporal horns of the lateral ventricles. The third ventricle is usually slit-like but in cases of hydrocephalus and obstruction will become round and distended. The fourth ventricle is in the posterior fossa below the level of the tentorium cerebelli and is usually sickle-shaped. The bone of the cranium is brilliant white on CT scans. Just like ordinary X-rays, the tissues that are relatively impenetrable to the rays are recorded as white on the final film and tissues that allow the rays to pass through are darker in colour.

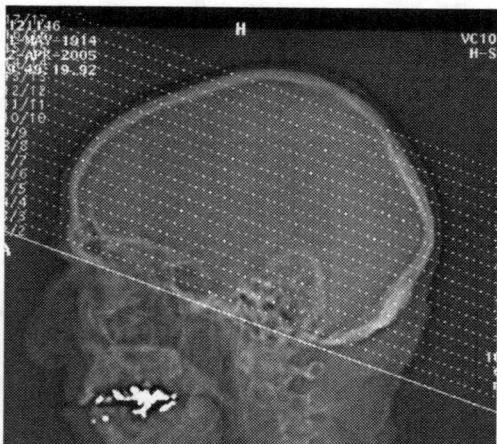

Figure 1. *Note how the CT scan contains a topogram or scout view in the top left hand corner which is a lateral view of the skull with lines running through it. These lines have numbers and the slices that follow are axial images and have corresponding numbers on them so that we can identify through which part of the cranium they were taken. The bottom slices are small and have a lot of bone and very little brain in them as they are in the uppermost part of the cranium and as we travel through the brain, and move up the scan, the slices become progressively larger.*

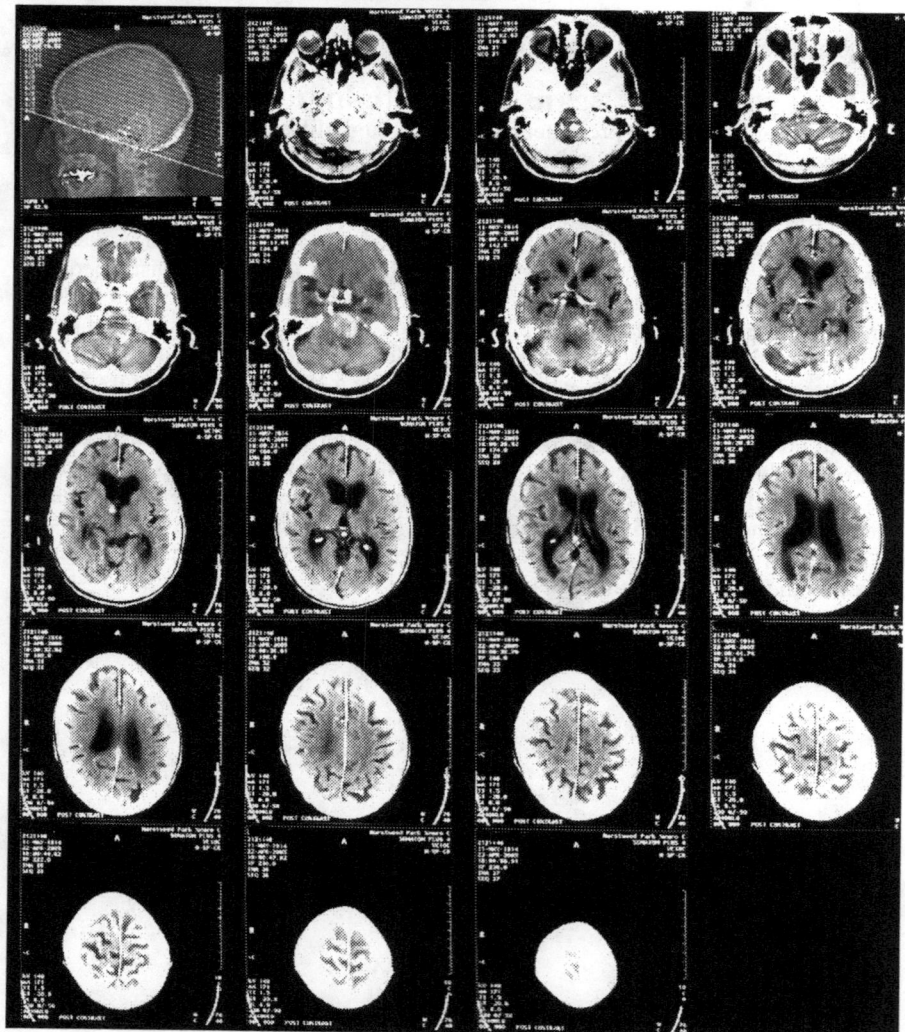

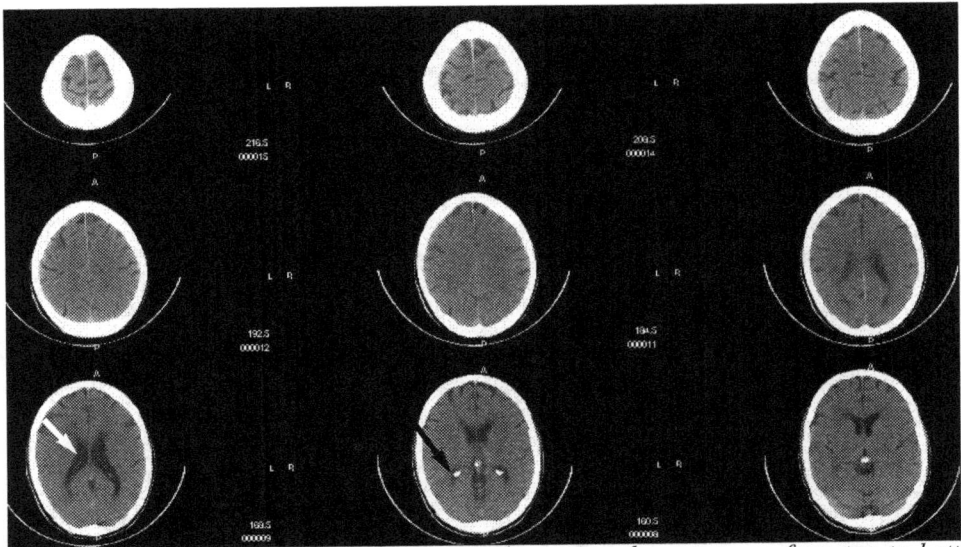

Figure 2. *Note how the size of the images changes as the cuts move from top to bottom through the cranial space. In this electronic image, the uppermost images correspond to the top of the cranium as opposed to the other way around on the hard copy seen in figure 1. Note the lateral ventricles as denoted by the white arrow and the white of the calcified choroid plexus in the trigone of the right lateral ventricle as denoted by the black arrow*
.

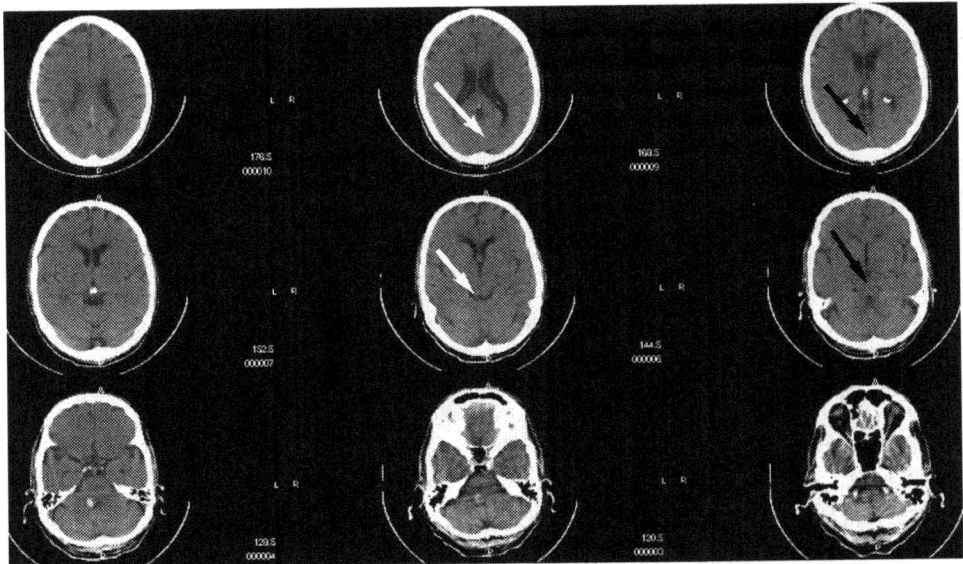

Figure 3. *Note the falx (top white arrow), denoting the supratentorial space and how on the next slice, the falx disappears and the top of the posterior fossa is demonstrated (top black arrow). Note the basal cisterns as demonstrated by the bottom white arrow and the brain-stem as denoted by the bottom black arrow. The basal cisterns have a fluid density as they contain CSF.*

129

Bone is dark on MRI (T1 WI and T2 WI) because of the calcium deposited in it. At the edges of the brain adjacent to the bone, there are fluid-filled spaces, the subarachnoid spaces, and these are the same colour as the ventricles (dark on CT scan and T1 WI and white on T2 WI) since both contain CSF.

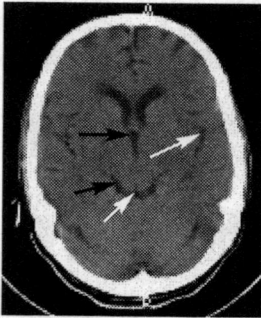

Figure 4. *This is an uncontrasted axial CT scan. The top black arrow indicates the slit like third ventricle, the bottom black arrow the ambient cistern, the bottom white arrow the quadrigeminal cistern and the top white arrow the sylvian fissure.*

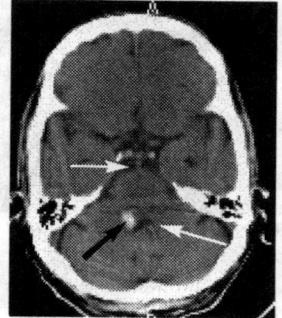

Figure 5. *This is an uncontrasted axial CT scan. The top arrows shows the pre pontine cistern and the bottom arrow the fourth ventricle, which in this case contains fresh blood (black arrow).*

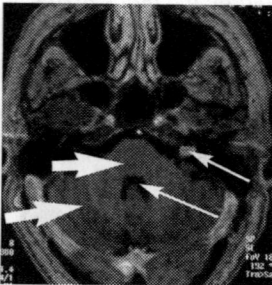

Figure 6. *This is a contrast enhanced axial T1 WI. The top thick arrow demonstrates the pons and the bottom thick arrow demonstrates the cerebellum. The top thin arrow demonstrates a small intracanalicular vestibular schwannoma in the cerebellopontine angle and the bottom thin arrow demonstrates the sickle shaped fourth ventricle.*

Just posterior to the third ventricle, the brain stem can be seen with the basal cisterns around it. These consist of the prepontine, ambient and quadrigeminal cisterns. The supratentorial space is separated from the infratentorial space by the tentorium cerebelli. In the supratentorial space you will see the two cerebral hemispheres seperated by the falx cerebrum. Immediately below the level of the tentorium, the falx is no longer visible and this is the anatomical space of the posterior fossa in which the cerebellum is housed. The cerebellum abuts the brain stem and the area between the brainstem and the cerebellum is called the cerebellopontine angle.

Some of the different structures of the brain seen on scans are the parenchyma consisting of white matter and grey matter, the subarachnoid spaces including the basal cisterns, the ventricular system, the substance of the cerebellum and then the bony vault and skull base surrounding the brain. T1 WI are excellent for demonstrating normal anatomy. In evaluating a patient's radiology, it is important to make sure that you know how many films have been done. A patient may have several sets of films; there may be three CT scan films, one for evaluation of the bone in which only bone windows were done and the brain had been factored out, one where soft tissue had been factored in without contrast and one where soft tissue had been factored in post contrast enhancement. The MRI will usually consist of several types of sequences with T2 WI and pre and post contrast T1 WI being the most common. The MRI will consist of not only axial cuts but also coronal and sagittal cuts. When putting the scans up onto the viewer, look in the right upper corner of each of the small images and identify the name of the patient. Ensure the scan is orientated the correct way around (if the name of the patient is not back to front or upside down, you are correct in your orientation). Ensure that the films you are looking at are for the correct scan date. Then try to find a "c" sign, the word "contrast", "gadolinium" or "gad" on the scan within the small square. This indicates that contrast had been administered.

When reading scans you need to have a system and be methodical. A useful system is to approach the scan from the outside inwards. Therefore, if we look at the large square of film that the scan is printed on, we start at the outside of the film and and look at the survey or scout image. This gives us a general idea of the way that the gantry of the scanner has been angled, by seeing the way that the lines go through the anatomical plane of the head and how many slices have been done. For instance, in the posterior fossa it is usual to do thinner cuts than in the rest of the brain. When presenting a scan you would start by saying "This is a contrasted (or uncontrasted) axial, sagittal or coronal CT/MRI (T1 or T2 weighted) scan of (person's name) done on (date of scan) and the most striking abnormality is ......"
Progressing from the outside of the slice inwards, look firstly at the bone and, if you have a CT scan with bony windows, concentrate on these first. When looking at CT scans, be aware that there are several suture lines in the skull. The most obvious sutures are the lambdoid and the coronal suture. The coronal suture is seen about a third of the way back from the anterior part of the skull and the lambdoid suture is seen in the region of the posterior fossa cuts, see figure 7. MRI sequences are of little or no benefit when evaluating bone.

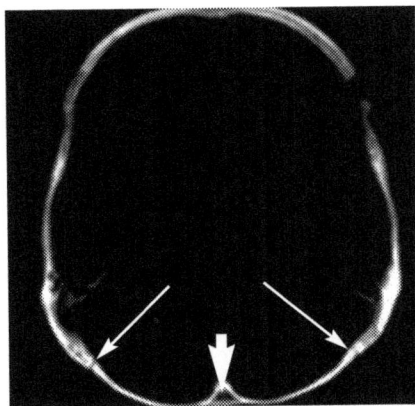

Figure 7. *This is a bone window of an axial CT scan. Both lambdoid sutures are indicated with the thin white arrows and the internal occipital protuberance with the thick white arrow. Note the burrhole in the left frontal region.*

Then, as far as the substance of the cerebrum is concerned, try to look for asymmetry. The sulcal pattern is a useful adjunct in this as a mass lesion in a hemisphere may flatten the sulcal pattern on that side. The sulci can be seen best on the convexity of the brain, at the top half, in the first few cuts from the vertex downwards. When identifying lesions on a scan it is important to be able to describe them. You need to describe whether the lesion is homogenous or not. There might be a central necrotic or cystic component with the lesion having hetereogeneous appearance of both solid tumour and cyst or it may be a homogenous (uniform density), solid tumour. Does the lesion have an irregular or regular outline, does it

131

enhance with contrast and is there any associated oedema or mass effect? Having carefully studied the cerebral hemispheres, it is important to then focus on the ventricular system.

Hydrocephalus and ventriculomegaly

Any dilatation of the ventricular system or asymmetry should be noted. When the ventricles are dilated, it may be due to brain atrophy (hydrocephalus ex vacuo) and in this case the sulcal pattern will be enlarged as well as the basal cisterns. Alternatively, it could be due to hydrocephalus, in which case the ventricles become larger but the sulcal pattern and the basal cisterns become smaller due to the compressive effect of the ventricles. It is important to differentiate between communicating and non-communicating hydrocephalus. A basic rule is that if all four the ventricles are large then the ventricles are all communicating with each other and it is therefore communicating hydrocephalus. If there are one or two ventricles that are large and the rest are small then it is non-communicating hydrocephalus. For instance, a colloid cyst of the third ventricle will block off the foramina of Monroe and will cause both lateral ventricles to distend. The fourth ventricle which is not in communication with the lateral ventricles, due to an obstruction at the level of foramen of Monroe, will be normal in size, and this a non-communicating pattern of hydrocephalus. In communicating hydrocephalus, the obstruction is outside of the ventricular system and it can either be because the subarachnoid spaces and cisterns are obliterated, the outlet foramina are obstructed or because there is decreased absorption by the arachnoid villae.

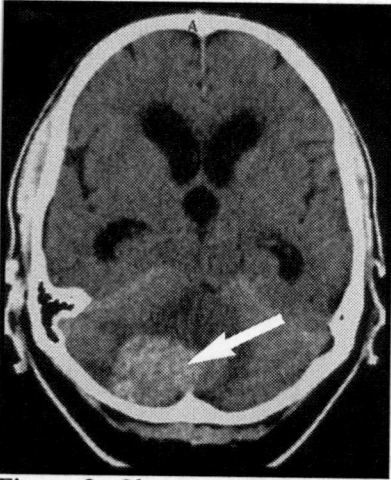

Figure 8. *Obstructive hydrocephalus. This is an uncontrasted axial CT scan. There is a haemorrhage in the posterior fossa (arrow) which is obstructing the fourth ventricle leading to obstructive hydrocephalus with dilatation of both anterior and temporal horns of the lateral ventricles and also dilatation of the third ventricle.*

When evaluating the posterior fossa, it is important to note that the vermis is usually of a different colour than the two cerebellar hemispheres. It can be easy to confuse the normal appearance of the vermis with that of a tumour. In patients presenting after a head injury it is important to evaluate the skull base for fractures. These are seen best on the bony cuts of the CT scan, which should be performed in all traumatic cases.

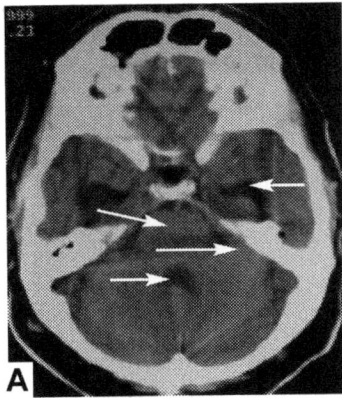

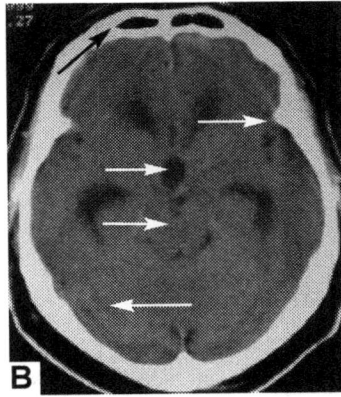

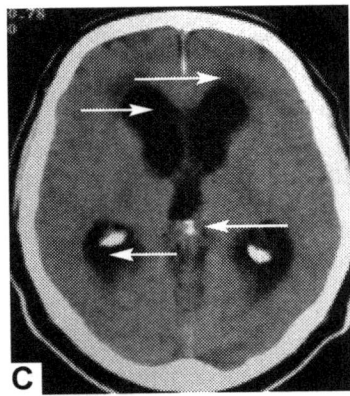

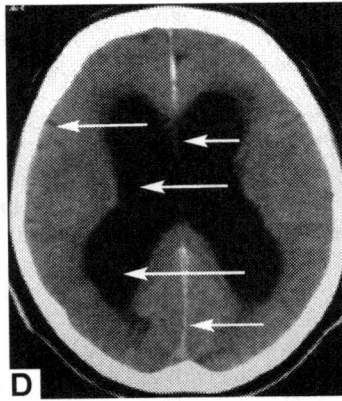

Figure 9.*These are uncontrasted axial CT scans. In these images communicating hydro-cephalus is depicted with dilatation of all the ventricles and the arrows are described from top to bottom; A: The top arrow demonstrates the dilated temporal horn of the left lateral ventricle, the next arrow demonstrates the pons, the next arrow demonstrates the left petrous part of the temporal bone and the last arrow shows the dilated fourth ventricle; B: The top arrow demonstrates the frontal air sinus, the next arrow the top part of the sphenoid ridge of the left temporal bone, next arrow demonstrates the dilated third ventricle, the next arrow the midbrain and the last arrow demonstrates the folia of the right cerebellar hemisphere; C: The top arrow demonstrates periventricular lucency due the increased hydrostatic pressure of CSF in the ventricle, the next arrow demonstrates the dilated frontal horn of the right lateral ventricle, the next arrow demonstrates the pineal gland and the next arrow the trigone of the right lateral ventricle containing choroid plexus; D: The top arrow depicts a cerebral sulcus, the next the septum pellucidum, the next demonstrates the body of the right lateral ventricle, the next the occipital horn of the right lateral ventricle and the last arrow demonstrates the falx cerebri.*

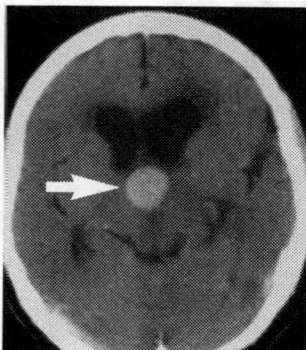

Figure 10. *Obstructive hydrocephalus. A colloid cyst of the third ventricle blocks both the foramina of Monroe bilaterally leading to obstructive hydrocephalus of the lateral ventricles.*

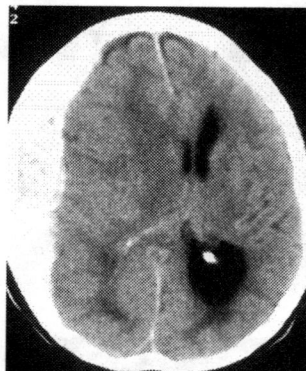

Figure 11. *Obstructive hydrocephalus. This is an uncontrasted axial CT scan. The acute subdural haemorrhage on the right has caused midline shift and trapped the frontal and occipital horns of the left lateral ventricle leading to dilatation and hydrocephalus.*

Trauma

A CT scan is the preferred investigation for cranial trauma. It does not require MR compatible ventilators or instruments, is simple, fast and widely available. The images are very sensitive for acute haemorrhage as well as cerebral oedema. CT scans are also the preferred imaging modality for evaluating bone and is an excellent tool for diagnosing fractures of the skull base, skull vault and facial bones. In trauma, the main categories of pathology are skull fractures, diffuse brain injury, intracerebral haemorrhages and extra-axial haemorrhages.

Skull fractures

The telltale sign of a skull fracture on a CT scan is usually overlying soft tissue swelling or disruption of the soft tissue with gas in the tissue. Fractures may be linear or depressed, comminuted or simple. Depressed fractures are frequently associated with dural tears and underlying intracerebral haemorrhages. Base of skull fractures may be difficult to identify, as they can often be hairline cracks. Fluid in the mastoid air cells or in the frontal sinus (opacification of the sinus) is frequently an indication of a skull base fracture with an associated dural tear and CSF leak. Intracranial air is another indication of a dural tear.

Diffuse brain injury

Diffuse brain injury (DBI) is part of a wide spectrum ranging from concussion to severe diffuse axonal injury. The hallmark of diffuse brain injury is pinpoint haemorrhage. These occur due to acceleration -deceleration and rotational forces imparted to the brain with subsequent tears in the white matter tracts, leading to pin point haemorrhages. They are usually found at the grey – white matter interface.

There are three grades of DBI:

Grade 1 – diffuse point bleeds throughout the brain.
Grade 2 – as above with point bleeds in the corpus callosum and
Grade 3 – as grade 2 with point bleeds in the dorsal mid-brain.

These 3 grades correlate well with prognosis and mid-brain haemorrhages are usually associated with a poor prognosis. Acute subdural haematomas are frequently associated with DBI as the rotational forces and acceleration - deceleration forces can lead to the draining veins suspended between the dura and the cortical surface being torn with subsequent haemorrhage into the subdural space.

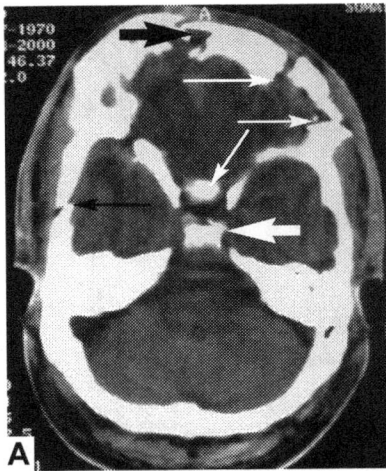

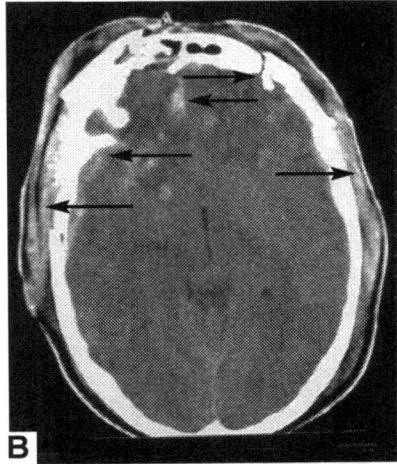

Figure 12. *These are uncontrasted axial CT scans. These images depict severe cranial trauma. A: The top 3 arrows depict a comminuted fracture of the frontal bone involving the frontal air sinus, the lower black arrow depicts a fracture of the right temporal bone, the angled arrow shows the tuberculum sellae and the thick white arrow the dorsum sellae B: The top arrow demonstrates a linear fracture of the frontal bone, the next demonstrates frontal lobe haemorrhagic contusions, the next a thin acute subdural haematoma and the last two arrows demonstrate extracranial soft tissue swelling secondary to traumatic impacts.*

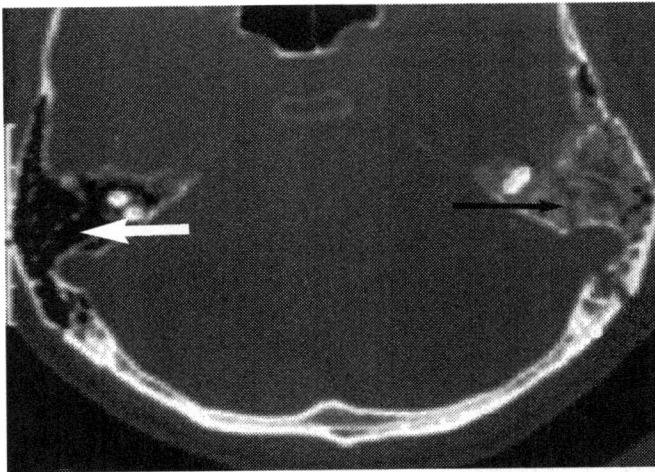

Figure 13. *This is the bone window of an axial CT scan. The black arrow depicts a transverse fracture of the petrous part of the temporal bone. This base of skull fracture has opacified the mastoid air cells on the left. The normal black appearance of the right sided mastoid air cells (thick arrow) is because they are filled with air whereas the white opacified air cells on the right are filled with fluid secondary to the fracture.*

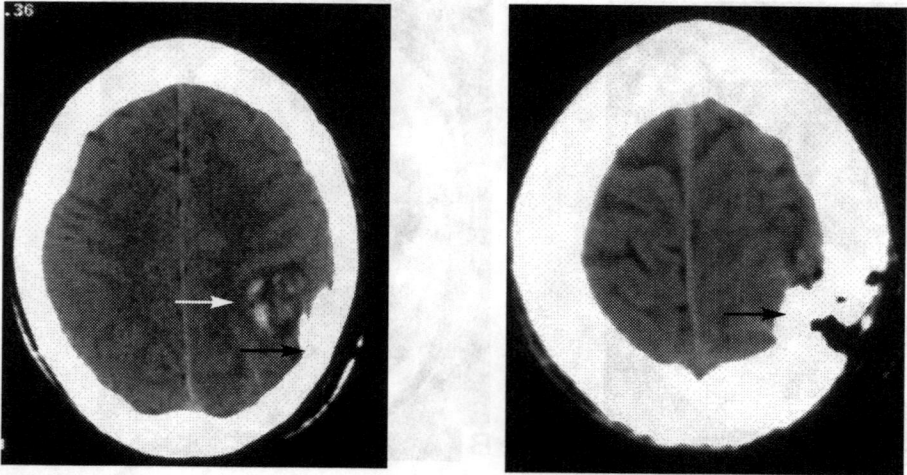

Figure 14. *These are uncontrasted axial CT scans. A comminuted, depressed fracture is depicted on these two axial slices (black arrows) with an underlying haemorrhagic contusion (white arrow). This is a typical example of focal brain trauma.*

Diffuse Injury Grade	CT appearance	Mortality
I	Normal CT scan	9.6%
II	Basal cisterns not effaced and midline shift < 5mm	13.5%
III	Cisterns compressed or absent and midline shift < 5mm	34%
IV	Shift > 5mm but no mass lesion of >25 cm^3 present	56.2%

Table 1. *The Marshall classification.*
(Marshall LF, Bowers-Marshall S, Klauber MR et al. A new classification of head injury based on computerised tomography. J Neurosurg 75 (Suppl):S14-20, 1991)

Intracerebral haemorrhage

We frequently see coup and contrecoup injuries where the impact side (coup side) as well as the opposite side (contrecoup side) demonstrates traumatic brain damage. This may for instance happen when a person falls onto the back of their head. The patient will have focal soft tissue swelling over the occiput with some focus of pathology there, frequently an intracerebral haemorrhage with some associated subarachnoid haemorrhage. Also the brain then moves forward and rubs over the rough surface of the orbital roof in the anterior cranial fossa and the frontal lobe poles impact against the inner skull leading to bifrontal contusions. There are frequently associated bitemporal contusions as the anterior poles of the temporal lobes collide with the sphenoid ridge, which forms the anterior border of the middle cranial fossa. These are devastating injuries and with longterm sequelae. These contusions quite often "blossom" as they enlarge and have associated oedema, usually about a week after the injury. Other intracerebral haemorrhages, called haemorrhagic contusions, can be larger versions of the pinpoint bleeds in diffuse brain injury and are caused by the same mechanism.

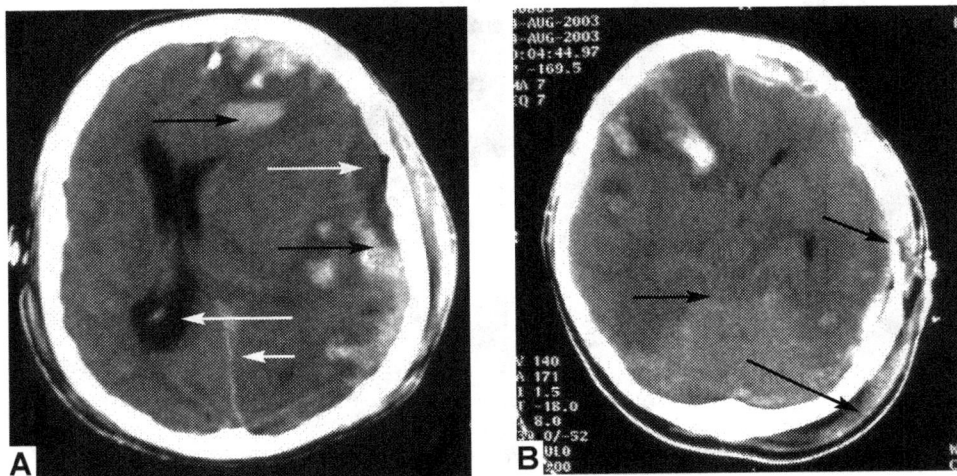

Figure 15. *These are uncontrasted axial CT scans. Both images depict severe diffuse brain injury. Note how on the left the hemisphere has swollen up and is herniating across the midline. A: The top arrow depicts a haemorrhagic contusion and several of these can be seen throughout both hemispheres, the next arrow demonstrates a hyperacute component of an acute subdural haematoma where the blood is so fresh that it has not yet had the time to clot and become hyperdense. It is important not to confuse this with a chronic subdural haematoma which has the same density. The next arrow demonstrates the clotted component of the acute subdural haematoma, the next arrow demonstrates the trapped ventricles due to midline shift and the last arrows demonstrates a parafalcine acute subdural haematoma. B: The top arrow shows a skull fracture. The next arrow demonstrates obliteration of the basal cisterns due to brain swelling. The last arrow demonstrates the widespread soft tissue swelling secondary to focal impacts. In this case the haemorrhagic contusions, acute subdural haematoma and parafalcine subdural haematoma point towards a diffuse brain injury with acceleration-deceleration and rotational forces and the skull fracture to a focal, impact type injury. This is typical for motor vehicle accidents where there is a combination of these mechanisms of injury.*

Extra-axial collections

Subdural and extradural collections may be difficult to tell apart. Subdural collections are usually craggy, irregularly shaped and depress the underlying brain. Epidural (extradural) haemorrhages are bicrescentic or biconvex lesions that strip the dura away from the bone. On CT scans both are white in the acute phase. In the hyperacute phase, before the blood has had a chance to clot, these lesions are darker than the brain and hypodense. Following the acute phase, the blood lyses and turns into deoxyhaemoglobin and bilirubin and it becomes more serous. The colour on CT scans changes to become more grey and eventually it becomes dark, very much the same density as the CSF. This happens over a couple of weeks. There is definite clinical significance in differentiating between a subdural and extradural haemorrhage. A subdural haemorrhage may sometimes continue to bleed but far more so, extradural haematomas have the propensity to do this. This gives rise to 'the talk and die' phenomenon where patients arrive in the hospital awake (the lucid interval) but then subsequent

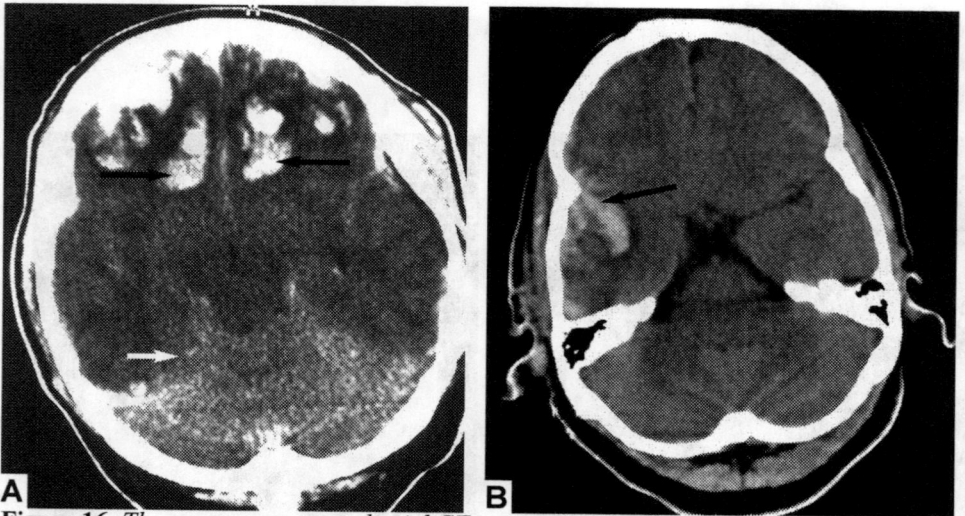

Figure 16. *These are uncontrasted axial CT scans. A: Note the severe bilateral haemorrhagic contusions (black arrows) and note the difference in density between the area of the tentorium cerebelli and the rest of the brain (white arrow). It can be difficult to tell whether this is due to ischaemia in the frontal and temporal lobes or is just the different imaging characteristics of the dura (tentorium cerebelli) and the brain parenchyma. These contusions are usually caused when the brain moves forward over the rough surface of the anterior cranial fossa; B: The movement of the brain cause the parenchyma of the frontal and temporal lobes adjacent to the Sylvian fissure to collide with the sphenoid ridge of the temporal bone, causing haemorrhagic contusions and in this case a small acute subdural haematoma (black arrow).*

ly deteriorate due to ongoing haemorrhage from the ruptured vessel on the dural surface leading to increased haematoma formation and brain compression. When evaluating these lesions it is important to note their location, how big they are and what their effects are on the brain. When reporting these lesions, especially to a senior colleague, state the location of the haemorrhage and on how many cuts it can be seen on the CT scan as this indicates the total volume of the clot. CT scans are usually performed in 7 or 8mm cuts (the vertical distance between the slices) in the supratentorial area and therefore a haemorrhage that can be seen on 7 cuts is between 5-6cms high. When this is combined with the thickness of the clot you can get an estimate of how large it is. A haematoma 1 or 2 cm wide that can be seen on 4 or 5 cuts would be judged to be a large haematoma. It is sometimes difficult to visually separate the haematoma from the bone (since both are white) and if looking at the scans on the CT workstation it can be useful to change the settings of the scan (ask the radiographer to help you) and this frequently demonstrates the interface between the bone and the blood. Using Hounsfield units are also useful. It is important to look at the effect on the underlying brain and a midline shift of 5mm or more is significant. An extra-axial collection in the temporal lobe has much more clinical effect than a collection on the convexity as the temporal lobe is situated adjacent to the midbrain and even small haematomas can cause compression of the midbrain. It is easy to see the edge of the tentorium cerebelli at the medial border of the temporal lobe and it is possible to see herniation of the brain tissue (uncus) through this hiatus with subsequent compression of the brainstem. Acute extradural haematomas usually result from injury to the anterior or posterior branches of the middle meningeal artery. However, fractures associated with venous sinuses can also lead to extradural haematomas caused by a venous bleed rather than an arterial source. Venous extradural haematomas are more common in children. Subdural haematomas can also be interhemispheric or be found on the surface of the tentorium cerebelli.

Figure 17. *This is an uncontrasted axial CT scan and it demonstrates an acute extradural haematoma with typical biconvex shape. This is because the dura is stripped away from the brain by the haematoma. These haematomas usually do not cross the suture lines.*

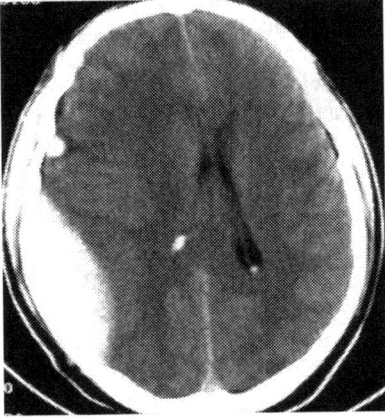

Figure 18. *This is an uncontrasted axial CT scan and it demonstrates an acute subdural collection with typical crescenteric shape. Note the marked midline shift as in figure 17 above.*

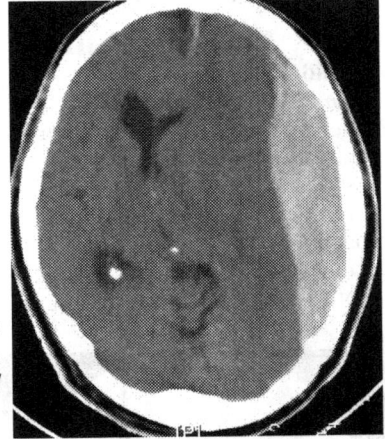

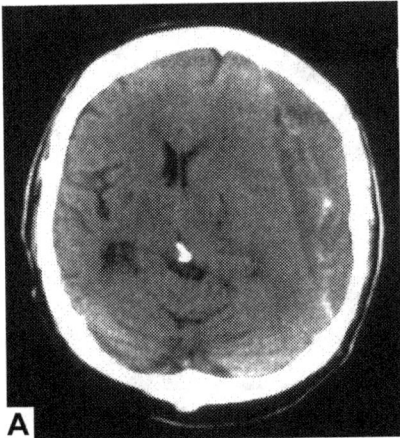

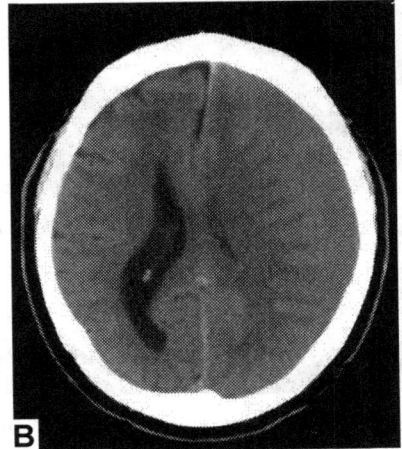

Figure 19. *These are uncontrasted axial CT scans. A: This chronic subdural haematoma is hypodense to brain. B: In this scan the subdural haematoma is isodense to brain making it very difficult to diagnose. It is the midline shift in these cases that make the diagnosis. The most difficult scenario is that of bilateral isodense subdural haematomas where there is no midline shift. In these cases, the ventricles will usually appear compressed and the basal cisterns and the sulci are also compressed.*

Brain tumours

Brain tumours can be either primary or secondary (metastasis). The administration of contrast medium greatly improves the CT sensitivity and specificity for tumour diagnosis. Enhancement with contrast may either represent blood-brain barrier breakdown or tumour neo-vascularity. Because of disruption of the normal cyto architecture in brain tumours, the blood-brain barrier does not remain intact and this allows seepage of contrast out of the vascular system. Similarly, the fast growing tissue of malignant tumours requires new blood vessels to feed the rapidly growing cells and this will lead to contrast enhancement at the area of the tumour. This is because tumours have more blood vessels and therefore more contrast density/intensity than the surrounding normal brain. Tumours are divided into intra-axial (within the neural axis that is the parenchyma of the brain or the spinal cord limited by the pia mater) and extra-axial tumours (outside of the neural axis and therefore outside the brain parenchyma and pia mater).

Primary brain tumours
(Low grade) astrocytoma
CT scan
Homogenous and frequently difficult to discern from brain
No contrast enhancement
Little surrounding oedema
MR scan
Homogenous and hypointense on T1 WI
Hyperintense on T2 WI
No contrast enhancement

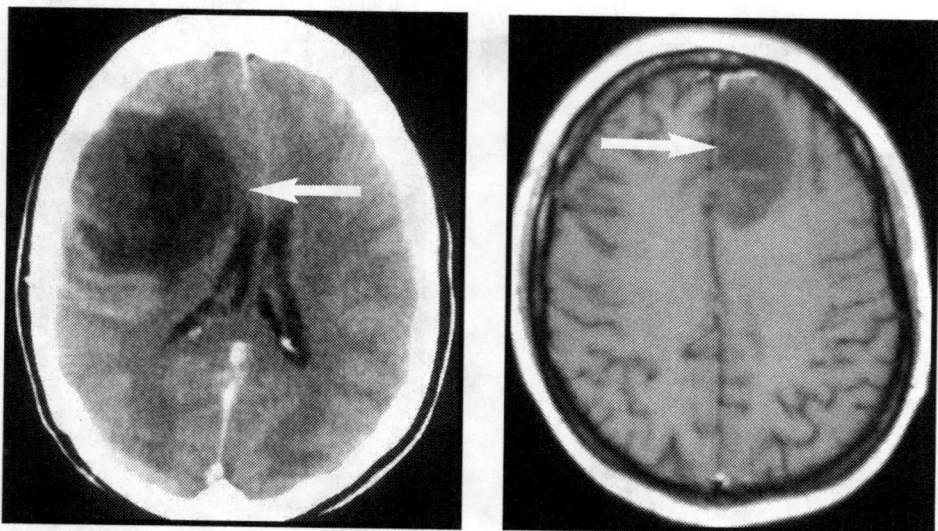

Figure 20. *The image on the left is a contrast enhanced axial CT scan and the image on the right is a contrast enhanced axial T1 WI. The hypodensities (arrows) on both scans are typical of low grade astrocytomas, as is the fact that they do not enhance.*

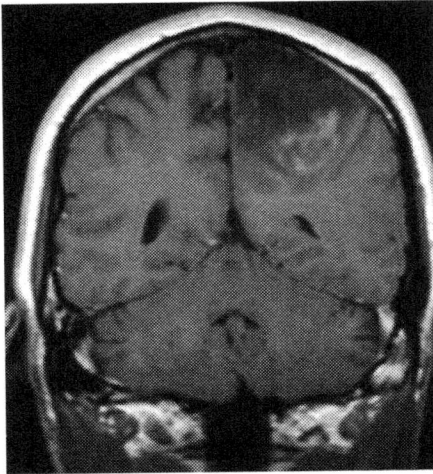

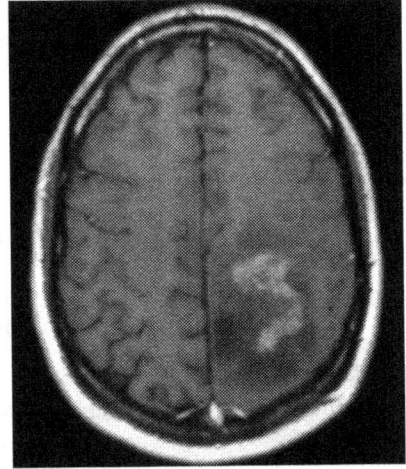

Figure 21. *Anaplastic astrocytoma. The scan on the left is a contrast enhanced coronal T1 WI and the scan on the right is a contrast enhanced axial T1 WI. The lesions are also hypodense on CT and hypointense on T1 WI like the low grade astrocytomas but, unlike the low grade astrocytomas, enhance with contrast.*

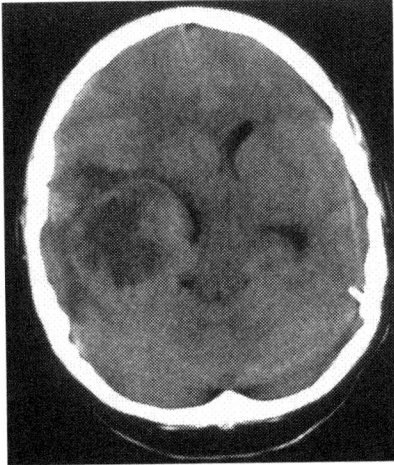

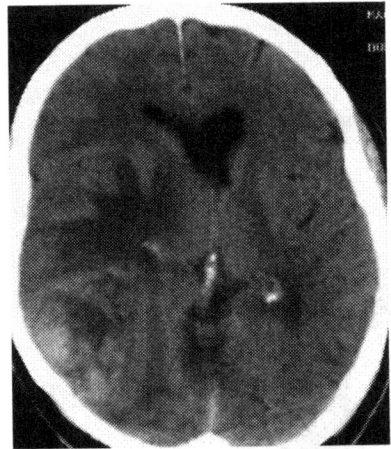

Figure 22. *Glioblastoma. The image on the top left is an uncontrasted axial CT scan and the image on the top right is a contrast enhanced axial CT scan. The image on the right is a contrast enhanced axial T1 WI. Glioblastomas have central necrosis, are irregular and craggy with strong heterogeneous enhancement and have surrounding oedema.*

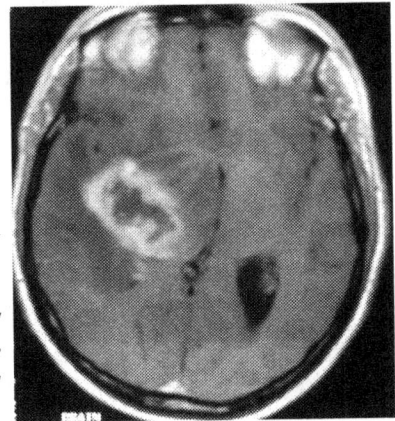

Anaplastic astrocytoma
As for low grade astrocytoma but less homogenous, may have contrast enhancement

Glioblastoma Multiforme
CT scan
Heterogeneous with a hypodense centre
Strong but heterogeneous and irregular contrast enhancement
Surrounding oedema
Calcification indicates likely transformation from low grade.
MR scan
Heterogeneous and hypo/isointense on T1 WI
Hypointense centre on T1 WI (necrosis)
Strong and heterogeneous enhancement with contrast
Hyperintense on T2 WI
Surrounding oedema on T2 WI and FLAIR
The most important differential is that of an abscess which is usually round, thin walled and may be multiple

Pilocytic astrocytoma (mostly in children)
CT scan
Discrete solid or mixed solid/cystic mass found in the cerebral hemispheres or vermis
Hypo/iso dense to brain
No surrounding oedema
Calcified in 20%
Solid component enhances strongly
MR scan
Solid component hypo/isointense on T1 WI
Strong and heterogeneous enhancement with contrast
Solid component and cyst hyperintense on T2 WI, cyst does not suppress with FLAIR (abnormal fluid)

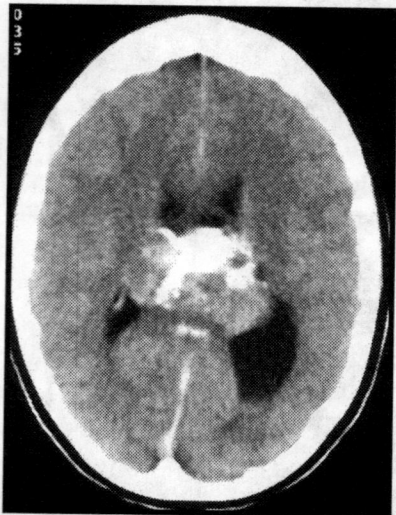

Figure 23. *Pilocytic astrocytoma. In this uncontrasted axial CT scan, this tumour has calcificied regions denoting a slow growth pattern These tumours are isodense or hypodense to brain and enhance strongly with contrast administration.*

Oligodendrogliomas (oligodendrocytes and glial cells)
CT scan
Hypo/isodense
Most are calcified
Variable enhancement
MR scan
Hypo/isointense on T1 WI
Half enhance with contrast.
Hyperintense on T2 WI

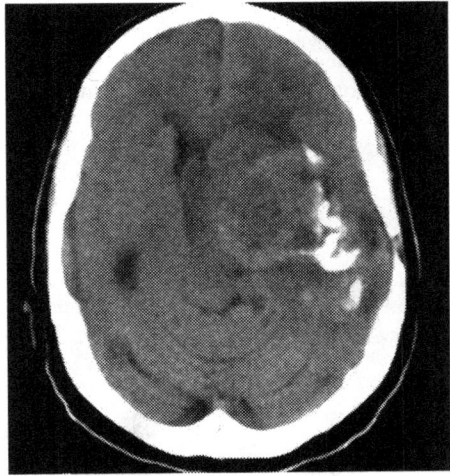

Figure 24. *Oligodendroglioma. In this uncontrasted axial CT scan, this tumour demonstrates calcification and is isodense to brain. In this case there was minimal contrast enhancement.*

Ependymoma
Posterior fossa (small children)
CT scan
Floor of fourth ventricle and cerebello-pontine angle
Isodense to brain
Half are calcified
Variable enhancement
Hydrocephalus
MR scan
Hypointense on T1 WI
Half enhance with contrast.
Isointense on T2 WI
Variable enhancement
Hydrocephalus

Supratentorial (older children and adults)
CT scan
Parenchymal or intraventricular mass
Heterogenous
Half are calcified
Hydrocephalus (in intraventricular tumours)
Variable enhancement
MR scan
Hypointense on T1 WI
Isointense on T2 WI
Variable enhancement
Hydrocephalus (in intraventricular tumours)

Meningiomas
CT scan
Mostly hyperdense
Calcification in 25%
Strong, homogenous enhancement
Associated bony changes such as osseous hypertrophy
MR scan

143

Isointense or slightly hyper intense on T1 WI
Isointense on T2 WI, surrounding oedema in half with decreased signal intensity on T2 if there is calcification.
Strong, homogenous enhancement, dural tail (origin from dura can be seen)

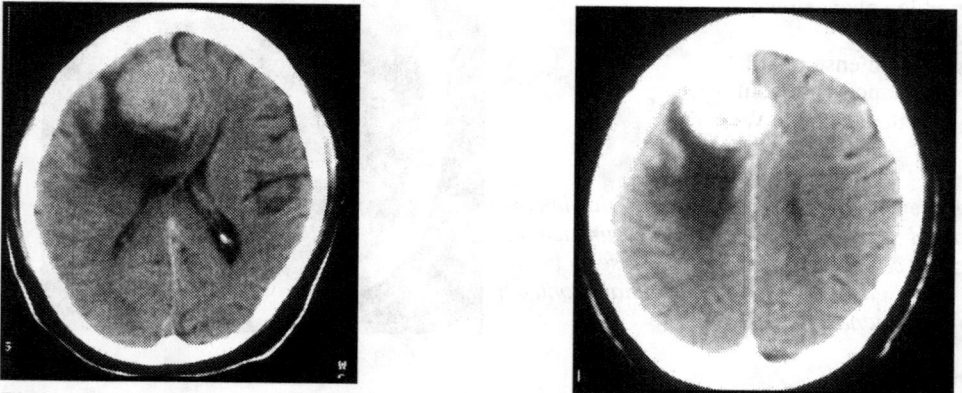

Figure 25. *Meningioma. The scan on the left is an uncontrasted axial CT scan of the brain and the scan on the right a contrast enhanced axial CT scan. The meningioma clearly demonstrates attachment to the dura of the falx, has a lot of surrounding oedema and enhances brilliantly with contrast.*

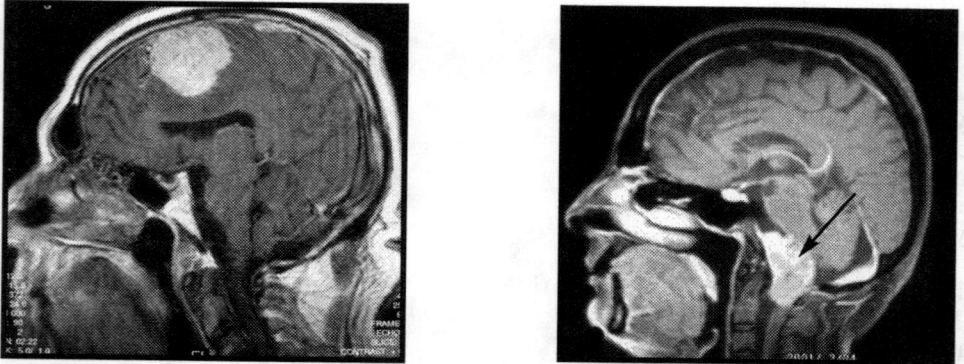

Figure 26. *The image on the left is a sagittal T1 WI following contrast administration. This also clearly demonstrates a dural attachment and brilliant contrast enhancement of the same meningioma as seen above. The image on the right is a contrast enhanced saggital T1WI scan and demonstrates a skull base meningioma occupying a large part of the foramen magnum (arrow).*

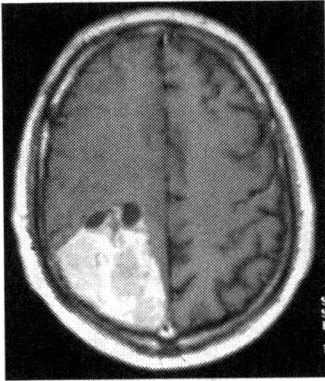

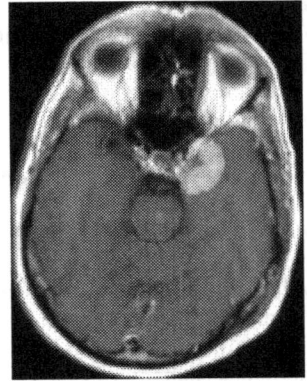

Figure 27. *The image on the left is a contrast enhanced axial T1 WI of the brain, demonstrating dural attachment and vivid enhancement of this convexity meningioma. The image on the right is a contrast enhanced axial T1 WI which clearly shows a meningioma of the left cavernous sinus.*

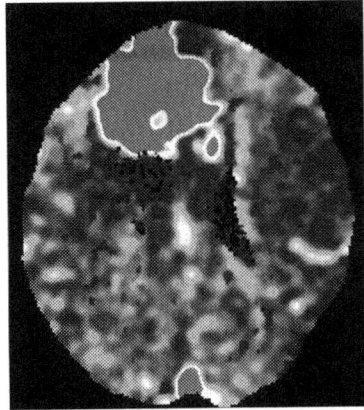

Figure 28. *This image demonstrates a dynamic perfusion CT scan which is performed using pixel density and transit time to measure flow and volume. It clearly demonstrates high flow and high blood volume within the same tumour as seen in figure 25.*

Primary central nervous system lymphoma
CT scan
Mostly hyperdense
Frequently in periventricular location
Moderate, homogenous enhancement
MR scan
Isointense on T1 WI
Isointense on T2 WI (hyperintense on FLAIR)
Strong, homogenous enhancement

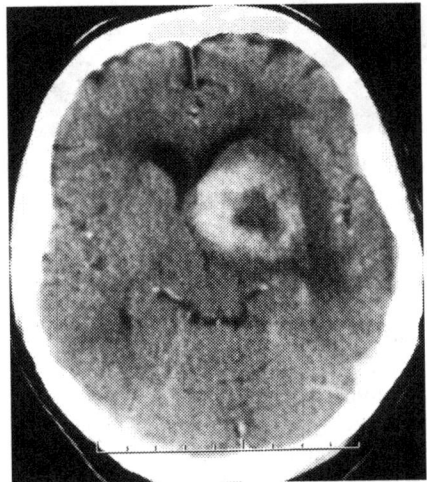

Figure 29. *Lymphoma. This uncontrasted axial CT scan demonstrates a high density periventricular lesion. Note the central area of necrosis and associated oedema.*

145

Intracranial cyst-like lesions
Dermoid cyst (located in midline)
CT scan
Hypodense (density of fat)
Does not enhance
MR scan
Hyperintense on T1 WI (hypointense on STIR)
Heterogenous on T2 WI
No enhancement

Epidermoid cyst (located in midline and cerebello-pontine angle)
CT scan
Hypodense (density of CSF)
May have some calcification
Does not enhance
MR scan
Hypointense on T1 WI
Hyperintense on T2 WI
Does not suppress on FLAIR sequence

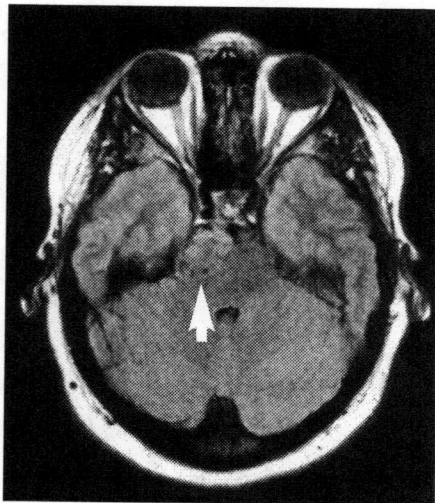

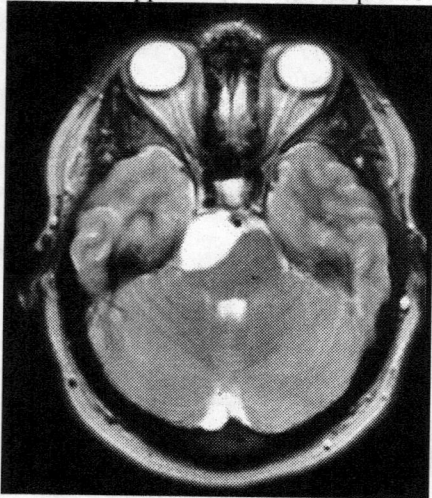

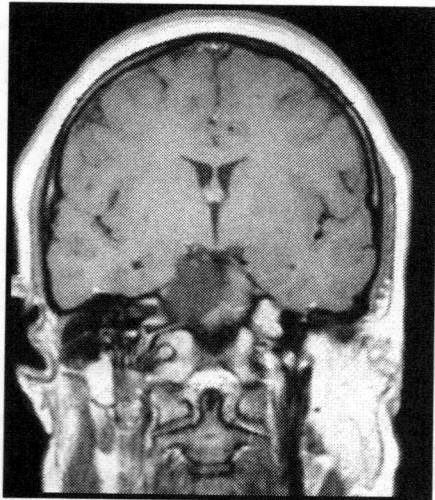

Figure 30. *The image on the left is an axial T2 WI and demonstrates an epidermoid cyst in the right cerebellopontine angle. Note that it is brightly intense on this image. A FLAIR image will have a similar intensity. The image on the top right is a T1 WI axial scan and the image on the bottom right is a coronal T1 WI. Note that the same lesion is hypointense on these images. It would not enhance on contrast enhanced images.*

Colloid cyst of the third ventricle
CT scan
Mostly hyperdense, can be isodense
Obstructive hydrocephalus
Does not enhance
MR scan
Variable on T1 WI and T2 WI
Does not enhance

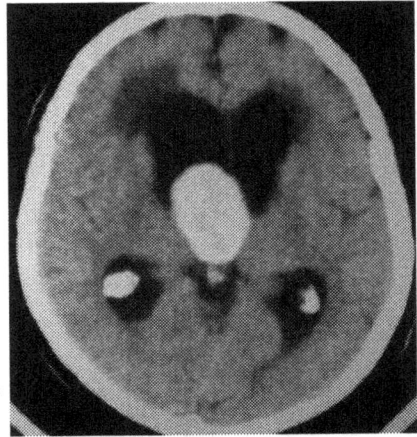

Figure 31. *Colloid cyst. This image is of an uncontrasted axial CT scan of the brain demonstrating a typical hyperdense lesion in the third ventricle with obstructive hydrocephalus.*

Arachnoid cysts (Sylvian fissure, basal cisterns, CPA)
CT scan
Mostly CSF density
Obstructive hydrocephalus
Does not enhance
MR scan
Same intensities as CSF
Does not enhance
Suppresses with FLAIR (used to discern from epidermoid cysts which do not suppress)

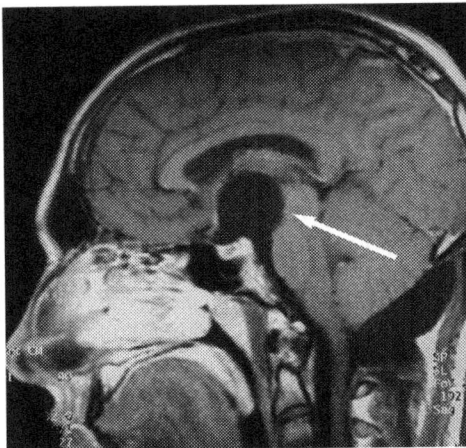

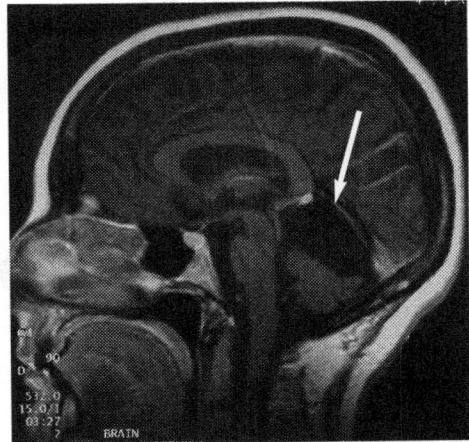

Figure 32. *These are uncontrasted sagittal T1 WI scans. The scan on the left demonstrates a suprasellar arachnoid cyst. the image on the left demonstrates an arachnoid cyst in the posterior fossa.*

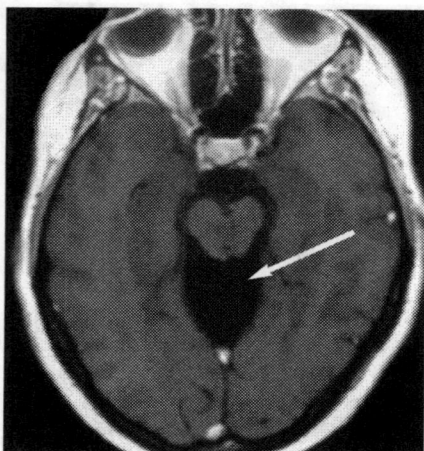

Figure 32a. *This image is an axial T1 WI demonstrating an arachnoid cyst of the posterior fossa. Note the CSF density of the lesion.*

Pituitary region tumours
Microadenomas (<1cm)
CT scan
Not seen, may be seen following contrast
MR scan
Variable on T1 WI and T2 WI
May enhance

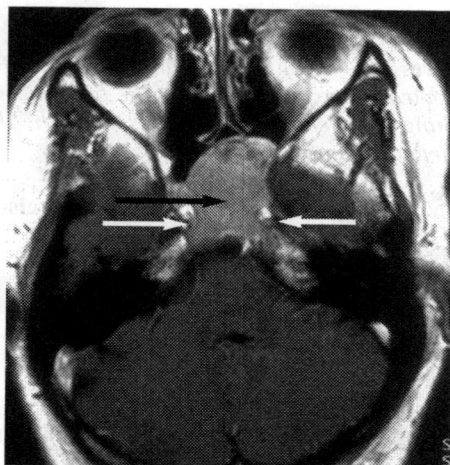

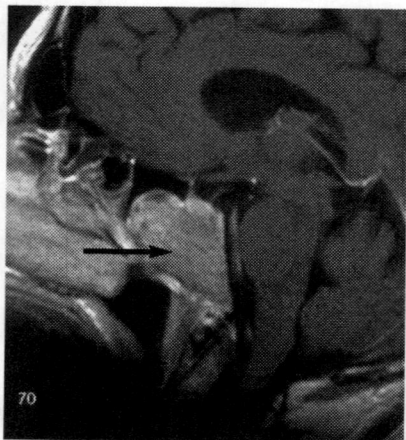

Figure 33. *The image on the left is a sagittal contrast enhanced T1 WI and the image above is an axial contrast enhanced T1 WI. Both show a pituitary macroadenoma (black arrows) with the axial image showing involvement of the cavernous sinuses bilaterally (white arrows).*

Macroadenomas (>1cm)
CT scan
Mostly isodense
Cysts/necrosis common
Usually enhances
May show signs of erosion and have extra sellar extension
MR scan
Isointense to gray matter on T1 WI and T2 WI
Usually enhances
Extra sellar extension may occur
Always look for haemorrhage

Craniopharyngiomas

CT scan
Mostly cystic
Calcified
Enhances
MR scan
Variable on T1 WI and T2 WI
Tend to erode the posterior clinoid
Hydrocephalus

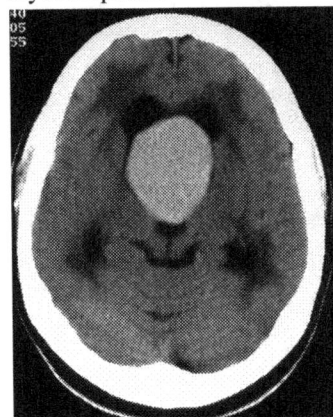

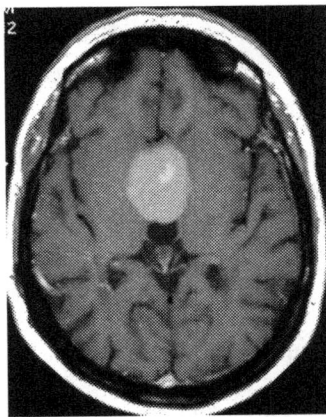

Figure 34. *The image on the left is a contrast enhanced axial CT scan and the image on the right is an unenhanced axial T1 WI. The craniopharyngioma enhances with contrast on the CT scan and is naturally hyperintense on the T1 WI because of the high lipid content of the tumour.*

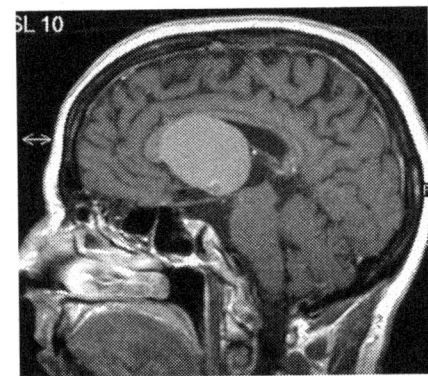

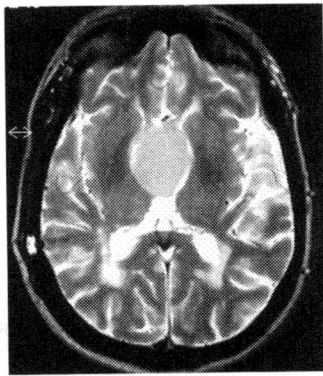

Figure 35. *The image on the left is an unenhaced sagittal T1 WI and the image on the right is a T2 WI axial scan of the brain. Note how the craniopharyngioma is hyperintense on both due to its high lipid (T1 WI) and fluid content (T2 WI)*

Neuronal tumours
Central neurocytomas (intraventricular)

CT scan
Mixed solid/cystic
Heterogeneous
Calcified in 50%

Enhances heterogeneously
MR scan
Isointense T1 WI
Hyperintense T2 WI
Inhomogeneous
Enhances heterogeneously
Hydrocephalus

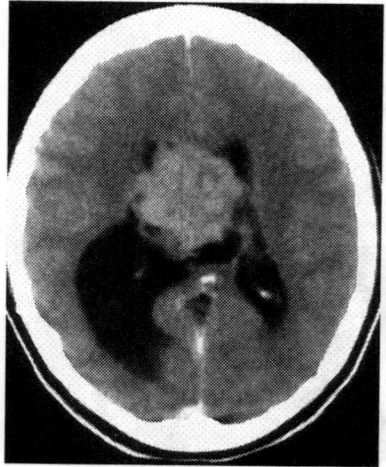

Figure 36. *This unenhanced axial CT scan of the brain demonstrates a central neurocytoma. These lesions are frequently heavily calcified and enhance with contrast and are histologically similar to oligodendrogliomas.*

Pineal region tumours
Germinoma (lesion infiltrates and displaces the pineal gland)
CT scan
Iso/hyperdense lesion at the posterior aspect third ventricle (pineal region)
Hydrocephalus
Enhances strongly
MR scan
Iso/hypointense T1 WI
Hyperintense T2 WI
Inhomogeneous
Enhances strongly and heterogeneously

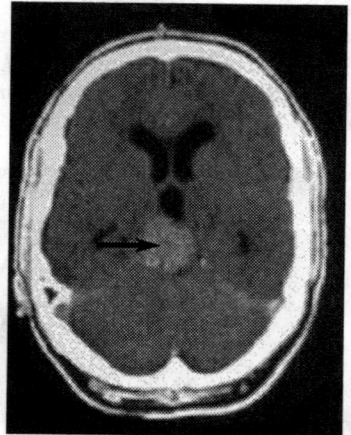

Figure 37. *Germinoma. This is an unenhanced axial CT scan. Tumours of the pineal region can be very difficult to tell apart as they all share some features. However, this lesion demonstrates infiltration and destruction of the pineal which is typical for germinomas.*

Pineal parenchymal tumours (lesion grows from inside out, displacing pineal circumferentially)
Pinealocytoma
CT scan
Iso/hypodense posterior aspect third ventricle (pineal region)
Does not enhance
Hydrocephalus
MR scan
Iso/hypointense T1 WI
Hyperintense T2 WI
Well delineated
Enhances strongly

Pinealoblastoma
CT scan
Heterogeneous lesion
Enhances heterogeneously
Hydrocephalus
MR scan
Iso/hypointense T1 WI
Hyperintense T2 WI
Poorly delineated
Enhances strongly
Demonstrates local infiltration

Tumours of the posterior fossa
Hemangioblastoma (Association with Von Hippel-Lindau disease)
CT scan
Low density cyst
Enhancing mural nodule
Sometimes solid enhancing tumour
MR scan
Iso/hypointense T1 WI
Hyperintense T2 WI
Nodule enhances strongly

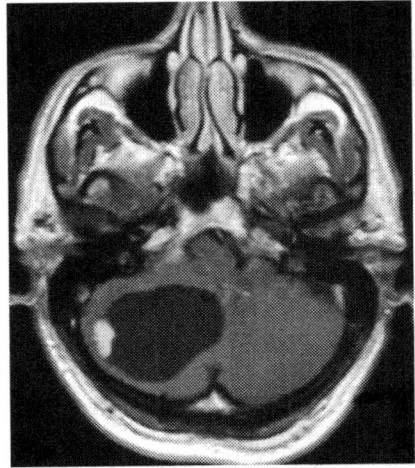

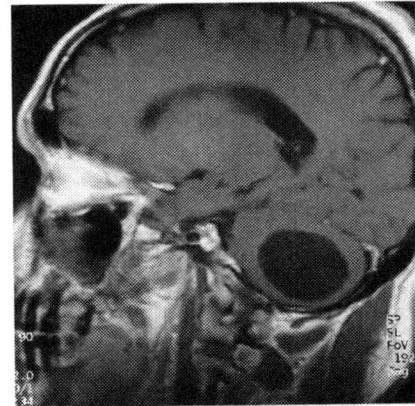

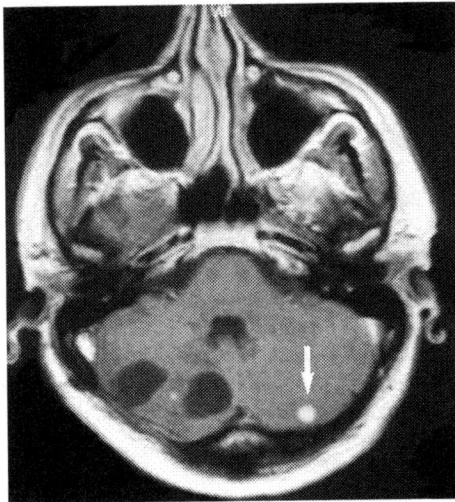

Figure 38. *These are contrast enhanced T1 WI. The top image is a T1 WI demonstrating the classical appearance of a hemangioblastoma. Note the large cyst with an enhancing mural nodule. The bottom right image is a sagittal scan of the same lesion. The image on the left is an axial contrast enhanced T1 WI from a different patient and demonstrates multiple hemangioblastomas. There is also a nodule in the left cerebellum without an associated cyst (arrow).*

Medulloblastoma (Primitive neuro-ectodermal tumour of post fossa)
CT scan
Hyperdense, solid
Midline posterior fossa
Associated hydrocephalus common
Enhances fairly uniformly
MR scan
Midline homogenous posterior fossa tumour

151

Iso/hypointense T1 WI
Isointense T2 WI
Enhances
Drop metastasis (seeding through CSF)

Astrocytoma (see glial tumours)

Skull base tumours
Chordoma
CT scan
Hypodense mixed cystic and solid
Midline location
Commonly calcified
Bony destruction
Enhances heterogeneously
MR scan
Iso/hypointense T1 WI
Isointense T2 WI
Enhances heterogeneously

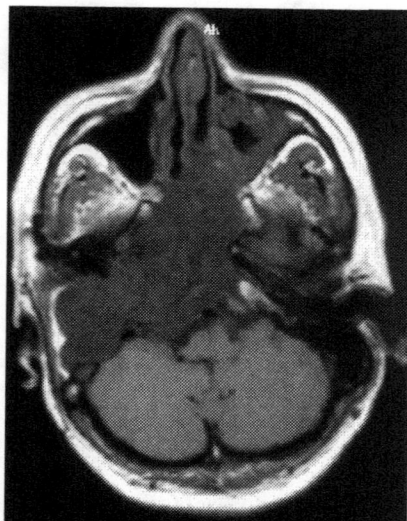

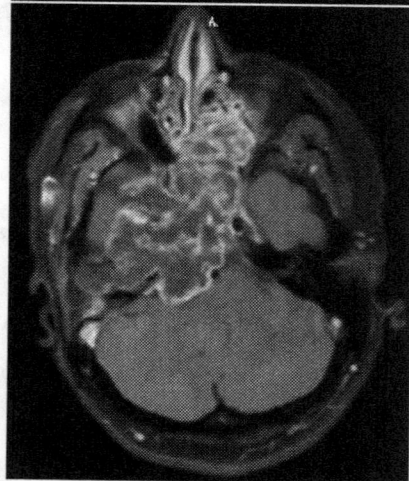

Figure 39. *The image on the top is an unenhanced axial T1 WI and the image on the bottom is a contrast enhanced T1 WI demonstrating an extensive skull base chordoma. Note the strong but inhomogeneous enhancement of the tumour.*

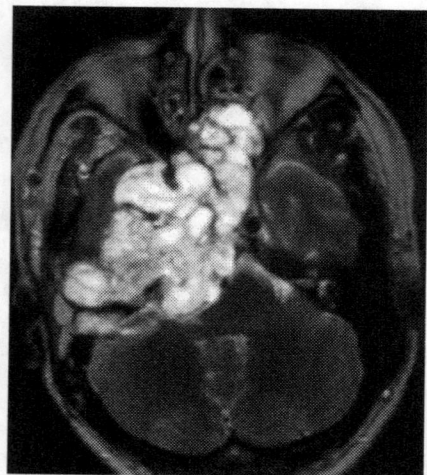

Figure 40. *This image is an axial T2 WI of the same patient and the high signal (and the low signal on the T1 WI) indicates the high fluid content of these tumours. The images demonstrate the highly aggressive infiltrative nature of these tumours.*

Vestibular Schwannoma
CT scan
Iso/hyperdense tumour in the cerebello-pontine angle
Solid or solid/cystic
Expanded internal auditory meatus

Enhances uniformly
MR scan
Iso/hypointense T1 WI
Hyperintense T2 WI
May be heterogenous/cystic components
Enhances strongly
Has a clear relation to the facial nerve on high-resolution scans

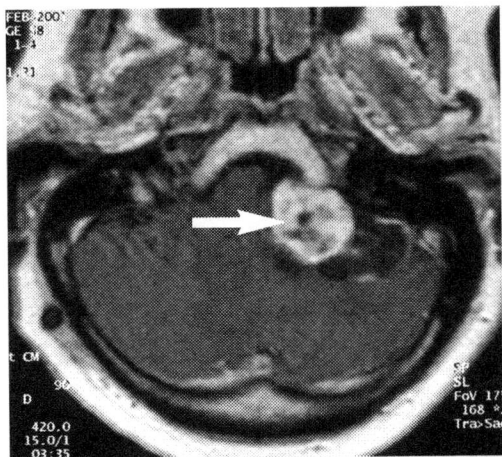

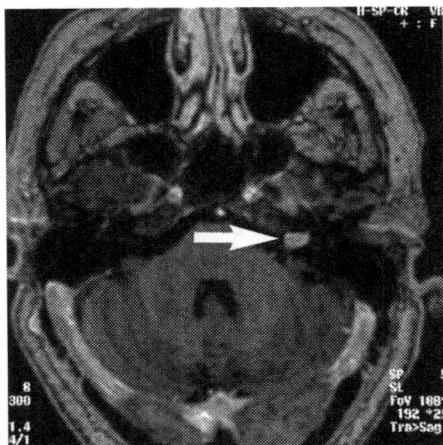

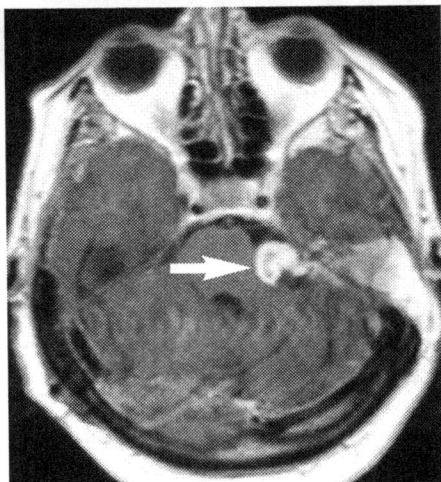

Figure 41. *These axial contrast enhanced T1 WI demonstrate different sizes of left sided vestibular schwannomas. The image top right demonstrates an intracanalicular schwannoma (white arrow). The image on the left demonstrates frank brainstem compression.*

Metastatic tumours
CT scan
Iso/hypodense tumour in parenchyma/dura
Severe surrounding oedema
Enhances strongly, frequently ring enhancing
MR scan
Iso/hypointense T1 WI
Hyperintense T2 WI
May have heterogeneous/cystic components
Enhances strongly
Severe surrounding oedema

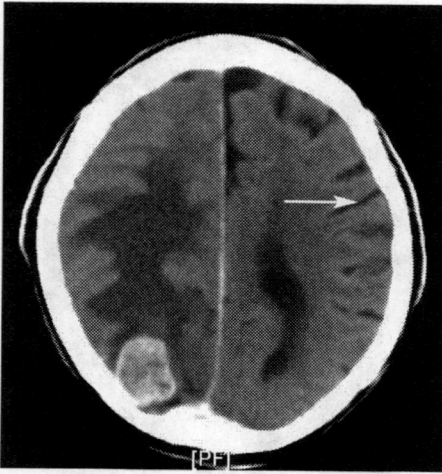

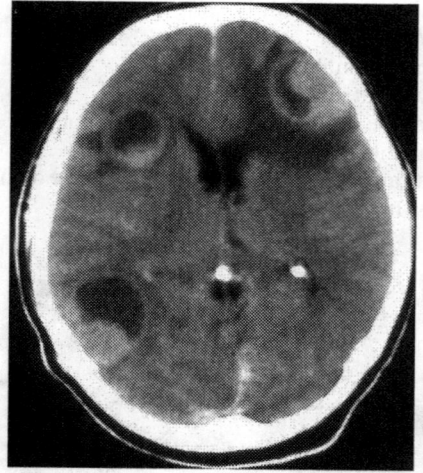

Figure 42. *These images are contrast enhanced axial CT scans of the brain. The image on the left demonstrates a single metastasis in the right occipital lobe with surrounding brain oedema and effacement of the sulcal pattern. See the normal sulci in the left hemisphere (arrow). The image on the right demonstrates multiple metastases with surrounding oedema.*

Vascular Pathology
Arterial infarct
CT scan
May see hyperdense vessel (thrombosis)
Hypodensity after 24 hrs
Can be seen within hours on perfusion CT scan
May have haemorrhagic transformation after 24-48 hours
MR scan
Loss of grey white differentiation on T1 WI
Hyperintense T2 WI
Enhances with contrast

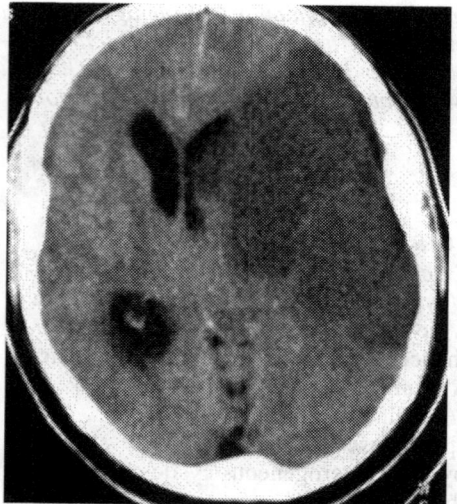

Figure 43. *This uncontrasted axial CT scan of the brain demonstrates an ischaemic infarct of the dominant left hemisphere in the middle cerebral artery distribution*

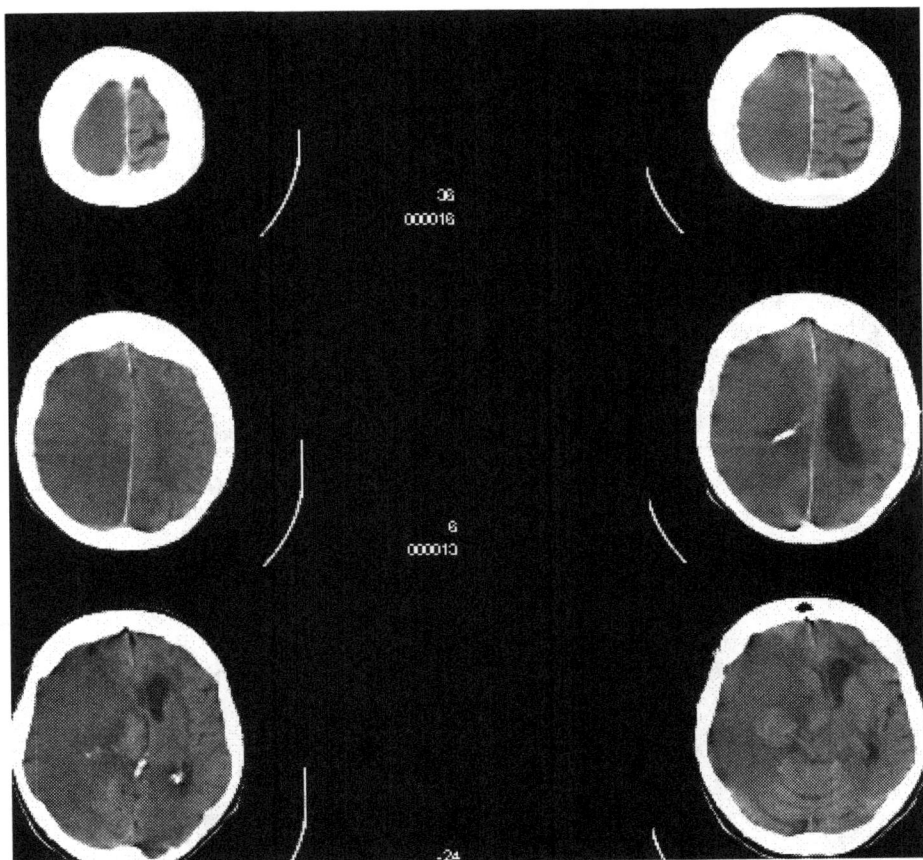

Figure 44. *This sequence of slices of an uncontrasted axial CT scan of the brain demonstrate an ischaemic infarct of the right, non dominant hemisphere in the distribution of the middle cerebral artery.*

Venous infarct
CT scan
Hyperdense sagittal sinus
Parenchymal petechial haemorrhages
Empty delta sign with contrast administration (enhancing dura around haematoma in confluence of sinuses)
MR scan
Haematoma seen in sinus
T1 WI in the acute stage isointense with brain, in the subacute stage hyperintense
Parenchymal swelling and haemorrhage, hyperintense on T2 WI

Spontaneous Haemorrhage
SAH (aneurysmal)
CT scan
Positive in 97% within 12 hours of haemorrhage and decreases to about 70% sensitivity on day 3.
Hyperdensity in basal cisterns and subarachnoid spaces.
Hydrocephalus (early hydrocephalus = dilated temporal horns, plump third ventricle)

Blood in occipital horns of lateral ventricles
May have subtle obliteration of Sylvian fissure
MR scan
Isointense with brain on T1 WI in the acute phase and hyperintense on T2 WI
Siderosis in the chronic phase is hypointense on T2 WI

Grade	Description
Fisher 0	Unruptured aneurysm
Fisher 1	No blood seen
Fisher 2	Diffuse blood and no vertical layers of blood > 1mm
Fisher 3	Clot and vertical layers of blood > 1mm
Fisher 4	Intracerebral haematoma or/and intraventricular blood

TABLE 2. *Fisher grading scale. This CT scan scale is used in SAH to predict vasospasm. The incidence of vasospasm is higher in Fisher 3 than 2, but lower in Fisher 4.*

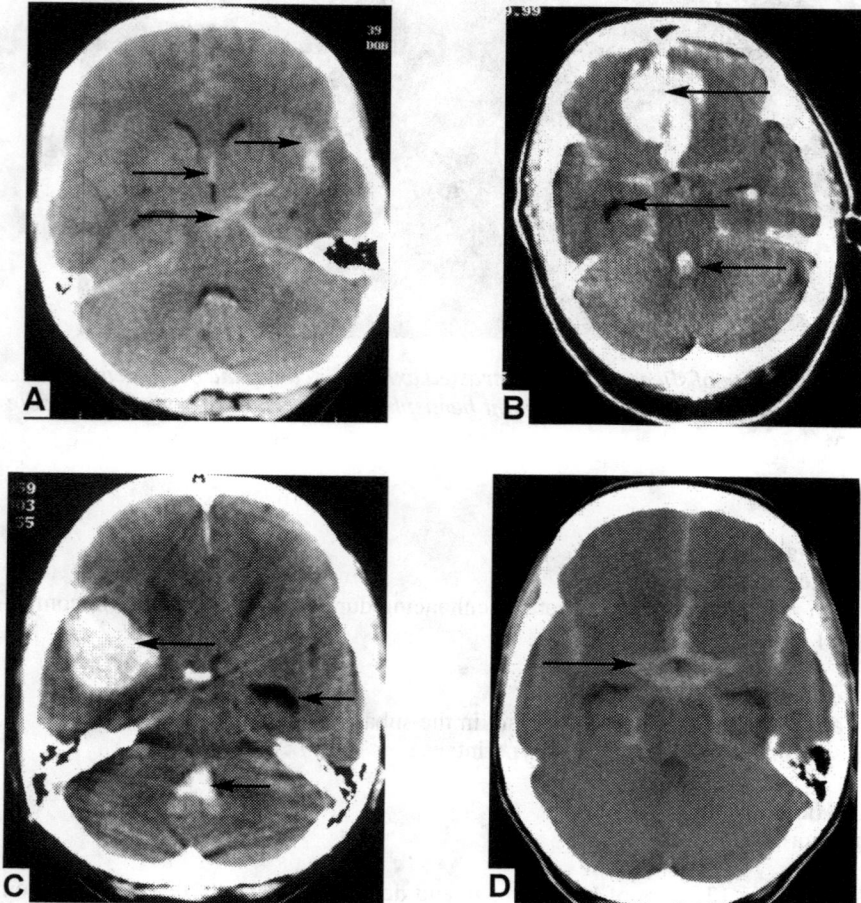

Figure 45. *See legend on opposite page.*

Figure 45. *(see opposite page) These images are uncontrasted axial CT scans demonstrating subarachnoid blood; A: The top arrow demonstrates fresh blood in the left Sylvian fissure, the next arrow demonstrates blood in the third ventricle and the last arrow demonstrates blood in the pre pontine cistern at the base of the brain;. B: The top arrow demonstrates an intraparenchymal haemorrhage secondary to an anterior communicating artery aneurysm. This is a pattern of blood indicative of this type of aneurysm. The next arrow demonstrates the dilated temporal horn of the right lateral ventricle and the last arrow demonstrates blood in the fourth ventricle; C: The top arrow demonstrates an intraparenchymal haemorrhage in the right Sylvian fissure, the next arrow demonstrates a dilated temporal horn and the last arrow, blood in the fourth ventricle; D: This image demonstrates the star shaped haemorrhage in the basal cisterns and the interhemispheric and Sylvian fissures that is classically associated with SAH.*

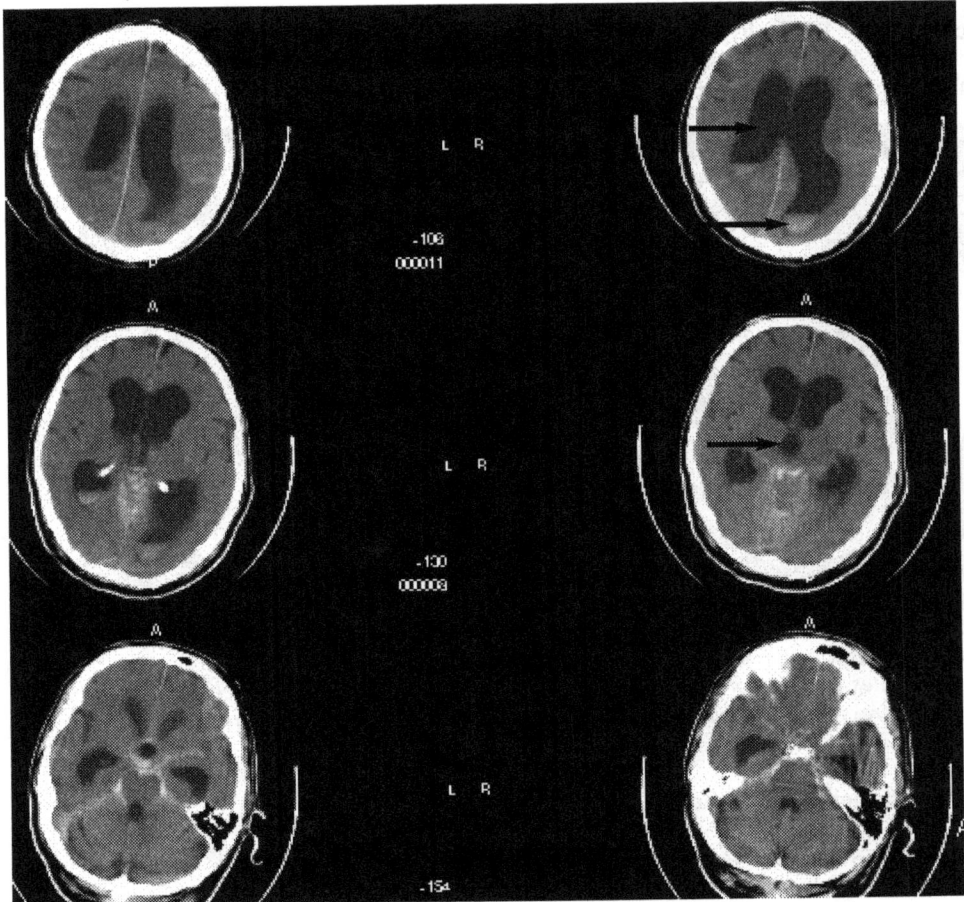

Figure 46. *This sequence of images are a selection from an uncontrasted axial CT scan demonstrating SAH. Notice how the classic star shape subarachnoid distribution of blood is seen in this sequence, also the associated hydrocephalus (top arrow) and blood in the ventricular system (second arrow). The whole of the ventricular system is dilated with the lateral ventricles, the third ventricle (bottom arrow) and the fourth ventricle dilated, indicating communicating hydrocephalus.*

Parenchymal hypertensive haemorrhage
CT scan
Hyperdense mass (clotted blood)
Seen in several sites including putamen, insula, brainstem, posterior fossa
MR scan
Depends on age of clot
In T1 WI – remember 'Big Great White Bear!'
Hyperacute, within hours - Black (hypointense)
Acute stage, less than 3 days - Grey (isointense),
Subacute stage, 3 to 14 days - White (hyperintense),
Chronic stage, more than 14 days - Black (hypointense)

In T2 WI – remember 'Bear, What Bear?'
Acute stage – Black (hypointense)
Subacute – White (hyperintense)
Subacute stage and chronic stages – Black (hypointense)

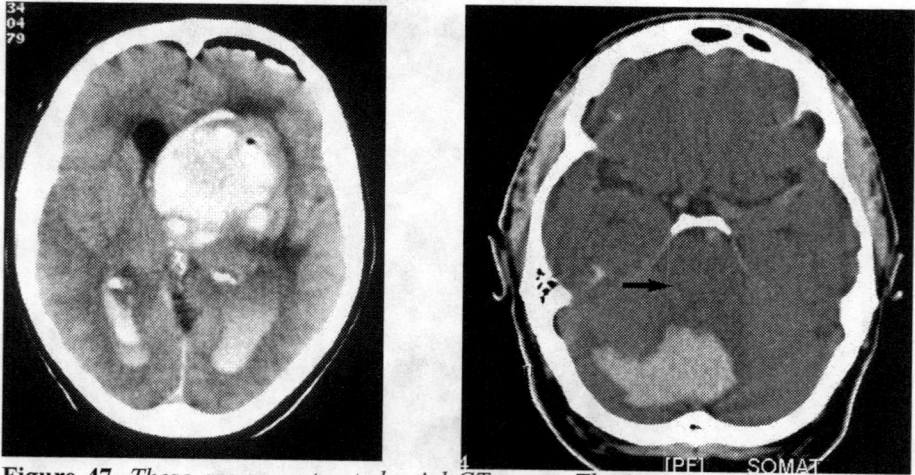

Figure 47. *These are uncontrasted axial CT scans. The image on the left demonstrates a spontaneous parenchymal intracerebral haemorrhage in the region of the left basal ganglia and internal capsule with extension into the ventricular system. The image on the right demonstrates a posterior fossa spontaneous intraparenchymal intracerebellar haemorrhage with compression and occlusion of the basal cisterns (arrow) and fourth ventricle.*

Vascular anomalies
AVM (arteriovenous malformation)
CT scan
Hyperdense serpentine vessels
Enhances strongly with contrast
MR scan
Flow voids on T1 WI, enhances strongly with contrast
Flow voids on T2 WI

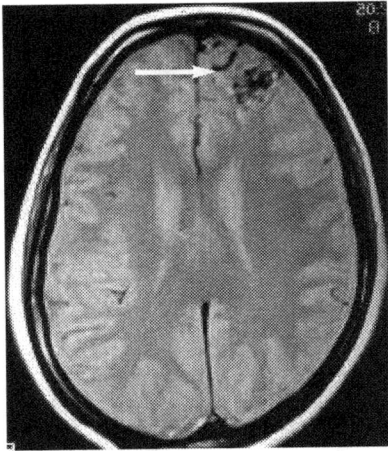

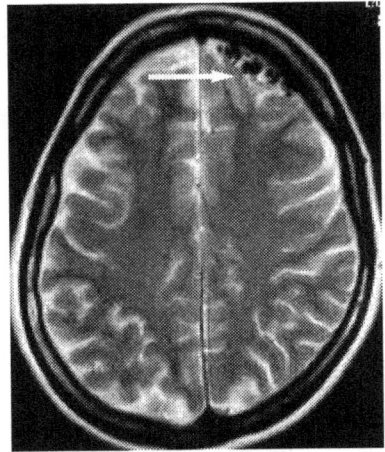

Figure 48. *The image on the left is an uncontrasted axial T1 WI and the image on the right an axial T2 WI. They both demonstrate the serpentine flow voids (arrows) associated with an arteriovenous malformation.*

Cavernous Malformation (multiple in > 50%, also called cavernoma)

CT scan
Small hyperdense mass
Little or no enhancement
MR scan
'Popcorn' lesion - multi lobulated
Variable intensity depending on age of haematoma with hypointense, siderotic rim on T2 WI
Little or no enhancement

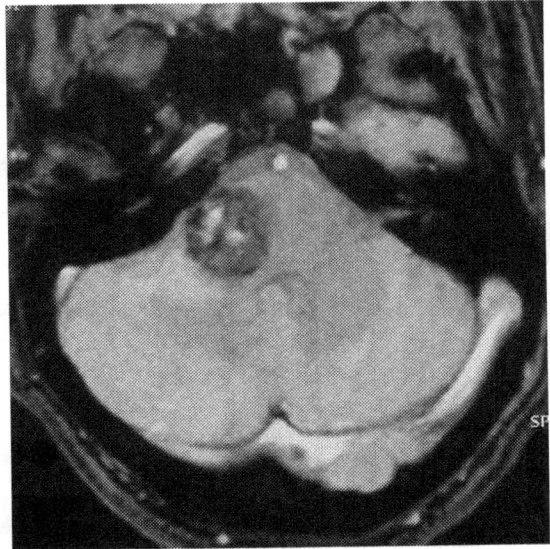

Figure 49. *This is an axial T2 WI. This brainstem cavernoma demonstrates the typical 'popcorn' appearance and has a siderotic, black ring around it.*

Venous angioma
CT scan
Usually normal
Small enhancing mass
MR scan
Variable intensity depending flow and on age of associated haematoma
Caput medusae lesion with several veins draining to single large vein

159

Infection

Empyema

CT scan (can miss lesion)
Can be subdural or extradural
Enhancing rim
Frequently spreads from infection in mastoids and facial sinuses
MR scan (much more sensitive, especially coronal cuts)
More intense signal than CSF on T1 WI
Enhances strongly
Underlying brain hyperintense on T2 WI due to reactive, oedematous brain

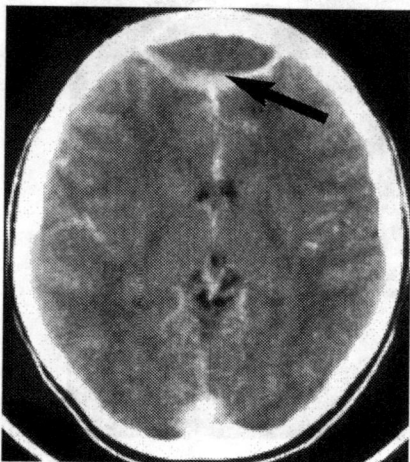

Figure 50. *Empyema. This contrast enhanced axial CT scan of the brain (right) demonstrates a frontal extradural empyema (arrow).*

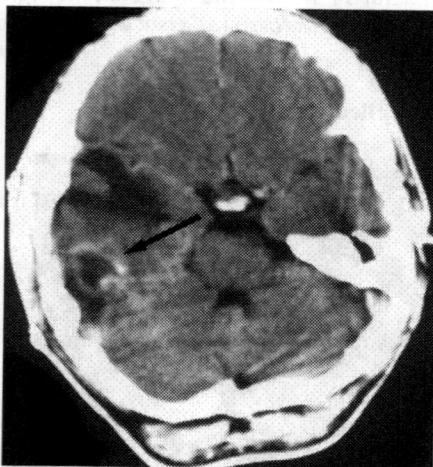

Figure 51. *Cerebritis. The image below is that of an uncontrasted axial CT scan and the image on the left is that of a contrast enhanced axial CT scan. Both demonstrate cerebritis and early abscess formation. Note the oedema and the irregular enhancement (arrow) with central necrotic area.*

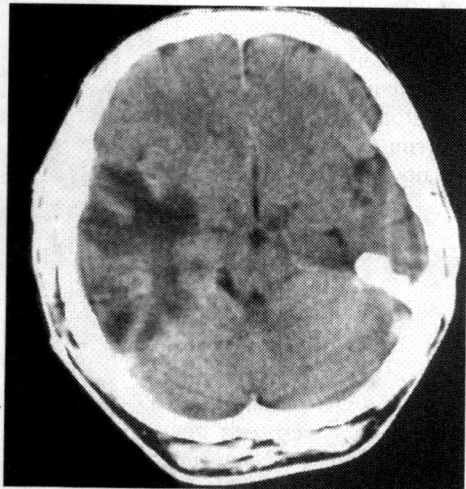

Cerebritis

CT scan
Hypodensity, surrounding oedema
Enhances strongly but inhomogenously with contrast
MR scan
Hypodense, inhomogeneous on T1 WI
Hyperintense T2 WI
Enhances with contrast

Abscess

CT scan
Central hypodensity
Capsule, thinnest on the aspect facing the ventricle
Capsule enhances strongly and uniformly
Surrounding oedema
MR scan

Central hypodense centre on T1 WI
Hyperintense T2 WI
Capsule enhances strongly and uniformly
Surrounding oedema

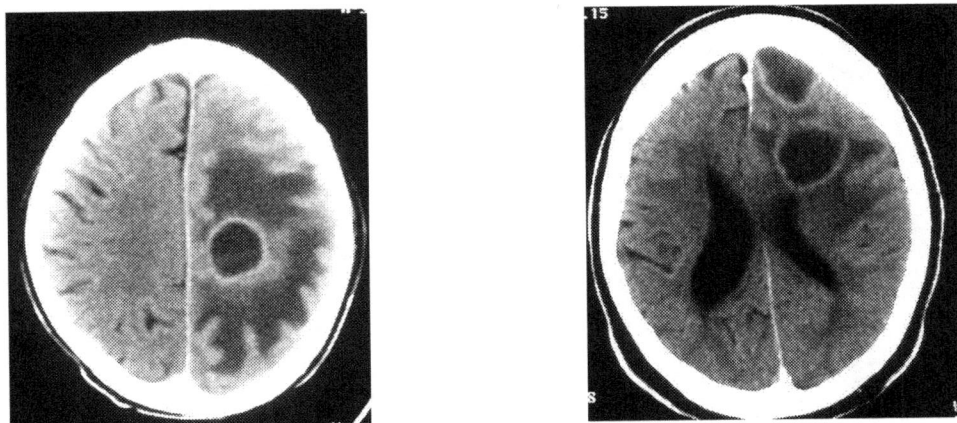

Figure 52. *These images are from axial contrast enhanced CT scans and the image on the left demonstrates a single abscess with associated oedema. The image on the right demonstrates two abscesses.*

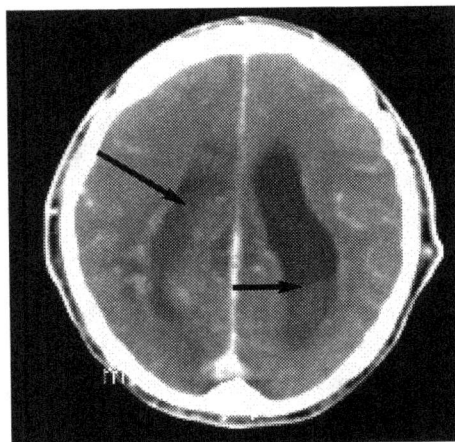

Figure 53. *This contrast enhanced axial CT scan of the brain demonstrates severe intracranial infection. The image demonstrates ventriculitis with pus in the right lateral ventricle leading to a cast in the ventricle (top arrow) as well as pus in the left lateral ventricle as demonstrated by the fluid-fluid level (bottom arrow).*

6

INTERPRETATION OF SPINAL IMAGING

W Adriaan Liebenberg

Contents

Normal appearances of spinal MR imaging

Clearing C-spine X-rays following trauma

Degenerative conditions
Rheumatoid arthritis
Spinal stenosis
Disc herniation

Spinal tumours

Extradural compartment
Primary tumours
Bony tumours and cartilage producing tumours of the spine
Osteoid osteoma
Osteoblastoma
Osteochondroma
Lymphoproliferative tumours
Solitary plasmacytoma
Multiple myeloma
Lymphoma
Tumour of notochordal origin
Chordoma
Metastatic tumours

Intradural, extramedullary compartment
Meningioma
Schwannoma
Myxopapillary ependymoma

Intramedullary compartment
Ependymoma
Astrocytoma
Paraganglioma
Haemangioblastoma

Cysts
Arachnoid cyst
Dermoid cyst
Epidermoid cyst
Perineural cyst (Tarlov cyst)
Synovial cyst
Neurenteric cyst

Infection
Osteomyelitis
Epidural empyema (abscess)
Discitis
Tuberculosis of the spine

Vascular pathology
Abnormal vasculature
Dural arteriovenous fistula
Arteriovenous malformation
Cavernous angioma
Spinal cord infarct
Subdural haematoma
Epidural haematoma

Normal appearances of the spine on MR imaging
Vertebrae
Vertebral bodies are hyperintense compared to spinal cord on T1 WI with the marrow (containing fat) being more intense than the rest of the vertebra. The vertebrae are of a slightly higher intensity that the intervertebral discs on T1 WI. The hallmark of pathology in vertebrae is a decrease on T1 WI and an increase of intensity on T2 WI due to the increased water content associated with most pathology and the displacement of the normal marrow.

Neural foramina
When evaluating sagittal MR scans as in figure 1, the scout view will orientate you as to whether the image is to the right or the left of the midline. The upper portion of the neural foramen contains fatty connective tissue with the nerve root located in the inferior portion of the foramen. The nerve root will be displaced in lateral disc protrusions and may be displaced upwards, displacing the fatty tissue.

Intervertebral disc
Healthy discs in young patients have a high water content and therefore are hypointense on T1 WI and relatively hyperintense on T2 WI. As patients get older, the discs dehydrate or they may dehydrate secondary to pathological processes, becoming relatively hypointense on T2 WI compared to normal discs. The annulus fibrous appears as a hypointense signal on T1WI and T2 WI.

Spinal cord
All neural tissues demonstrate intermediate signal intensity (gray) on both T1 and T2 WI. CSF demonstrates hypointensity on T1 WI and is hyperintense on T2 WI.

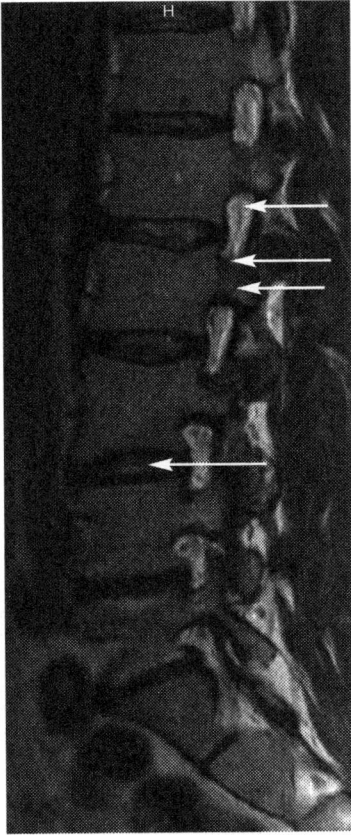

Figure 1. *This is a sagittal T2 WI of the lumbosacral spine. This image is taken off the midline, and in this case to the right of the spinal canal, and demonstrates the neural foramina, which are white due to the fatty tissue contained within them. The top arrow points toward the top of a neural foramen and the next arrow to the bottom. Note that this arrow points directly at the nerve as it lies in the inferior part of the foramen. The third arrow points directly at a pedicle. The last arrow points at an intervertebral disc.*

Clearing C-spine X-rays following trauma

The following three views are essential and mandatory:

Lateral c-spine film demonstrating the C7-T1 junction clearly and demonstrating the upper border of T1. If this is not possible with a normal lateral film, then a swimmers view should be performed (one arm above the head).

A-P view

Open mouth view demonstrating the odontoid process.

The following sequence is useful in clearing the cervical spine:

Alignment – Assess the alignment of the anterior vertebral line, the posterior vertebral line and the spinolaminar line. More than 3.5 mm subluxation is abnormal. At C2/C3 there may be a normal physiological subluxation of up to 3mm, especially in children. Subluxation of up to 50% of the width of the vertebral body signifies unifacet dislocation and a subluxation of more than this signifies a bifacet dislocation, which is usually accompanied by widening of the interspinous spaces.

Angulation – angulation of more than 11 degrees between two adjacent vertebrae is indicative of a fracture or ligamentous injury and potential instability.

The diameter of the spinal canal – anything less than 14 mm is indicative of impending spinal cord compression.

Examination of the pre vertebral soft tissue shadow - from C1 to C4 the soft tissue should be maximally half the width of a vertebral body and below C4 it should be maximally equal to the width of a vertebral body (5mm at C2 and 17 - 22 mm at C6).

The distance between the skull base and the atlas should not exceed 5mm as this can be indicative of atlanto – occipital dissociation.

The vertebral bodies should be examined to ascertain that there are no compression fractures or burst fractures.

The intervertebral discs are not visible on plain x-rays or CT scans but they can be examined by looking at the disc spaces between the vertebrae which demonstrate the anatomy of the (invisible) discs. Therefore a narrowing of one disc space will imply that there has been compression, and possibly herniation, of an intervertebral disc. If there is an associated neurological deficit without a fracture or dislocation, an MR scan will demonstrate the anatomy of the disc and any related prolapse.

The odontoid peg should be examined on the open mouth view for fractures. The vertical line that separates the front teeth must not be confused with a fracture. On the lateral c-spine view there should not be more than 3mm between the dens and the atlas (atlanto-dens interval). More than this implies injury to the transverse ligament and more than 5mm implies disruption of this ligament.

Degenerative conditions

Rheumatoid arthritis

CT scanning may demonstrate C1/2 subluxation, cranial settling and dens erosions. MRI may demonstrate pannus formation and acquired spinal stenosis. Plain flexion and extension images as well as MR in flexion and extension are invaluable to demonstrate dynamic subluxations.

Spinal stenosis

Spinal stenosis is either congenital or acquired. Sagittal T2 WI demonstrates spinal stenosis well but the most useful image is the axial T2 WI. In the cervical spine, anterior compression of the spinal cord can be caused by prolapsed discs, osteophytic bars, ossification of the posterior longitudinal ligament, subluxation of the vertebrae and vertebral compression fractures. Posterior and lateral compression can be caused by hypertrophy of the ligamentum flavum and the facet joints. Damage to the cord is shown as hyperintensity on the T2 WI. In the lumbar spine the classic trefoil shape can be seen with the round canal taking on a triangular shape. There is usually encroachment due to facet joint hypertrophy as well as thickened ligamentum flavum. Added stenosis is caused by degrees of vertebral body subluxation and plain film extension and flexion views are important in identifying whether this is stable or not.

Disc herniation (prolapse)

The best images to evaluate the presence of disc herniation are the T2 WI as the CSF, being brilliantly white, contrasts well with the rest of the tissue and demonstrating a disc protrusion is easier than on T1WI where the intensity of the tissues are frequently quite similar. The best approach is to look at the sagittal T2 WI and pinpoint the pathology. Then use the axial T2 WI to evaluate the extent of the neural compromise. The T1 WI are good for evaluating the intervertebral foramina and looking at fine detail of the nervous structures. The sagittal and coronal images are useful for evaluating the lateral elements.

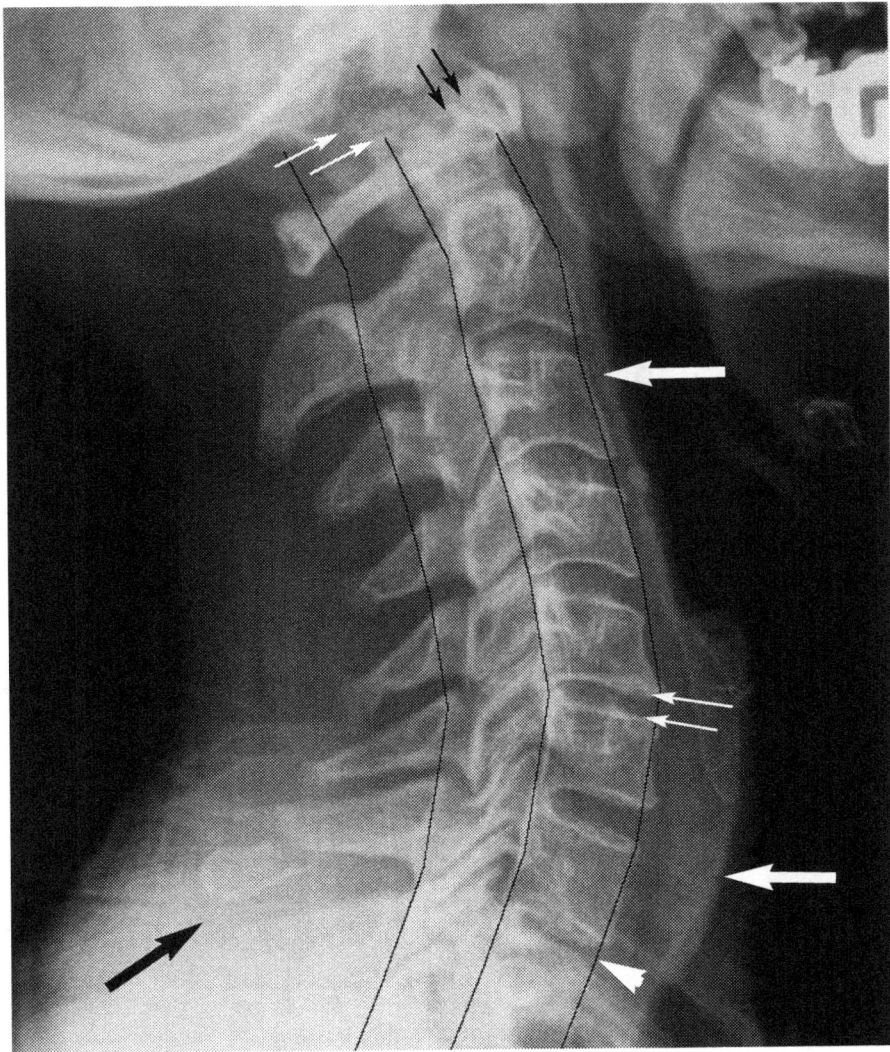

Figure 2. *This image depicts a lateral cervical spine x-ray. The two thin black arrows at the skull base demonstrates the atlanto-dens interval which should not exceed 3mm. The two thin white arrows demonstrate the space between the top of the atlas and the base of the skull which should not exceed 5mm. The top thick white arrow demonstrates the pre vertebral soft tissue shadow from C1 to C4 and the bottom thick white arrow the soft tissue below C4. The soft tissue from C1 to C4 should be maximally half the width of a vertebral body and below C4 it should be maximally equal to the width of a vertebral body (5mm at C2 and 17 - 22 mm at C6). The bottom two thin white arrows point toward a narrowed C5/6 disc space. MRI confirmed a C5/6 disc prolapse. The thick white arrow head points at the top edge of T1 which must always be seen. The thick black arrow points toward a clay shoveler's fracture (avulsion fracture of the tip of the spinous process). Note the three lines (anterior vertebral line, the posterior vertebral line and the spinolaminar line) demonstrating the alignment of the cervical spine.*

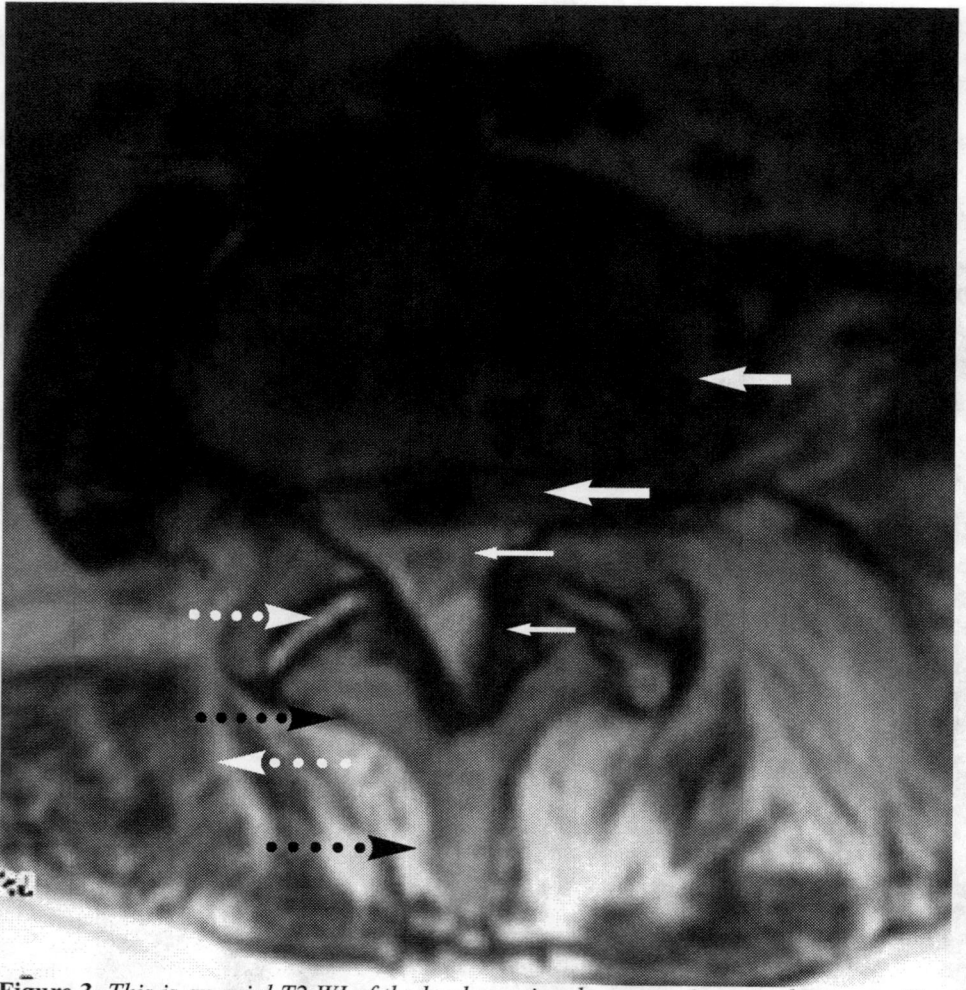

Figure 3. *This is an axial T2 WI of the lumbar spine demonstrating spinal stenosis. The top thick white arrow demonstrates the intervertebral disc. The next thick white arrow demonstrates a broad, flat central disc prolapse. The top thin white arrow demonstrates the compressed cauda equina, which takes on a trefoil shape. The bottom thin white arrow demonstrates the thickened and hypertrophied ligamentum flavum that is a main contributing factor in spinal stenosis. The top dashed white arrow demonstrates the facet joint, the bottom dashed white arrow demonstrates the paraspinal muscles, the top dashed black arrow demonstrates the lamina on the right-hand side and bottom dashed black arrow demonstrates the spinous process.*

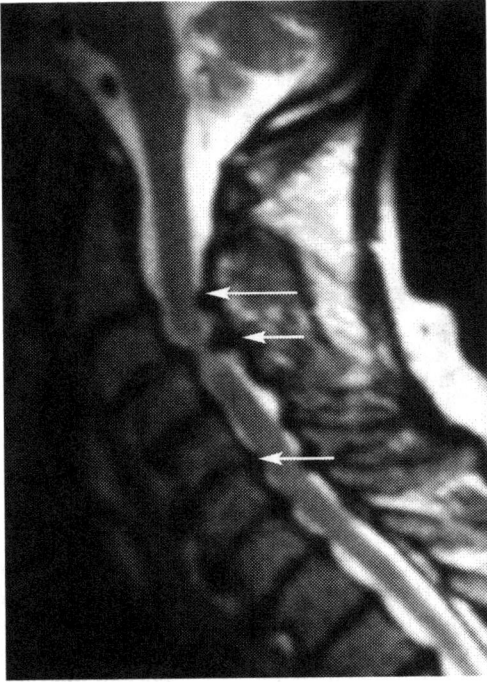

Figure 4. *This is a sagittal T2 WI of the cervical spine in a patient with severe cervical spondylosis and clinical quadri spasticity. The top arrow is pointing at a thickened area of ligamentum flavum, as is the next arrow down. The third arrow points toward anterior compression from a disc-osteophyte complex. Note how this patient has both severe anterior and posterior compression of the spinal cord. The intervertebral discs have associated bony osteophytes which are hard and require extensive drilling at the time of surgery. The decision as to whether a decompression is done from an anterior or posterior approach is based on where the compression is and how many levels are affected. Up to three levels may be decompressed from anterior with anterior cervical discectomies or corpectomies. A posterior approach via laminectomy is usually performed for extensive disease. Flexion and extension X-rays are useful to decide whether fusion is required at the same time.*

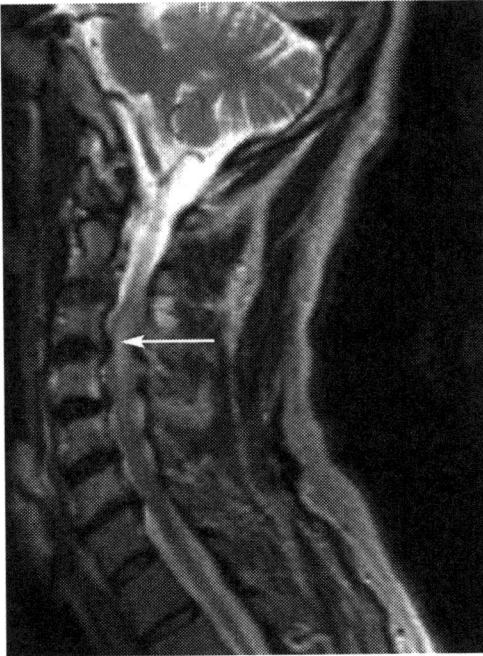

Figure 5. *This sagittal T2 WI of the cervical spine in a different patient from above, also demonstrates severe cervical spondylosis. The arrow is pointing towards associated signal change in the cord, which is a poor prognostic sign.*

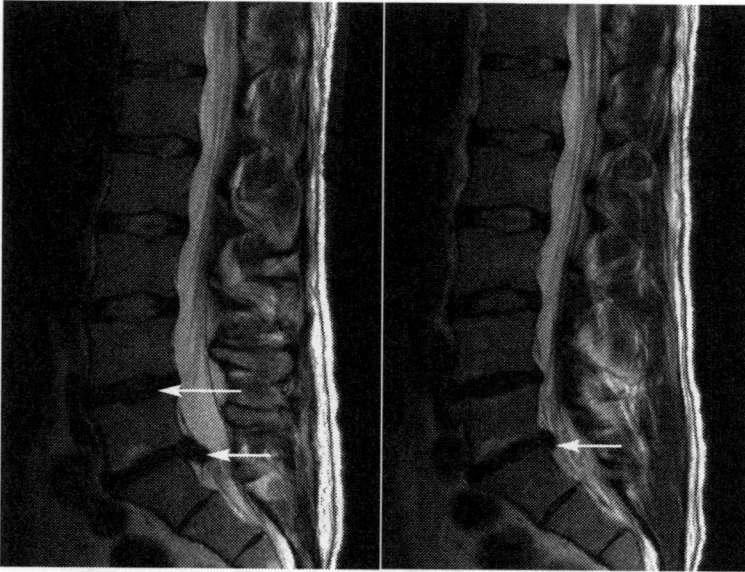

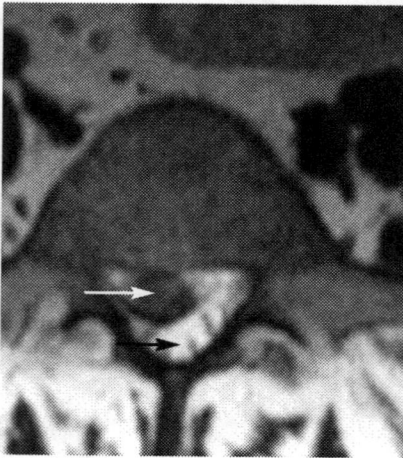

Figure 6. *The top images are sagittal T2 WI and the image on the left is an axial T2 WI of the same patient. The top arrow on the top left image demonstrates a degenerative intervertebral disc. Note how the intensity has changed from the normal intervertebral discs above it. This lower intensity is due to a lower water content of this damaged disc. The next arrow down shows a large downward extrusion of an intervertebral disc. The image top right is an image slightly towards the right of the midline compared to the image on the left. Note how the herniated segment appears smaller. This is because this is a mostly central disc prolapse as is demonstrated in the image on the left by the white arrow. The black arrow demonstrates the cauda equina which is compressed by the disc fragment*

Spinal tumours

Extradural compartment

PRIMARY TUMOURS

Bony tumours and cartilage producing tumours of the spine
Osteoid osteoma
CT scan
Hypodense nucleus, with surrounding sclerosis, may have associated calcium
Lesion is less than 1.5 cm in diameter
May enhance with contrast
MR scan
Hypointense on T1 WI and hyperintense on T2 WI
Calcium leads to hypointensity on both T1 and T2 WI sequences.

Osteoblastoma

CT scan

Hypodense nucleus, may have associated calcium, surrounding sclerosis as in osteoid osteoma

Lesion is more than 1.5 cm in diameter

It is an obviously expansile lesion

May enhance with contrast

Evidence of infiltration and destruction

MR scan

Hypointense on T1 WI and hyperintense on T2 WI

Surrounding oedema and may have soft tissue component

Osteochondroma

CT scan

A sessile bony outcrop with a cartilage cap

The cap may contain calcium

MR scan

On T1 WI a hyperintense centre (marrow) surrounded by a hypointense rim (cortex) and hypointense/isointense cap (cartilage).

On T2 WI an isointense centre (marrow) surrounded by a hypointense rim (cortex) and a hyperintense cap (cartilage)

Lymphoproliferative tumours

Solitary plasmacytoma

CT scan

Solitary lytic destructive lesion with collapse of the vertebra

May have soft tissue mass

Does not enhance

MR scan

Solitary lesion, hypo/isointense on T1 WI

Involves posterior elements with vertebral collapse

Moderate enhancement after gadolinium on T1 WI

Heterogeneous signal on T2 WI

Multiple myeloma

MR scan

This is a multifocal disease of the marrow of vertebrae with patchy involvement demonstrated on T1 WI as hypointense areas and on T2 WI as hyperintense areas.

Moderate enhancement after gadolinium on T1 WI

Lymphoma

CT scan

Homogeneous epidural mass

Enhances homogeneously with contrast

May present as lytic osseous lesion with associated soft tissue mass

MR scan

Homogenous epidural mass isointense on T1 WI with intense, homogeneous enhancement after contrast administration and hyperintense on T2 WI

May appear with characteristics as above but in the intramedullary space

May present as osseous lesion, hypointense on T1 WI with contrast enhancement and hyperintense on T2 WI

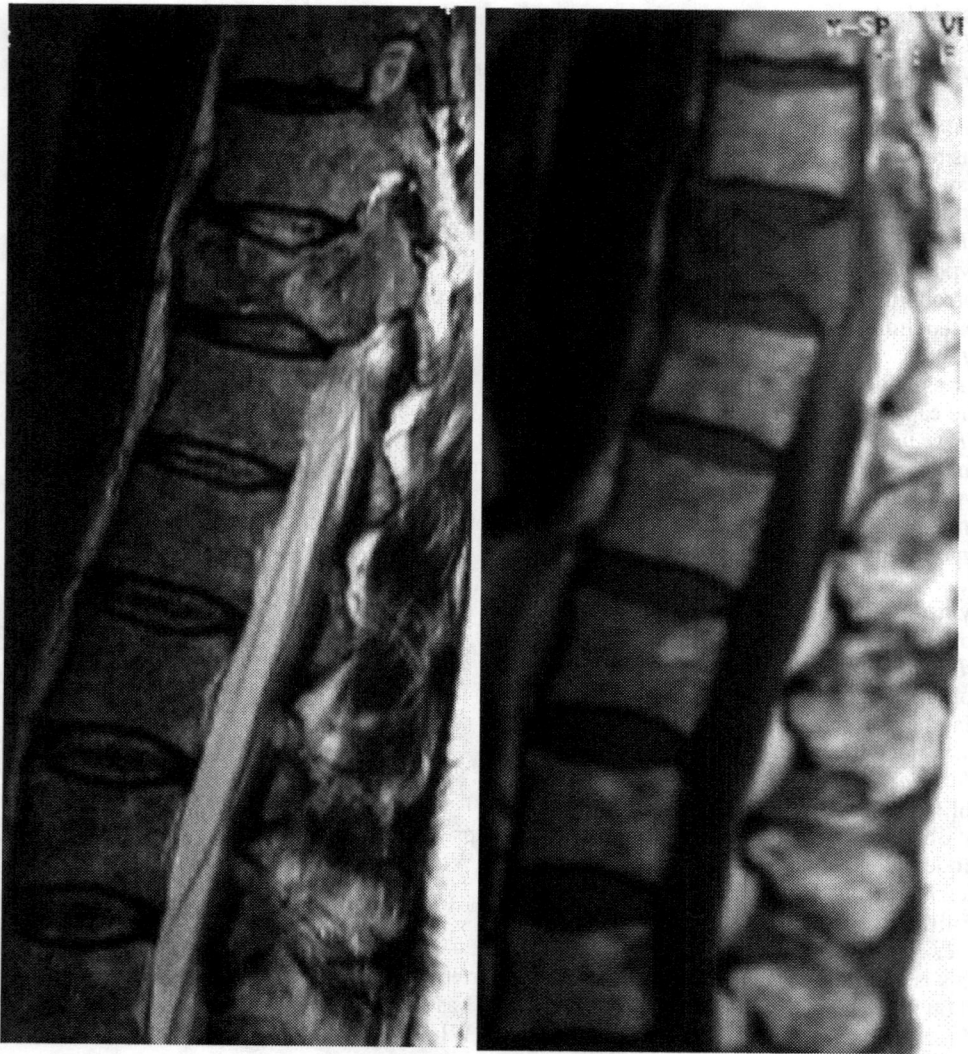

Figure 7. *The image on the left is a sagittal T2 WI of the thoracic spine and the image on the right is a sagittal T1 WI of the thoracic spine, both demonstrating a multiple myeloma lesion. Note how this lesion is centered on the anterior aspect of the vertebral body and extends into the spinal canal. The lesion is isointense to slightly hyperintense on T2 WI and hypointense on T1 WI*

Tumours of notochordal origin
Chordoma
CT scan
Destructive lytic lesion with associated soft tissue mass
Contains calcium and sclerotic elements
Enhances heterogeneously with contrast
MR scan
Heterogenous mass, hypointense on T1 WI with heterogeneous enhancement after contrast and hyperintense on T2 WI

METASTATIC TUMOURS (prostate, breast adenocarcinoma, lung adenocarcinoma, renal cell carcinoma and gastric carcinoma)
CT scan
Lytic, permeative lesion found mostly in posterior vertebral body but also pedicle and rest of vertebral body
May have associated soft tissue mass and may enhance with contrast.
MR scan
Disc sparing involvement of the vertebrae with vertebral destruction and may be associated with vertebral body collapse
On T1 WI the tumours are hypointense to bone and enhancement is variable
On T2 WI the tumours are hypo/isointense to marrow.

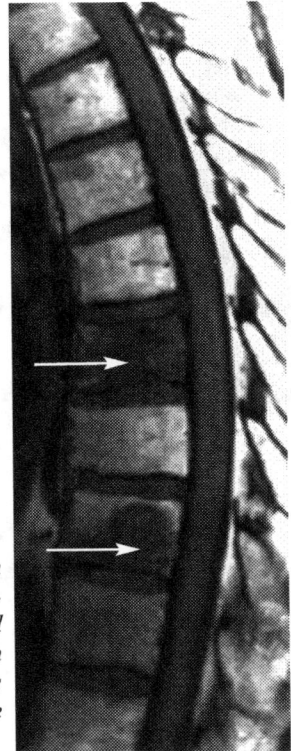

Figure 8. *This is a sagittal T1 WI of the thoracic spine which demonstrates two thoracic metastatic lesions. These vertebrae are darker in colour because the disease process has led to an increased water content of the affected vertebrae. Both vertebrae are still intact and have not lost their integrity. It is common for the vertebrae to collapse. Note the sparing of the relatively avascular intervertebral discs.*

173

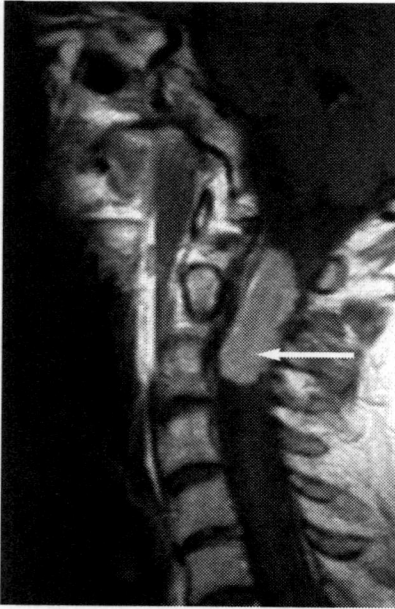

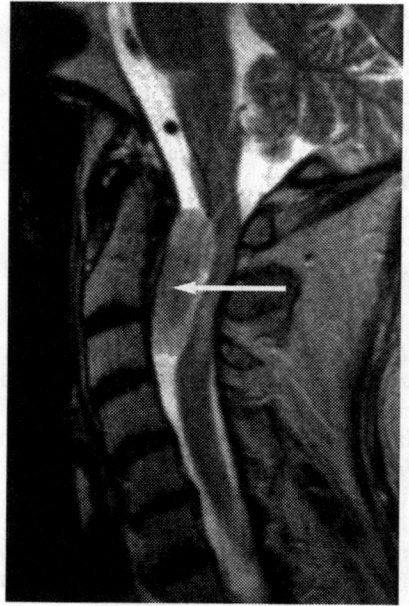

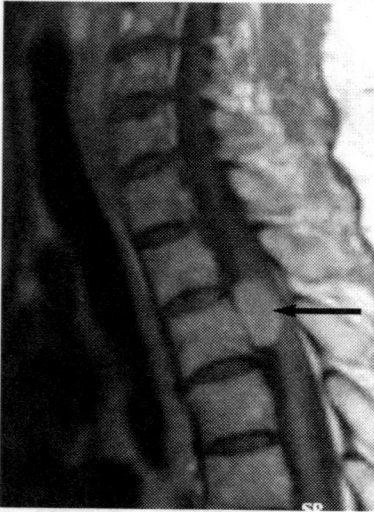

Figure 9. *The image on the top left is a sagittal contrast enhanced T1 WI of the cervical spine and the image top right is a sagittal T2 WI of the cervical spine. Both demonstrate a meningioma. Note how the meningioma is hyperintense to spinal cord following contrast enhancement and hyperintense to cord on the T2 WI. On T1 WI pre contrast these lesions are usually iso/hypointense to the tissue of the spinal cord. The image on the left is a sagittal T1 WI with contrast enhancement demonstrating a meningioma in the thoracic spinal canal.*

Intradural, extramedullary compartment

Meningioma
CT scan
Iso/hyperdense mass that enhances homogeneously with contrast
MR scan
Isointense to cord on T1 WI with intense homogeneous enhancement following contrast administration
Iso/hyperintense on T2 WI

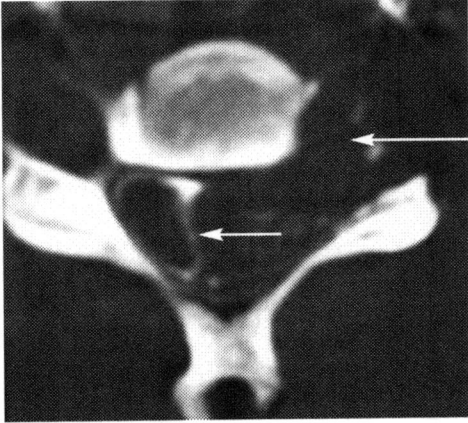

Figure 10. *This axial CT scan of the cervical spine demonstrates a neurofibroma that is extending through an expanded neural foramen on the left (top arrow). The spinal cord is completely pushed over to the other side (bottom arrow) and the neurofibroma fills nearly the whole of the spinal canal.*

Schwannoma
MR scan
Isointense to cord on T1 WI with intense homogeneous enhancement
Hyperintense on T2 WI
May have dumbbell extension through neural foramina

Myxopapillary ependymoma (arises in the conus medullaris or filum terminale)
CT scan
There may be evidence of spinal canal widening or pedicle erosion in the area of the conus
MR scan
This is frequently a heterogeneous lesion. They are usually isointense to cord on T1 WI with intense and well-delineated homogeneous enhancement and hyperintense on T2 WI There is an 80% incidence of associated cysts either within the tumour, rostral or caudal cysts at the poles of the tumour or reactive dilatation of the central canal.

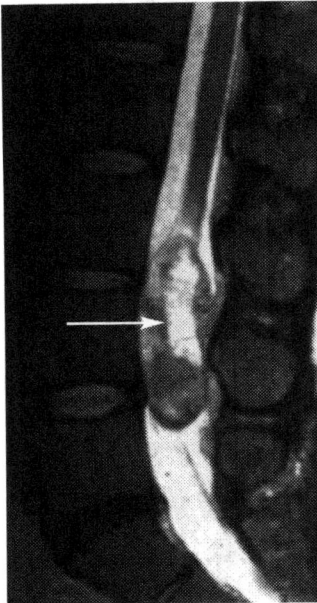

Figure 11. *This sagittal T2 WI of the lumbosacral spine demonstrates a myxopapillary ependymoma of the conus medullaris. Note the heterogeneous appearance and the hyperintense cyst fluid (arrow). This lesion expands the cord circumferentialy outwards.*

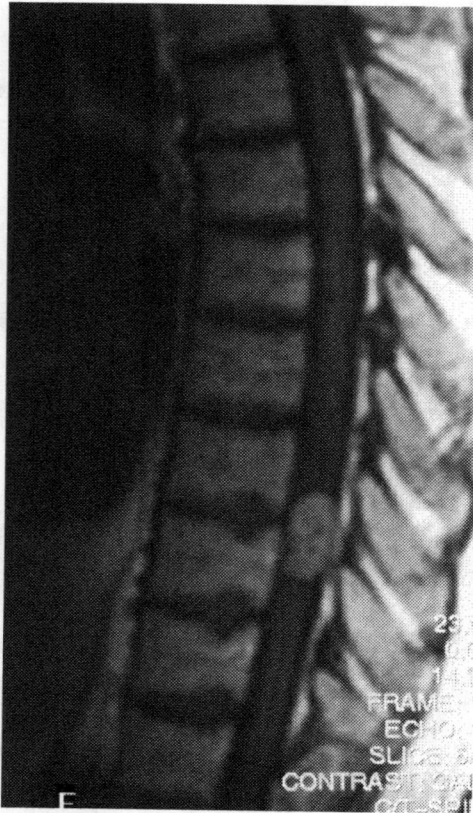

Figure 12. *This is a contrast enhanced T1 WI demonstrating a neurofibroma of the thoracic spine. Note how these lesions are very similar in appearance to the intraspinal meningiomas.*

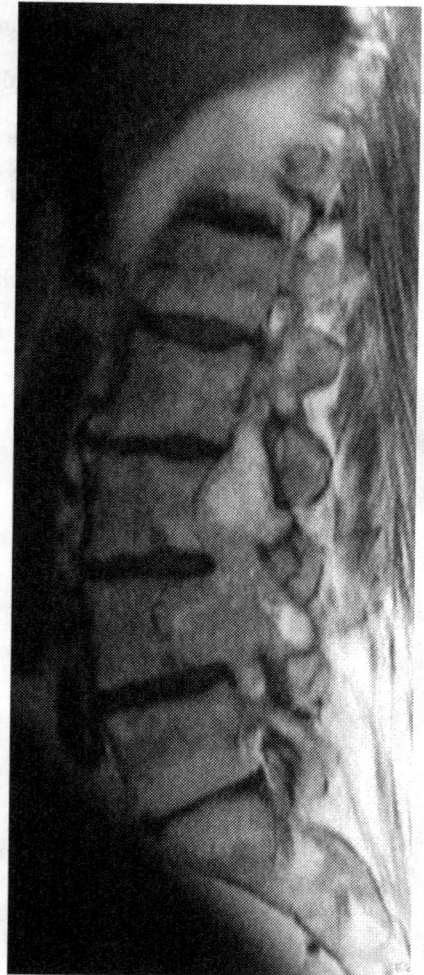

Figure 13. *This sagittal T2 WI of the lumbosacral spine demonstrates a heterogeneous hyperintense lesion. This paraganglioma proved to be extremely vascular at surgery*

Ependymoma (55% of intramedullary tumours)
CT scan
There may be evidence of spinal canal widening or pedicle erosion
MR scan
Isointense to cord on T1 WI with intense and well-delineated homogeneous enhancement (much better than the patchy enhancement seen with astrocytomas of the cord). Hyperintense on T2 WI, may be heterogeneous. Since they arise from the ependyma that lines the central canal, they are usually centrally located.

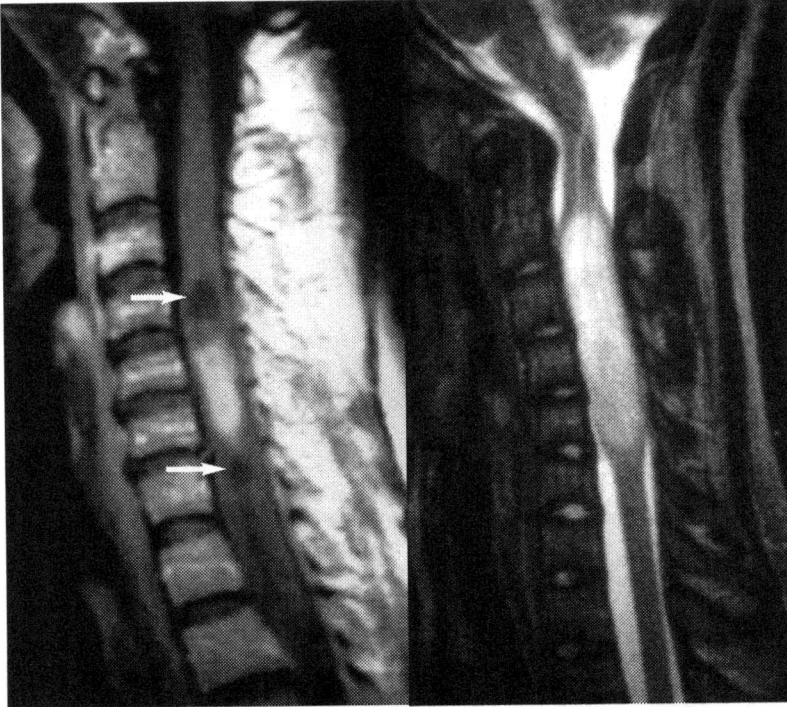

Figure 14. *The image on the left is a sagittal contrast enhanced T1 WI of the cervical spine that demonstrates an ependymoma. Note the two polar cysts as demonstrated by the two arrows. The lesion enhances homogeneously and intensely with contrast. The image on the right is a sagittal T2 WI of the cervical spine and demonstrates an ependymoma. It is homogeneous and hyperintense with good demarcation and is seen to expand the cord.*

Astrocytoma (30% of intramedullary tumours)
CT scan
There may be evidence of spinal canal widening or pedicle erosion
MR scan
Expanded cord that may have cystic component on T1 WI with variable signal intensity and variable enhancement and is hyperintense on T2 WI. These lesions appear very similar to the ependymomas. They arise from the parenchyma of the cord and are more eccentrically located than ependymomas.

Paraganglioma

CT scan

There may be evidence of spinal canal widening or pedicle erosion

MR scan

Well delineated mass hypo/isointense on T1 WI with intense homogeneous enhancement
Hyperintense on T2 WI

Haemangioblastoma

CT scan

There may be evidence of spinal canal widening or pedicle erosion

MR scan

Well delineated cystic mass hypo/isointense on T1 WI with enhancing nodule.
Hyperintense on T2 WI. May have associated syringomyelia.

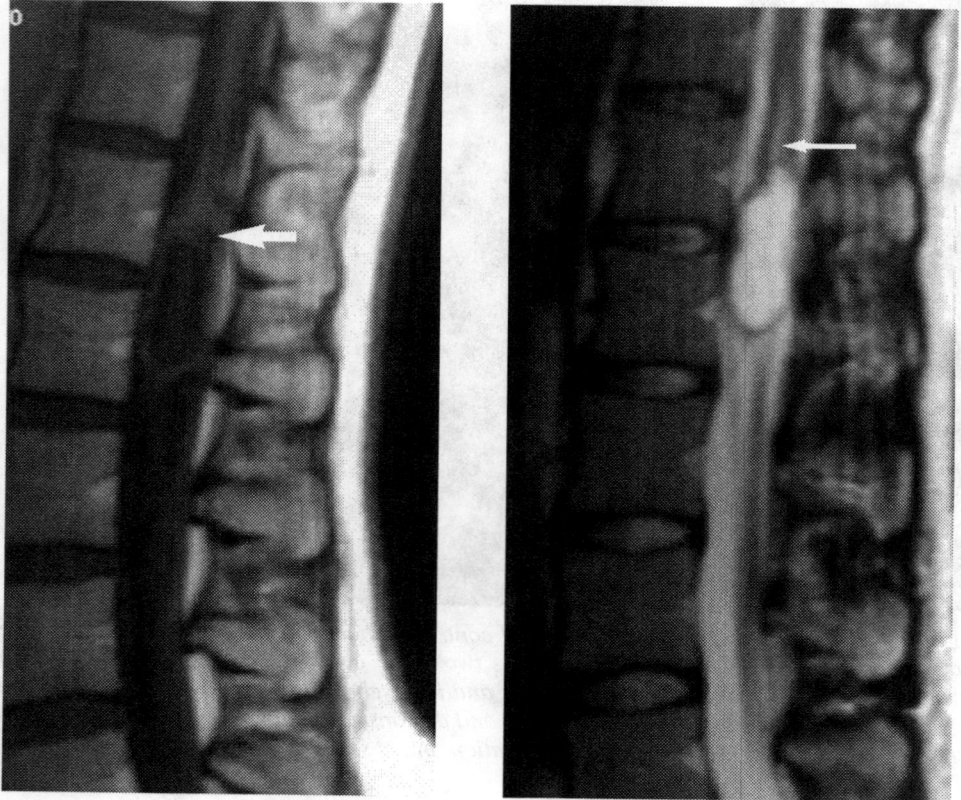

Figure 15. *Haemangioblastoma. The image on the left is a sagittal uncontrasted T1 WI of the thoracic spine and the image on the right is a sagittal T2 WI of the thoracic spine. Note the cystic mass with the mural nodule (thick arrow). This nodule enhanced with the administration of contrast. Note the associated syringomyelia (thin arrow).*

178

Cysts

Arachnoid cyst

MR scan
Extramedullary mass in either intra – or extradural space, CSF density (hypointense on T1 WI and hyperintense on T2 WI)
No contrast enhancement
Supresses on FLAIR images

Dermoid cyst (located in midline)

MR scan
Hyperintense on T1 WI (hypointense on STIR)
Heterogenous on T2 WI
May enhance

Epidermoid cyst (located in midline)

MR scan
Hypointense on T1 WI
Hyperintense on T2 WI
Does not suppress on FLAIR sequence

Perineural cyst (Tarlov cyst)

MR scan
A cystic enlargement of the nerve root sleeve, collection of CSF between the endoneurium and perineurium of the nerve root
Well defined with CSF intensity – hypointense on T1 WI and hyperintense on T2 WI

Synovial cyst

MR scan
Outpouching from the facet joint
Well defined with variable intensity secondary to protein contents
Enhancing rim

Neurenteric cyst

MR scan
Intradural, extramedullary cyst or intramedullary cysts
Isointense or slightly hyperintense to cerebrospinal fluid on T1 WI and hyperintense on T2 WI (fluid containing a high protein content within the cyst)
Associated vertebral abnormalities
Focal atrophy of the cord secondary from chronic compressive effect

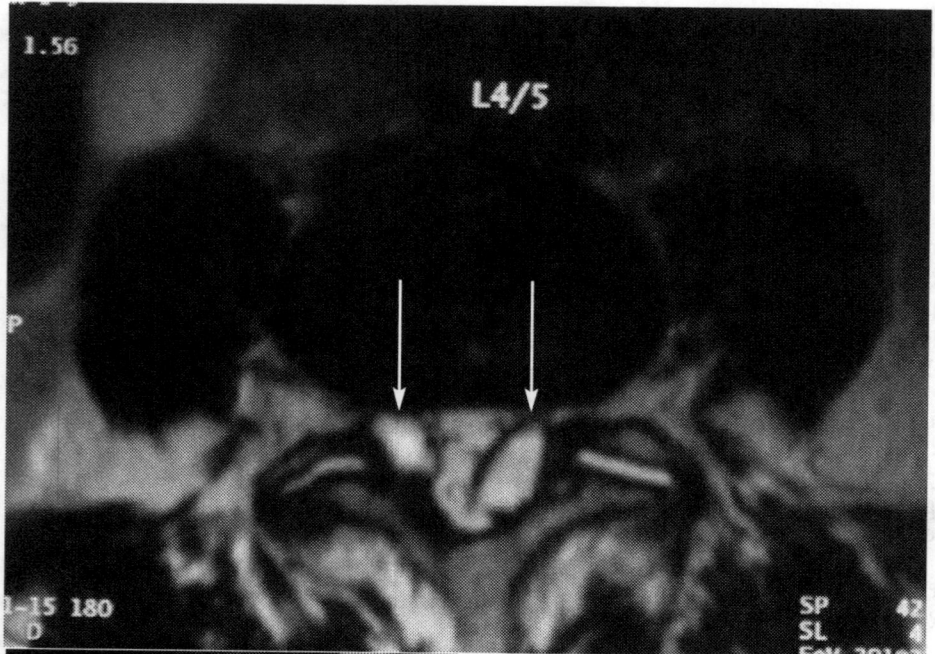

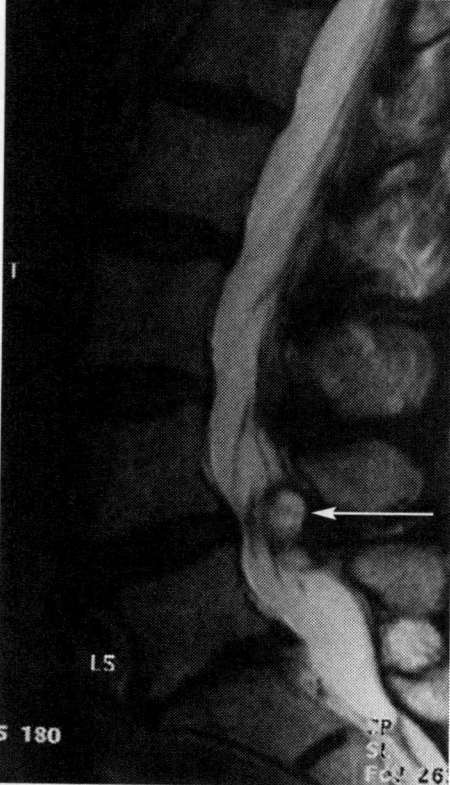

Figure 15a. *Synovial cysts. The image on the top is an axial T2 WI and the image on the left is a sagittal T2 WI. Note how the cysts are hyperintense and appear to arise from the facet joint.*

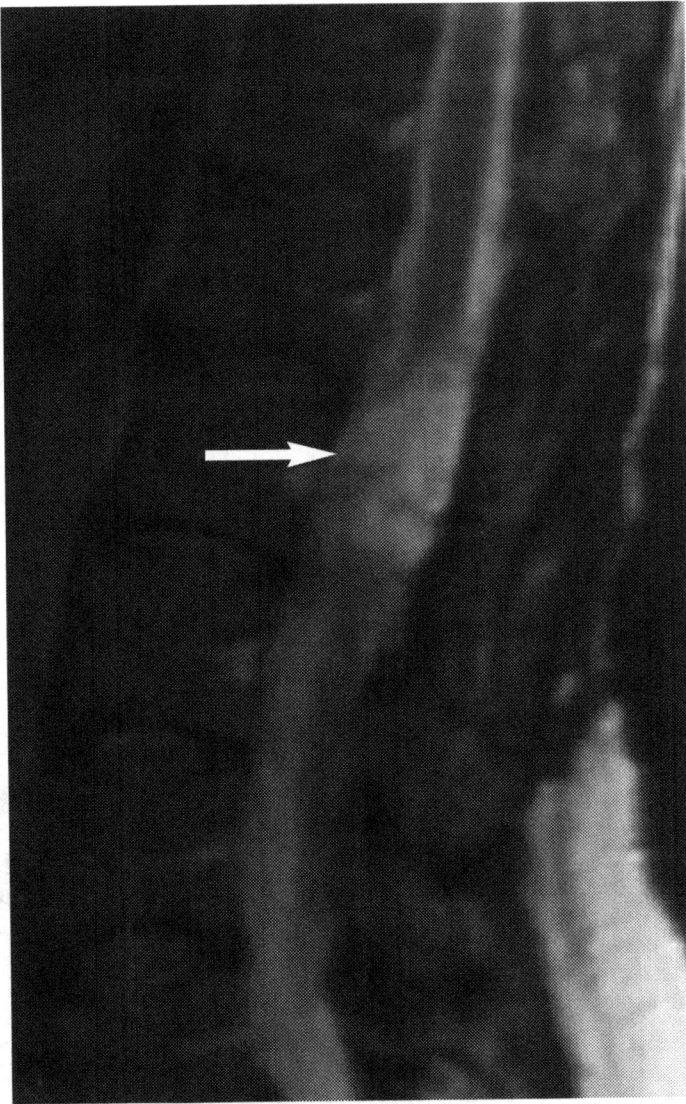

Figure 15b. *Dermoid cyst. The image is a sagittal T2 WI. Note how the cyst is hyperintense and heterogeneous. It would also be hyperintense on T1 WI. Fat suppression sequences like a STIR sequence will suppress the signal of the tumour.*

Infection
Osteomyelitis
Computer tomography is sensitive for detecting infection in the vertebrae, showing hypodensity at the site as well as frequently showing gas within the vertebrae. Associated discitis will lead to hypodensity of the infected discs. When there is healing of the lesions in the chronic phase the lesions become denser. On MRI scan there are low intensity changes on T1 WI and high intensity changes on T2 WI because of the increased water content and the lesions frequently enhance with contrast.

Epidural empyema (abscess)

MRI scanning of the spine is the imaging of choice showing a hypointense lesion on T1 WI that is hyperintense on T2 WI and enhances with contrast. The anterior located collections are almost always associated with discitis. Radionuclide scans are extremely sensitive and are usually the first imaging modality to detect these lesions.

Discitis

On imaging the disc appears hypointense on T1 WI and hyperintense on T2 WI, demonstrating a higher fluid content and may enhance with Gadolinium contrast administration.

Tuberculosis of the spine

Infection with *mycobacterium tuberculosis* starts in the vertebra or adjacent endplate and its hallmark is destruction of the vertebra and gibbus formation with collapse of the vertebra, whilst the integrity of the disc is maintained until quite late in the disease. On x-ray vertebral involvement with erosion kyphosis, with mostly involvement of the vertebrae and sparing the posterior elements is seen. There is frequently some soft tissue involvement with calcification. CT scans are quite useful in delineating the extent of the disease and demonstrating bony involvement and bony sequestra. MR may demonstrate as associated cold psoas abscess. Typically, the intervertebral disc is spared with the gibbus hypointense on T1 WI and hyperintense on T2 WI.

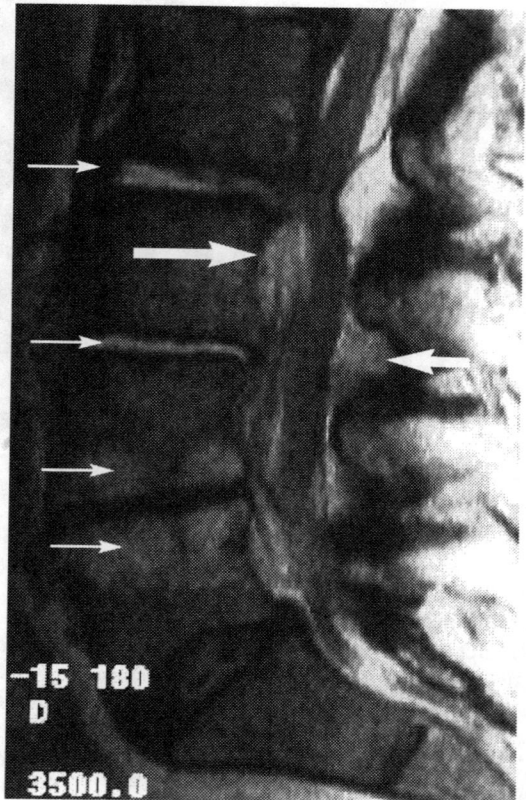

Figure 16. *This is a sagittal T2 WI of the lumbosacral spine. The two thick arrows demonstrate collections of pus, one anterior and one posterior of the cauda equina. The two top thin arrows demonstrate discitis with increased signal intensity. This is due to oedema associated with the infection of these disc spaces. The two bottom arrows demonstrate increased signal intensity in the vertebrae adjacent to the disc space signalling osteomyelitis.*

Vascular pathology

Abnormal vasculature

Dural Arteriovenous fistula (Type I AVM)

Usually located in the posterior intradural space either in or adjacent to the intervertebral foramen and is fed by a single arterial feeder entering the dural space through a dural root sleeve. On T1 WI the cord may be enlarged with multiple enhancing pial vessels and on T2 WI the cord is also enlarged with flow voids in the pia on the surface of the cord.

Arteriovenous malformation - Type II, III and IV (Type 1 is a dural AVF)

Type II has a nidus in the intramedullary space. Type III has an intramedullary nidus but with extramedullary extension and type IV is located ventrally, intra durally and perimedullary. Type II and III (intramedullary) demonstrate an enlarged cord and heterogenous signal on T1 WI and contrast enhancement. On T2 WI these are hyperintense and contain flow voids. Type IV demonstrates a ventral fistula with prominent flow voids on T1 WI and T2 WI demonstrates a hyperintense ventral lesion with flow voids.

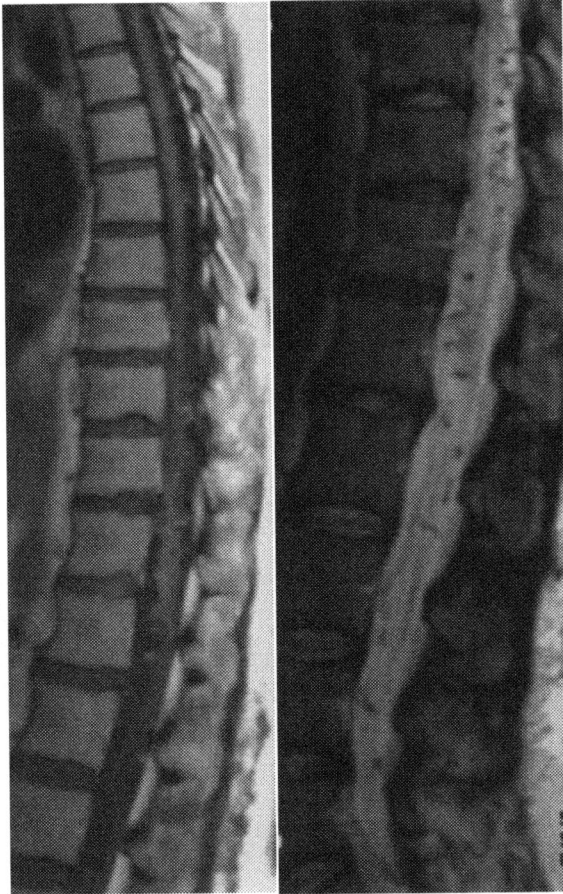

Figure 17. *The image on the left is a sagittal T1 WI and the image on the right is a sagittal T2 WI of the spine. Both demonstrate extensive flow voids from a arteriovenous malformation. The true nature of the vascular supply and drainage would be obtained from spinal angiography.*

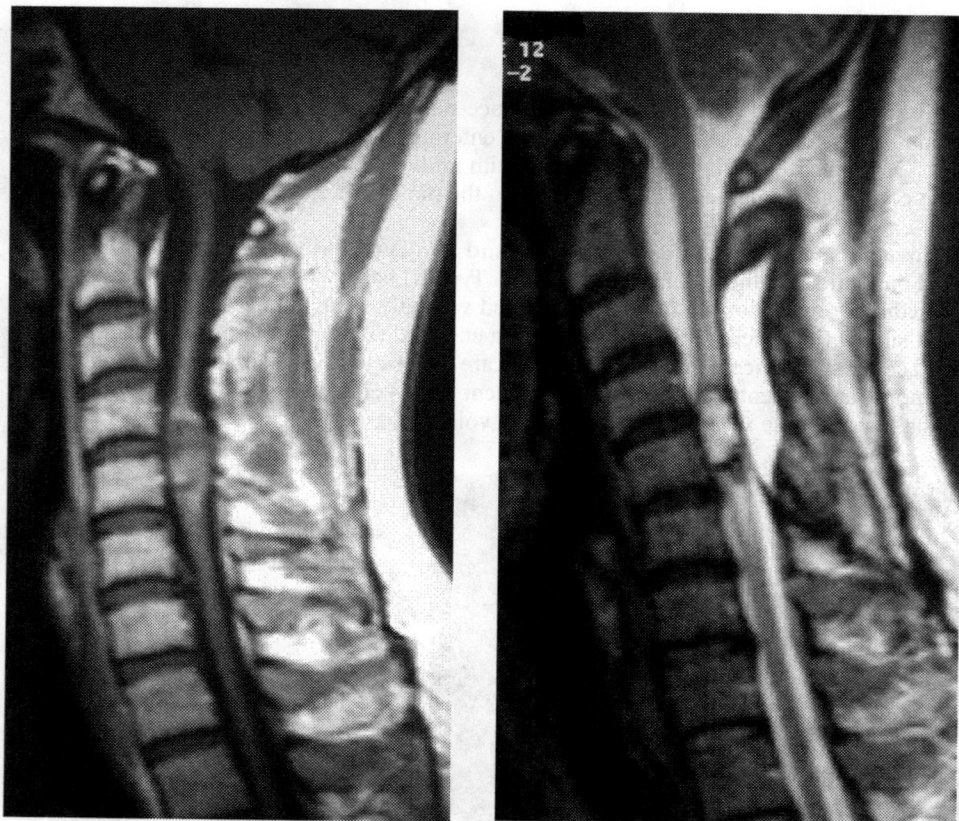

Figure 18. *Cavernoma. The image on the left is a sagittal contrast enhanced T1 WI of the cervical spine and the image on the right is a sagittal T2 WI of the cervical spine. Note the lobulated appearance of the lesion and the black, siderotic rim on the T2 WI.*

Cavernous angioma (cavernous malformation, cavernoma)
These intramedullary lesions have heterogenous signal on T1 and T2 WI with a hypodense ring (hemosiderin) on T2 WI.

Spinal cord infarct
The cord is usually slightly swollen but may be normal diameter and on T1 WI it usually has no features and on T2 WI is hyperintense to spinal cord. There may be a focal haemorrhagic conversion of the infarct.

Subdural haematoma
On CT scans these lesions are hyperdense in the acute and subacute phases. On MR scanning the intensity varies (see chapter 5) and it can be difficult to distinguish the blood from normal CSF. There might be some displacement of the cord that may be helpful in diagnosis.

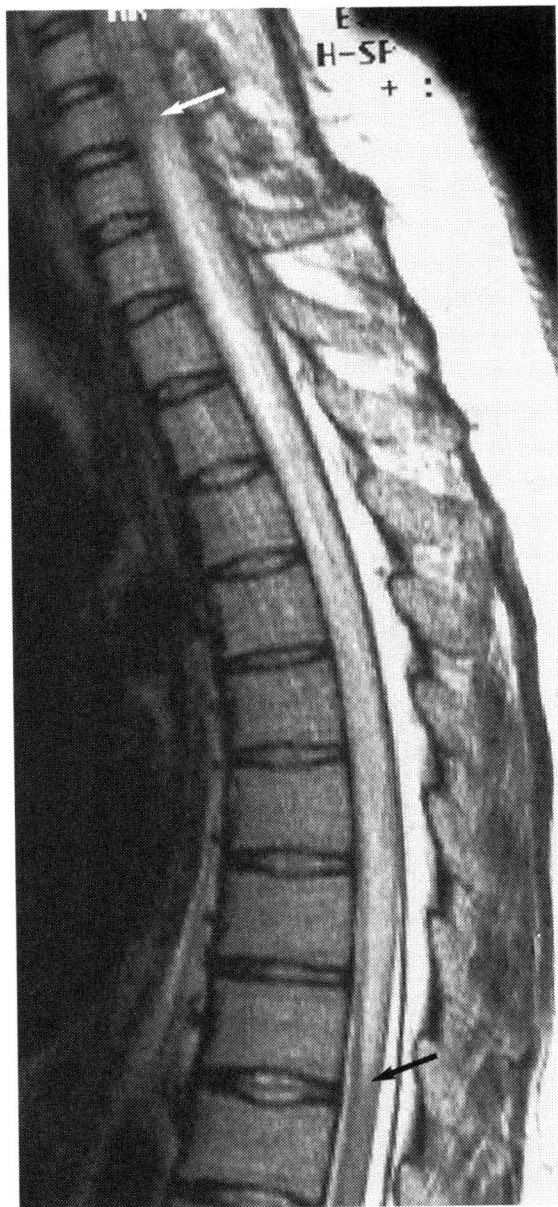

Figure 19. *This sagittal T2 WI demonstrates an extensive infarct of the spinal cord secondary to systemic hypotension. Note how the oedema associated with the infarction leads to a hyperintense signal on T2 WI.*

Epidural haematoma

On CT scans these lesions are hyperdense in the acute and subacute phases. On MR scanning the intensity varies according to the age of the lesion (see chapter 5). The location of the lesion in the extradural space helps with the diagnosis and it can be distinguished from an epidural abscess by the fact that it does not enhance with contrast and that there is no associated discitis or osteomyelitis.

7

NEURO ANGIOGRAPHY

J Zakier Hussain

Contents

Introduction
History of cerebral angiography
Standard projections

Cerebrovascular anatomy
The internal carotid artery
Anterior cranial circulation
The posterior cranial circulation
Extracranial circulation
The external carotid artery
Collateral circulation
Cerebral veins and the venous sinuses
Spinal cord blood supply

How to study a cerebral angiogram

Vascular malformation of the central nervous system

Preparation for cerebral angiography
Procedure of cerebral angiography
Spinal angiography
Intra-operative angiography
Wada test
Inferior petrosal sinus sampling

Complications of cerebral angiography

Conclusion

Introduction

Cerebral angiography studies both the intracranial and extracranial blood vessels that supply the brain and its related structures. This is done by selective catheterisation of an extracranial cervical vessel through a peripheral vessel and injection of contrast agent to opacify the vasculature for examination with x-rays. Similarly, spinal angiography evaluates the blood vessels of the spine. Together we refer to these investigations as neuro angiography. The diagnostic information obtained by this procedure, along with the clinical and other imaging studies can be used to plan or evaluate results of treatment. Additionally, interventional angiography is the endovascular treatment of vascular lesions via the traditional angiographic route.

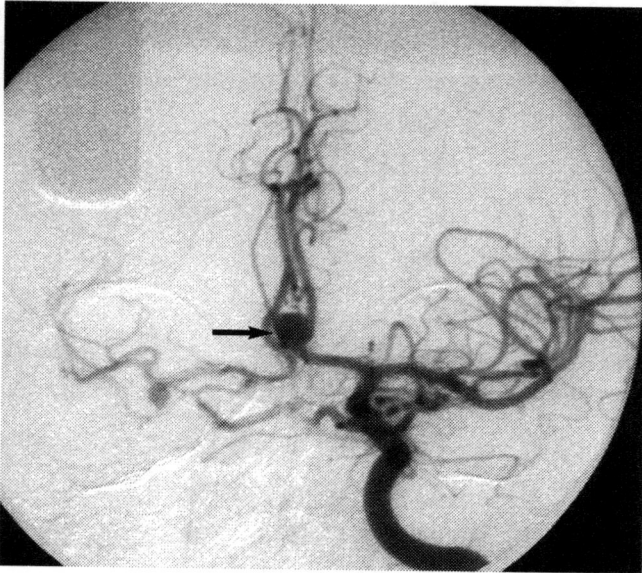

Figure 1. *This angiogram demonstrates an anterior communicating artery aneurysm (arrow) with good cross flow to the contralateral side.*

History of cerebral angiography

Wilhelm C. Roentgen invented X-rays in 1895. Following that, many developments emerged with the use of X-rays. Antonio de Egas Moniz (1874-1955), a neurologist from Portugal, was the pioneer of cerebral angiography. Moniz and his colleagues, Almeida Dias and Almeida Lima developed the early techniques of cerebral angiography, which they presented at the Societe de Neurologie in Paris in 1927. A 70% solution of strontium bromide was used as contrast on a surgically exposed *carotid artery*. Moniz performed rational and methodical studies to define the safe application of angiography. In 1933, he reported angiographic localisation of an intracranial aneurysm in a human. He shared the Nobel Prize in 1949 with Walter Hess in Medicine and Physiology for his pioneering work on prefrontal leucotomy in psychotic patients. In 1953, Seldinger popularised a percutaneous angiography technique where he used a styleted needle to puncture the artery through which a flexible metal guide wire was inserted and the needle removed. This was followed by rail-roading a polyethylene catheter over the wire. This formed the basis for vessel cannulation techniques. The modern neuro angiography machine allows precise depiction of normal and abnormal vessels and has improved markedly the understanding of the anatomy and pathophysiology of neurovascular lesions. It includes a mobile C-arm fluoroscopy unit the ability to record a rapid sequence of images. Rotational angiography with a work station capable of computing a three dimensional model are advantages. Digital subtraction road-mapping is helpful and bi-planar angiography is necessary if interventional procedures are to be performed. A power injector to inject contrast at a constant rate is also a useful adjunct in interventional neuroradiology especially when 3-D reconstruction is performed. Improved design of catheters and guide-wires, contrast agents and modern imaging technology has further increased the safety and efficacy of neuro angiography.

Standard projections

At least two radiographic projections are needed at right angles (frontal and lateral view) in every cerebral angiogram. Special views may be necessary for diagnosis and localisation of the abnormality.

Lateral view: The mid-sagittal plane of the skull is parallel to the plane of the image intensifier. The central ray is centred to a point 5 cm above the external auditory meatus, which is the location of the sella. The external auditory meatus should be superimposed as well as the floor of the sella and the orbital roofs.

Postero-anterior view (Caldwell's view): The tube is angled about 12 -15 degrees towards the patient's feet from the orbito-meatal line to obtain this view. The frontal projection is angled such that the roofs of the orbits are superimposed on the upper aspect of the petrous bones.

Towne's view: Antero-posterior view with 25-30 degrees caudal tilt from the orbito-meatal line would project the orbits low. This is a standard view for the posterior fossa.

Submento-Vertical or Water's view: This places the petrous ridge low. It is useful for basilar artery aneurysms and with a slight oblique view; the detangled internal carotid loops could be seen.

One image from the early arterial, late arterial, capillary, and venous phases is retained for filming. The rate is usually kept at three frames per second. Routine views for the vertebral injection include the lateral and frontal projections. In the frontal projection, the use of a greater angle than used for the carotid injection (steep Towne angle) allows better visualisation of the posterior circulation. While studying arteriovenous malformation the rate is increased to about six frames per second for a detailed study.

An arch aortogram using a 5F or 6F pigtail catheter in the left anterior oblique projection with 30-50 ml of contrast at a rate of 20-30 ml/s may be required in the case of proximal vessel stenosis, tortuosity or anatomic variations. Better images , however are obtained using selective catheterisation of the common carotid arteries with a Simmons II catheter.

Cerebrovascular anatomy

The three major branches arising from the aortic arch are the *innominate artery (brachiocephalic)*, left *common carotid artery* and left *subclavian artery*. The *innominate artery* divides at the level of the sternoclavicular joint into the right *subclavian artery* and the right *common carotid artery*. The *common carotid artery* divides into the *internal carotid artery* and *external carotid artery* (ECA) usually at C4-5 vertebral body level. The main arterial supply to the brain comes from the paired *carotid* and *vertebral arteries*.

The Circle of Willis described by Dr. Thomas Willis in 1664 is a nine-sided arterial anastomotic network. It has ten components that include the two *internal carotid arteries*, the two *posterior communicating arteries*, the *anterior communicating artery*, the two *anterior cerebral arteries,* the two *posterior cerebral arteries* and the *basilar artery.* It is the main source of collateral flow in the cerebral circulation. It is complete in only about 50% of individuals.

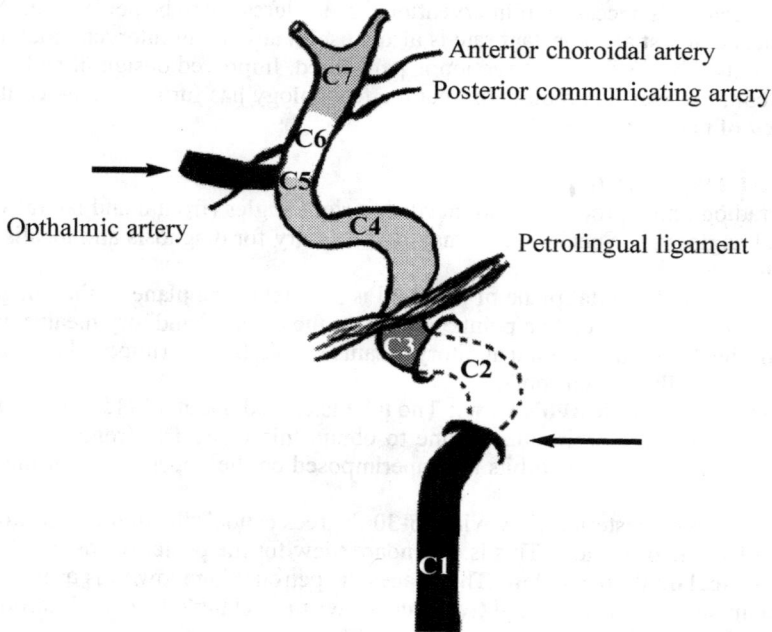

Figure 2. *The carotid artery and it's different segments. The top arrow demonstrates the clinoid process and the bottom arrow the carotid canal.*

The Internal carotid artery (ICA)

The cervical segment (C1) originates at the carotid bifurcation and terminates at the skull base as the ICA enters the carotid canal. The cervical segment has no branches. Initially it is situated posterolateral to the ECA but as it ascends, it lies medially.

The petrous segment (C2) lies within the petrous carotid canal and is surrounded by a venous and autonomic plexus. It has a vertical and horisontal segment with two branches, the carotico-tympanic artery and the vidian artery.

The lacerum segment (C3) starts from the foramen lacerum to the petro-lingual ligament. It has no branches.

The cavernous segment (C4) has a sinuous course within the cavernous sinus with a posterior ascending, horisontal and anterior vertical segment. The branches are the *meningo hypophyseal trunk* that supplies the pituitary through the *inferior hypophyseal artery*, the tentorium cerebelli through the *tentorial branch* and the clivus through the *clival branch*. The *capsular artery of McConnell* is an inconstant branch. The *inferolateral trunk* originates on the lateral surface of the horisontal segment and crosses the VIth nerve within the cavernous sinus. It's branches supply the dura of the cavernous sinus, gasserian ganglion and the third, fourth and sixth cranial nerves. It has important anastomoses with the *maxillary artery* and *middle meningeal artery.*

The clinoid segment (C5) is very short and has no branches. It lies between the proximal and distal dural rings.

The ophthalmic segment (C6) starts from the distal dural ring to the origin of *posterior communicating artery*. It's branches include the *ophthalmic artery* and *superior hypophyseal artery.*

The communicating segment (C7) starts from the *posterior communicating artery* origin to the bifurcation of the *internal carotid artery*. It's branches include the *posterior communicating artery* and *anterior choroidal artery.*

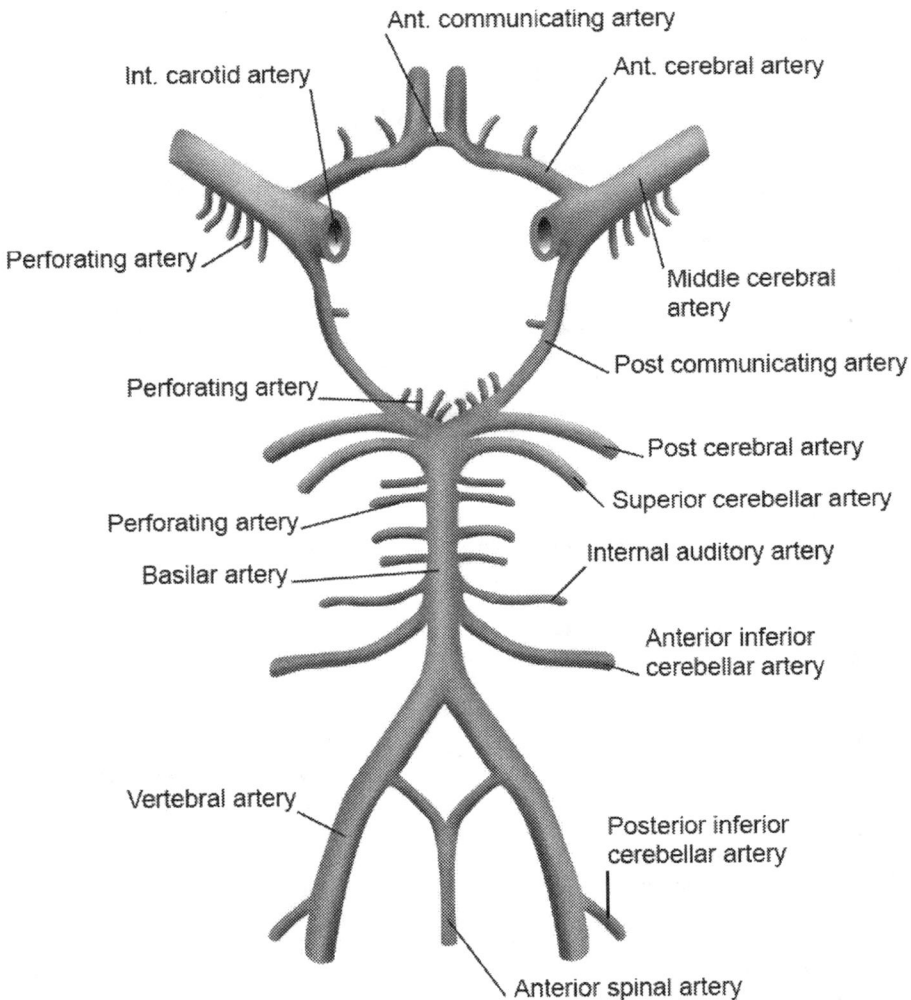

Figure 3. *Diagrammatic sketch of the circle of Willis.*
Posterior circulation - note that the posterior inferior cerebellar arteries originate from the vertebral arteries and the anterior inferior cerebellar arteries arise from the basilar artery. The anterior spinal artery is formed by a branch from each of the vertebral arteries. The basilar artery divides into two terminal branches, the two posterior cerebral arteries, just after giving of the two superior cerebellar arteries.
Anterior circulation - note how the carotid arteries divide into anterior cerebral arteries, supplying the medial halves of the hemispheres and the middle cerebral arteries, supplying the lateral halves of the hemispheres. The anterior communicating artery connects the two anterior cerebral arteries and the posterior communicating artery connects the posterior circulation to the anterior circulation.

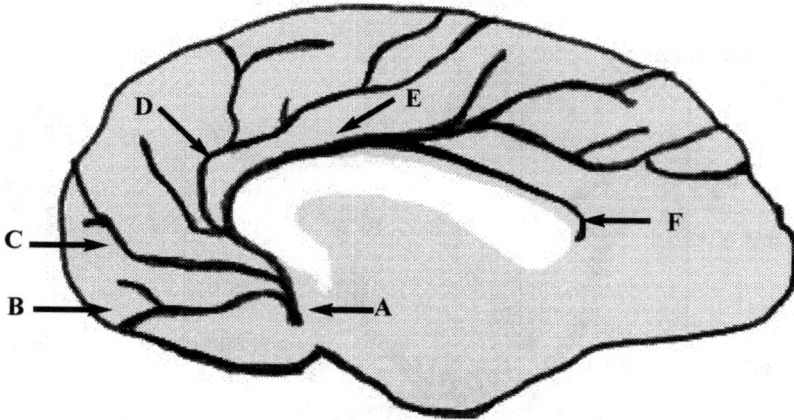

Figure 4. *This image demonstrates a diagrammatic representation of the anterior cerebral artery. A: Is the A 2 (post communicating segment) of the anterior cerebral artery; B: Is the orbitofrontal artery; C: Is the frontopolar artery; D: Is the callosomarginal artery; E: Is the pericallosal artery and F: Is the splenial branch.*

Anterior cranial circulation

The ***anterior cerebral artery*** is the smaller of the two terminal branches of the *internal carotid artery*. It is divided into:

The A1 segment, which is horisontal and extends from the *anterior cerebral artery* origin until the junction with *anterior communicating artery*. It's branches include the *medial lenticulostriate arteries* and *perforating arteries*, which supply the optic nerve and chiasm, anterior hypothalamus, septum pellucidum, medial anterior commissure, fornix and striatum.

The A2 segment is the *post-communicating artery* segment. It's main branch is the *recurrent artery of Heubner*, which runs back on the parent artery. It supplies the caudate nucleus, anterior limb of internal capsule, putamen and paracentral gyrus. The *orbito-frontal artery* runs along the floor of the anterior cranial fossa and supplies the gyrus rectus, olfactory bulb and medial aspect of orbital surface of the frontal lobe. The *fronto-polar artery* arises proximal to the origin of the *callosomarginal artery* and is directed to the medial aspect of the frontal lobe and supplies the superior frontal gyrus.

The A3 segment of the *anterior cerebral artery* starts beyond the corpus callosum. It gives rise to the *pericallosal artery* that passes in the cistern of the corpus callosum and its largest branch is the *calloso-marginal artery*. The *internal frontal* (*anterior, middle* and *posterior frontal arteries*), *paracentral* and *parietal branches* (*superior* and *inferior parietal arteries*) may arise from the *pericallosal* or *calloso-marginal arteries*.

The ***middle cerebral artery*** is the larger of the two terminal branches of the *internal carotid artery*. It is divided into 4 segments:

The M1 (sphenoidal segment) starts from the carotid bifurcation to the Sylvian fissure and runs horisontally. The *lenticulostriate* and *anterior temporal arteries* are important branches. The M1 segment is subdivided into pre-bifurcation and post-bifurcation segments.

The M2 segment (insular) turns 90 degrees into the Sylvian fissure lying on the insula where it branches.

The M3 segment (opercular) segment begins from the circular sulcus of the insula and terminates at the outer cortical surface of the Sylvian fissure.

The M4 segment (cortical) is the terminal branches on the surface of the cerebral hemisphere. The *orbito-frontal, prefrontal, precentral sulcal, centralsulcal, anterior parietal, pos-*

terior parietal, angular, tempero-occipital, posterior temporal and *intermediate temporal arteries* are the branches arising from the M3 and M4 segments.

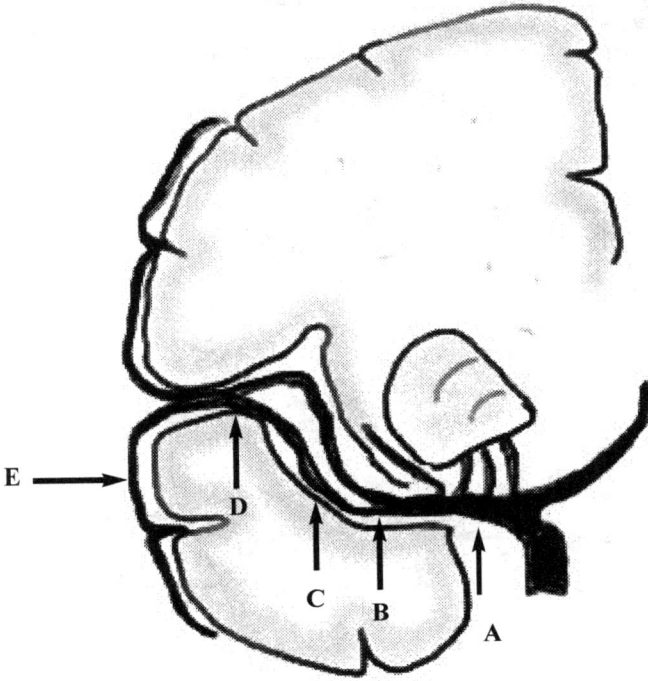

Figure 5. *This image demonstrates a diagrammatic representation of the middle cerebral artery. A: M1 segment prebifurcation; B: M1 segment post bifurcation; C: M2 segment; D: M3 segment; E: M4 segment*

The posterior cranial circulation

The *vertebral arteries* on each side are divided into 4 segments:

The **V1 (extra osseous)** segment extends in the foramen transversaria of the cervical verte-brae from the subclavian artery to the C6 foramen.
The **V2 (foraminal)** segment extends from the C6 foramen to the level of the C1 transverse foramen.
The **V3 (extra spinal)** segment extends from the atlas to the foramen magnum where it pen-etrates the dura.
The **V4 (intradural)** segment starts where the artery penetrates the dura at the foramen mag-

num to the junction with the contralateral vertebral artery to form the basilar artery.

The *vertebral arteries* have cervical branches that supply the deep cervical musculature and a spinal branch that supplies the spinal cord and the spinal canal. The meningeal branches include the *anterior meningeal artery*, which supplies the dura around the foramen magnum and the *posterior meningeal artery* that supplies the falx cerebelli. The intracranial branches include the *anterior spinal artery* and *posterior spinal artery, small perforating arteries* and the *posterior inferior cerebellar arteries.*

The *basilar artery,* formed by the union of the two *vertebral arteries,* divides into the two posterior *cerebral arteries* in front of the pons. The main branches are the *median* and *paramedian perforating branches, anterior inferior cerebellar arteries, superior cerebellar arteries* and the *posterior cerebral arteries.*

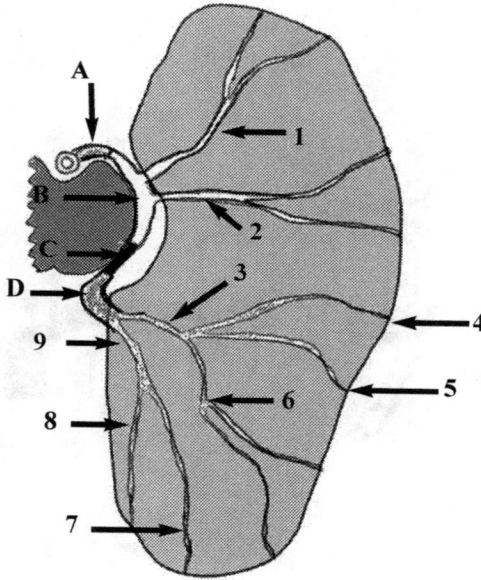

Figure 6. *Inferior aspect of the brain. The posterior cerebral artery originates from the basilar artery and has 4 segments. A: The P1 segment extends from the basilar bifurcation to the posterior communicating artery junction; B: The P2 segment extends from the posterior communicating artery to the posterior aspect of the midbrain and it runs in the crural and ambient cistern; C: The P3 segment extends from the quadrigeminal plate to the calcarine fissure within the perimesencephalic cistern and has no branches; D: The P4 segment is in the terminal part in the calcarine fissure and has two branches. The medial branch, the medial occipital artery (9) divides into the calcarine (8) and the parieto-occipital arteries (7). The lateral branch, the lateral occipital artery (3) gives rise to the anterior inferior (4), middle inferior(5) and posterior inferior temporal arteries (6). The anterior temporal (1) and posterior temporal arteries (2) are branches of the P 2 segment.*

The *posterior cerebral arteries* arise from the basilar bifurcation and are divided into four segments.

The P1 (pre-communicating) segment extends from the basilar bifurcation to the *posterior communicating artery* junction. It gives off perforating branches, which include the *thalamo-perforating, medial-posterior-choroidal artery, quadrigeminal plate branch* and *cerebral peduncle rami.*

The P2 (crural and ambient) segment extends from the *posterior communicating artery* to the posterior aspect of the midbrain and it runs in the crural and ambient cistern. The *thalamogeniculate, peduncular perforating arteries* and *lateral posterior choroidal artery* arises from this segment as well as the *anterior temporal artery, posterior temporal artery* and the *splenial branches.*

The P3 (quadrigeminal) segment extends from the quadrigeminal plate to the calcarine fissure within the perimesencephalic cistern.

The P4 (calcarine) segment is in the terminal part in the calcarine fissure and has two branches. The medial branch, the *medial occipital artery* divides into the *calcarine* and the *parieto-occipital arteries.* The lateral branch, the *lateral occipital artery* gives rise to the *anterior inferior, middle inferior* and *posterior inferior temporal arteries.*

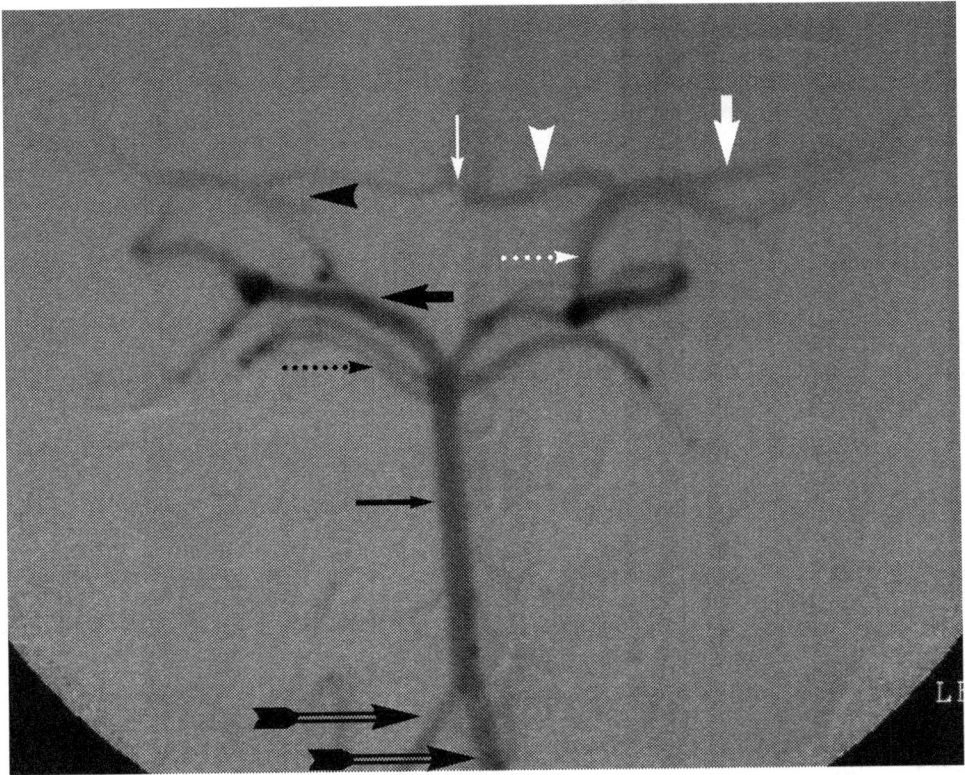

Figure 7. *The circle of Willis. This vertebral angiogram demonstrates the circle of Willis. Note the basilar artery (black arrow), right duplicated superior cerebellar artery (black dashed arrow), posterior communicating artery (white dashed arrow), anterior communicating artery (white arrow), right ICA (thick black arrowhead), right posterior cerebral artery (thick black arrow), A 1 segment of the left anterior cerebral artery (thick white arrow head) and middle cerebral artery (thick white arrow). Note how the basilar artery is formed by the two vertebral arteries (open arrows at the bottom).*

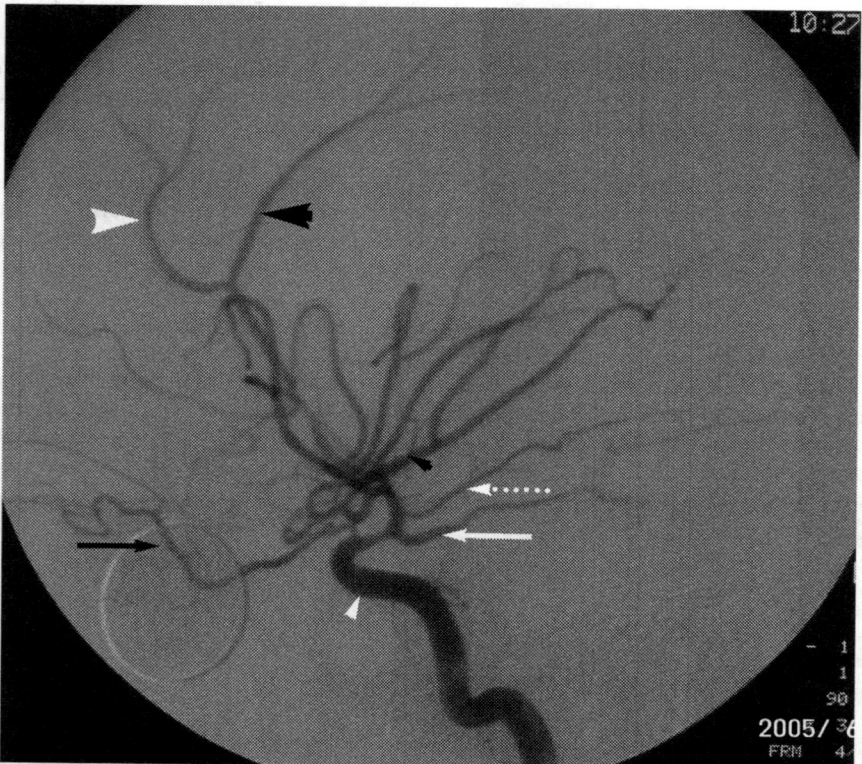

Figure 8. *This is the lateral view of an ICA angiogram demonstrating the ICA (white arrow head), the ophthalmic artery (black arrow), the posterior communicating artery (white arrow), the anterior choroidal artery (white dashed arrow), the middle cerebral artery (black arrow head), the pericallosal artery (thick black arrow head) and the callosomarginal artery (thick white arrowhead).*

An *internal carotid artery* to *basilar artery* anastomosis exists if the *embryonic arteries* such as the *persistent trigeminal artery* fail to involute. A *persistent trigeminal artery* is the commonest persistent *fetal artery* and its incidence varies from 0.1% to 0.6% in angiographic studies. It connects the pre cavernous segment of *internal carotid artery* with the *basilar artery* between the origins of the *superior cerebellar* and the *anterior inferior cerebellar artery*. The *persistent otic artery* is very rare and connects the petrous segment of *internal carotid artery* with the *anterior inferior cerebellar artery* after traversing the temporal bone, and exits through the internal auditory canal. The *persistent hypoglossal artery* is also rare and it joins the cervical *internal carotid artery* with the lower end of the *basilar artery* after passing through the hypoglossal canal. The *proatlantal intersegmental artery* originates from the dorsal aspect of the *internal carotid artery* at the C2-3 level and enters the foramen magnum to give rise to the *vertebral artery*. Sometimes it arises from the *external carotid artery* and joins the *vertebral artery* below C1. Dural collaterals with cortical vessels occur with progressive internal carotid occlusive disease.

Figure 9. *Persistent fetal arteries - see image on opposite page. A: Trigeminal artery; B: Otic artery; C: Hypoglossal artery; D: Proatlantal intersegmental artery*

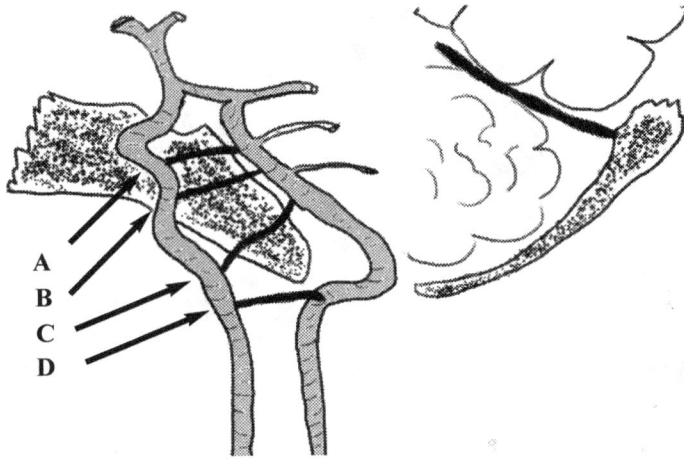

Figure 9. *Persistent fetal arteries - see legend on opposite page*

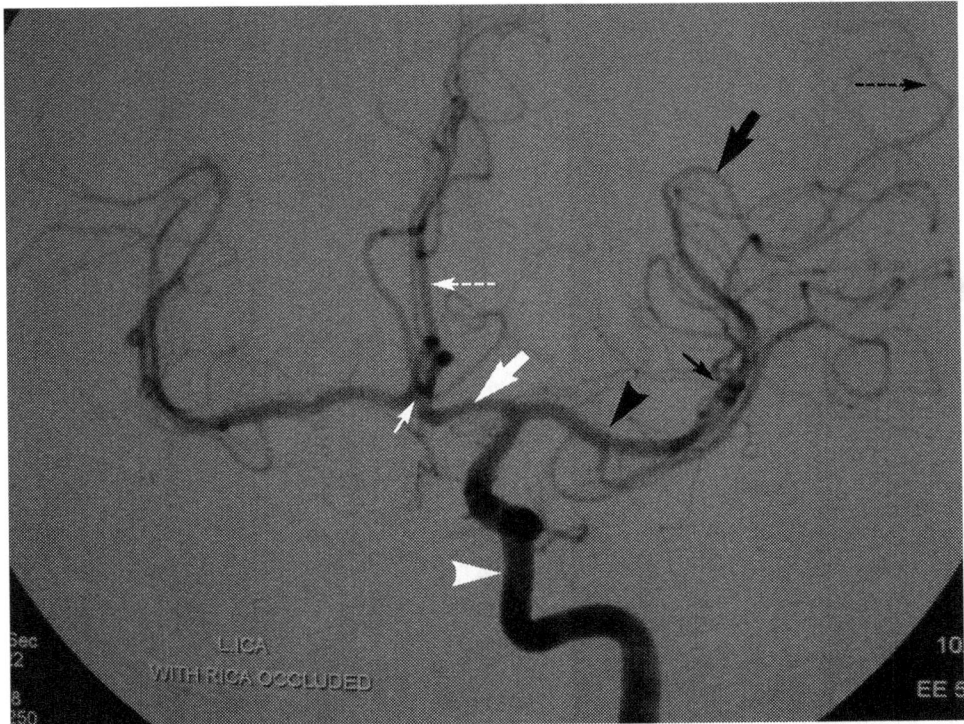

Figure 10. *This angiogram demonstrates an antero-posterior view of the left internal carotid artery (thick white arrow head) with cross compression of the right internal carotid artery. It demonstrates good flow across the anterior communicating artery (white arrow) to the opposite MCA and equal filling of both the ACA's at the same time. Note the A1 segment (thick white arrow), A2 segment (dashed white arrow), M1 segment (thick black arrow head), M2 segment (black arrow), M3 segment (thick black arrow) and M4 segment (dashed black arrow)*

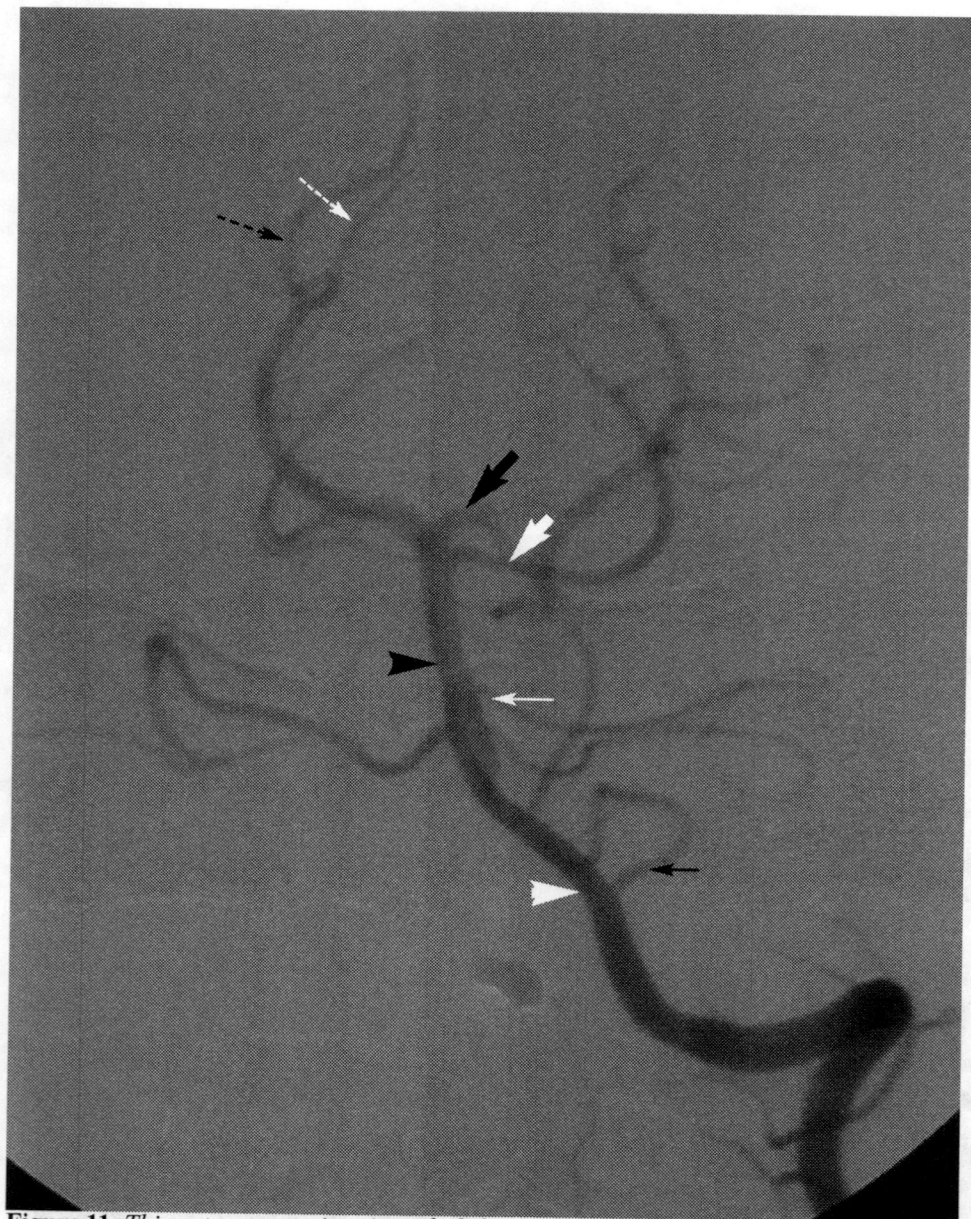

Figure 11. *This antero-posterior view of a left vertebral angiogram demonstrates the left vertebral artery (white arrow head), left PICA (black arrow), AICA (white arrow), the basilar artery (black arrow head), P1 segment of the PCA (thick black arrow), the superior cerebellar artery (thick white arrow), the parieto-occipital artery (black dashed arrow) and the calcarine artery (white dashed arrow).*

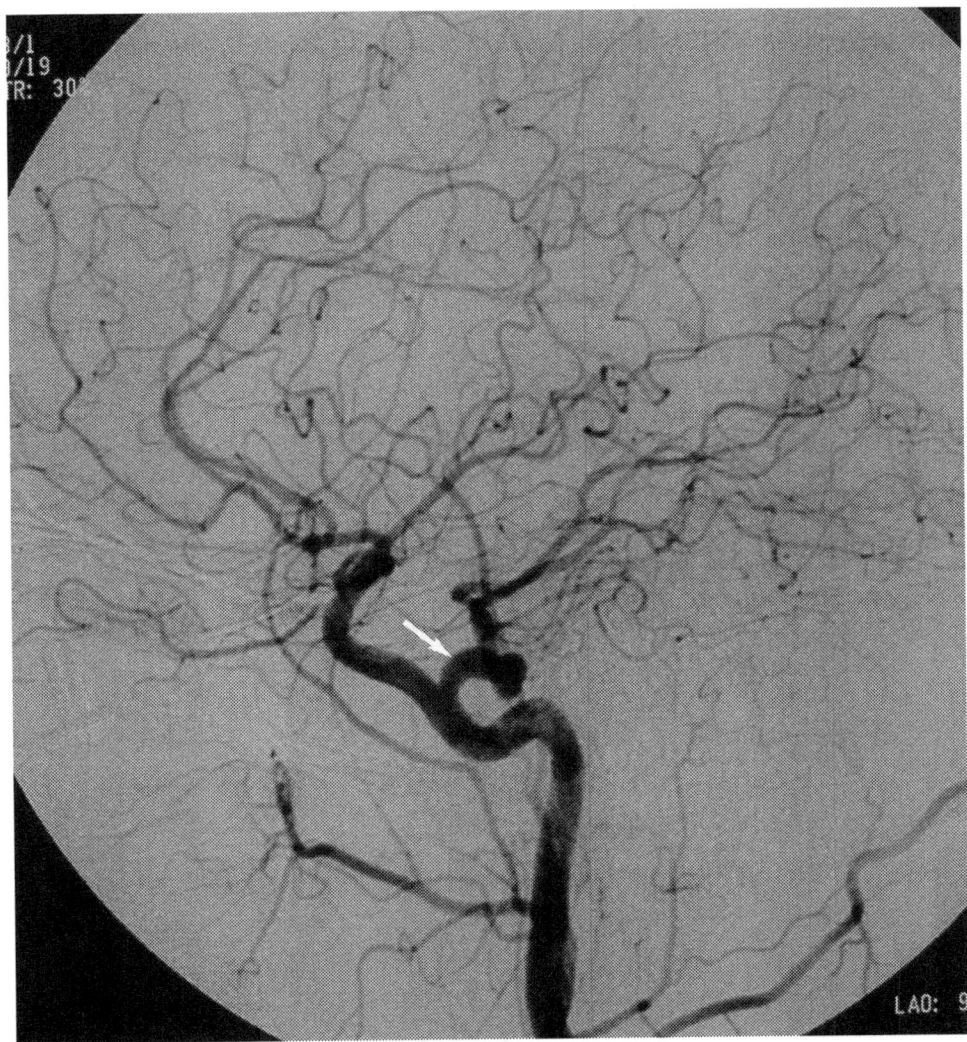

Figure 12. *This is a lateral view of an internal carotid angiogram and it demonstrates the filling of a persistent trigeminal artery (arrow) which connects the ICA with the basilar artery.*

Cerebral veins and the venous sinuses

Supratentorial veins

The supratentorial venous system is divided into the superficial and the deep group. In the majority of people, the superficial group of veins are the *superficial middle cerebral vein, the vein of Labbé* and the *vein of Trolard*. The *superficial middle cerebral veins* runs along the surface of the Sylvian fissure and curve medially to drain into the *cavernous sinus* or the *sphenoparietal sinus*. The *veins of Trolard* drain the *superficial middle cerebral vein* to the *superior sagittal sinus*. The *veins of Labbé* connect the *superficial middle cerebral vein to the transverse sinus*. There are also veins from the basal surface of the frontal, temporal and occipital lobes and these become prominent in cases of venous hypertension. The deep venous system originates in the *medullary veins*, which drain to the *subependymal veins* along the lateral ventricular wall and are paired. These aggregate into large tributaries such as the *septal veins, thalamostriate veins* and *internal cerebral veins*. The *septal vein* joins with the *thalamostriate vein* to form the *internal cerebral vein* behind the foramen of Monroe. The *thalamostriate veins* are formed by the confluence of the *anterior caudate veins* and *the terminal vein*. The *internal cerebral veins* unite with each other and with the *basal vein of Rosenthal* in the quadrigeminal cistern to form the *great cerebral vein of Galen*, which joins the *inferior sagittal sinus* to form the *straight sinus*. The *basal vein of Rosenthal* is formed from the confluence of the *anterior* and *deep middle cerebral veins* (veins that drain the insula and cerebral peduncles) and the *lateral mesencephalic veins*. It joins the ipsilateral *internal cerebral vein* and drain into the *vein of Galen*.

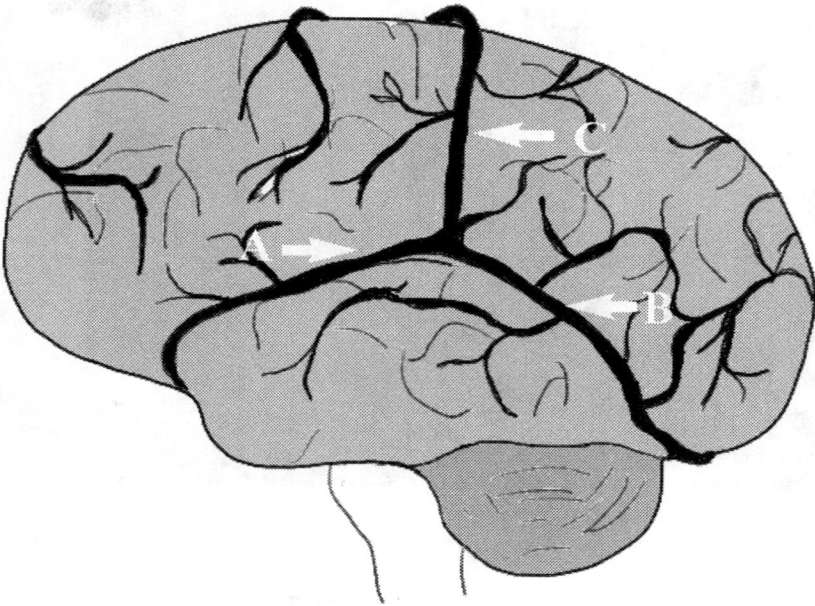

Figure 13. *The superficial venous drainage of the brain. A: Superficial middle cerebral vein; B: Vein of Labbé; C: Vein of Trolard*

Supratentorial venous sinuses

The *superior sagittal sinus* extends from the foramen caecum to the *torcular Herophili*. It drains the veins from the lateral and medial halves of the cerebral hemispheres. The *vein of Trolard* also drains to the *superior sagittal sinus*. The *torcular Herophili* is the confluence of the *superior sagittal sinus, straight sinus* and the *occipital sinus*. It ultimately drains into the *transverse sinuses*. The *inferior sagittal sinus* lies on the lower border of the falx and joins the *internal cerebral vein* to form the *vein of Galen*. The *straight sinus* drains the *vein of Galen* to the *torcular Herophili*. The *transverse sinuses* are found along the tentorium bilaterally and end in the bilateral *sigmoid sinuses*, which become the *internal jugular veins* in the jugular foramen. The *cavernous sinuses* lie on either side of the sella turcica and are the site of confluence of the intracranial and extracranial venous structures. Normal outflow from the *cavernous sinus* includes the *petrosal sinus, pterygo-maxillary sinus* via the *emissary veins, sphenoparietal sinus* and the *contra-lateral cavernous sinus* through the *inter-cavernous sinuses*. The *superior petrosal sinus* and *inferior ophthalmic vein* may be either afferent to or efferent from the *cavernous sinus*. The *sphenoparietal sinus* drains the *superficial sylvian vein* into the *cavernous sinus*. The *meningeal, uncal, orbital* and *inferior frontal veins* drain into the *sphenoparietal sinus*. Sometimes it may drain as a sinus called the *spheno-petrosal sinus* into the *superior petrosal sinus*.

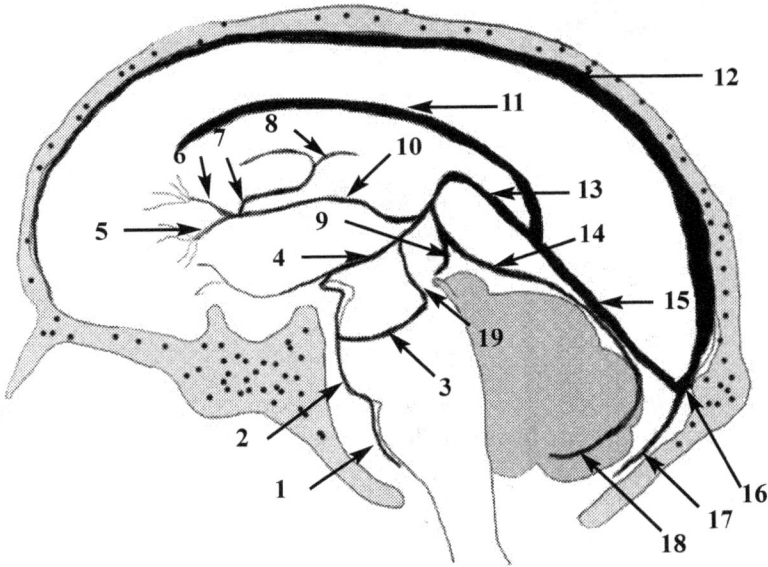

Figure 14. *The deep venous system, note that this is a schematic drawing and therefore dimensions are not true to life. 1: Anterior medullary venous plexus; 2: Anterior pontomesencephalic venous plexus; 3: Transverse pontine vein; 4: Basal vein of Rosenthal; 5: Septal vein; 6: Anterior caudate veins; 7: Thalamostriate vein; 8: Terminal vein; 9: Precentral cerebellar vein; 10: Internal cerebral vein; 11: Inferior sagittal sinus; 12: Superior sagittal sinus; 13: Vein of Galen; 14: Superior vermian vein; 15: Straight sinus; 16: Torcular Herophili; 17: Occipital sinus; 18: Inferior vermian vein; 19: Lateral mesencephalic vein.*

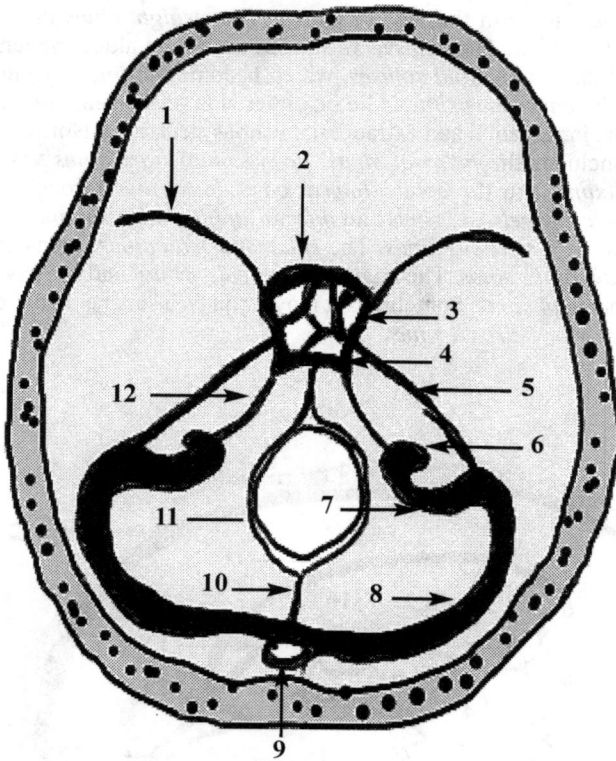

Figure 15. *Basal dural venous sinuses. 1: Sphenoparietal sinus; 2: Anterior intercavernous sinus; 3:Cavernous sinus; 4: Posterior intercavernous sinus; 5: Superior petrosal sinus; 6: Internal jugular vein; 7: Sigmoid sinus; 8: Transverse sinus; 9: Torcular Herophili; 10: Occipital sinus; 11: Marginal sinus; 12: Inferior petrosal sinus.*

Infra-tentorial veins and sinuses

The *sigmoid sinuses* are a continuation of the *transverse sinuses* and drain into the *internal jugular vein* on either side. It is the major outflow from the cranial cavity. The *occipital sinus* begins at the posterior margin of the foramen magnum and passes superiorly to the *torcular Herophili*. It drains into the torcular and is inconstant. It may connect to the sinus around the foramen magnum called the *marginal sinus* and drain directly to the neck veins. The *superior petrosal sinus* runs from the posterior aspect of the *cavernous sinus* to the *sigmoid-transverse sinus* junction. The *inferior petrosal sinus* runs from the posterior aspect of the *cavernous sinus* to the *jugular vein*. The posterior fossa veins are divided into the superior group, which contain the *precentral cerebellar vein, posterior mesencephalic veins,* and the *superior vermian vein,* which drain into the *vein of Galen.* The anterior group that contain the *anterior ponto-mesencephalic vein* and the *petrosal veins,* which drain into the *petrosal sinuses.* The posterior group, which contain the *inferior vermian veins,* drain into the *torcular Herophili* and the *transverse sinuses.*

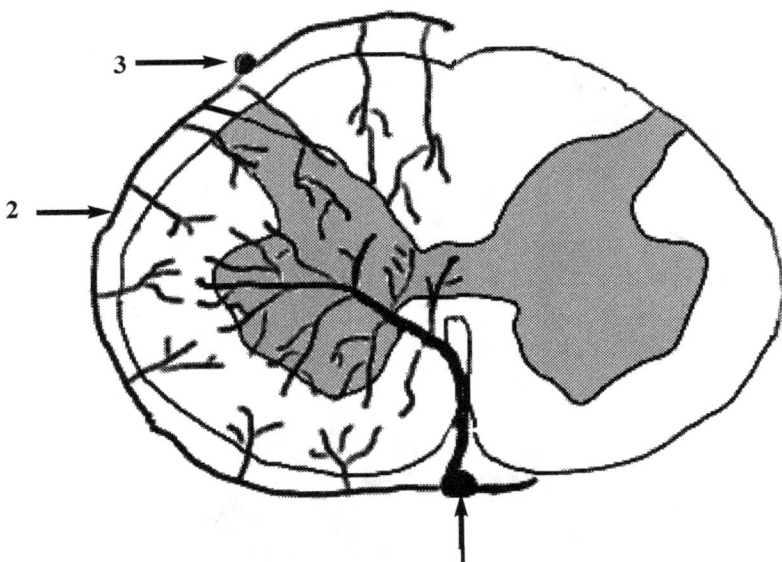

Figure 16. *Spinal cord blood supply. 1: Anterior spinal artery; 2; Arterial vasocorona; 3: Posterior spinal artery. Note how the anterior spinal artery supplies the anterior two thirds of the spinal cord and the paired posterior spinal arteries, the posterior third.*

Spinal cord blood supply

The spinal cord is supplied by an *anterior spinal artery* and two *posterior spinal arteries* that are branches of the *vertebral artery* and reinforced by multiple *radicular arteries*, which form the *anterior spinal artery* and the two *posterior spinal arteries*. The *radicular arteries* arise from neighbouring arteries at the level of each vertebral segment and accompany the nerve roots via the intervertebral foramina. The *anterior spinal artery*, coursing in the midline, usually originates in the upper cervical region, at the junction of the two descending *anterior spinal branches* of the *vertebral arteries*, and receives contributions from six to ten *anterior radicular arteries* throughout its length.

The paired posterolaterally located *posterior spinal arteries* arise as small branches of either the *vertebral* or the *posterior inferior cerebellar arteries*. Each *posterior spinal artery* receives contributions from ten to 23 *posterior radicular arteries*. The *anterior spinal artery* distributes blood to the anterior two thirds of the spinal cord, while each *posterior spinal artery* distributes blood to the ipsilateral posterior one third of the cord. The *artery of Adamkiewicz* may arise at any level between the fifth thoracic and the fourth lumbar arteries on either side, although it has a left-sided origin in 80% of individuals. The *artery of Adamkiewicz* has a large *anterior* and a smaller *posterior radicular branch*. On reaching the anterior aspect of the cord, the *anterior radicular branch* ascends a short distance and then makes a hairpin turn to give off a small ascending and a larger descending branch (in other words the terminal portion of the *anterior spinal artery*), which drops to the level of the conus medullaris, where it forms an anastomotic circle with the terminal branches of the two *posterior spinal arteries*. The cauda equina is accompanied and supplied by branches from the *lumbar, iliolumbar, lateral and median sacral arteries*; these branches also contribute to the anastomotic arterial circle around the conus medullaris.

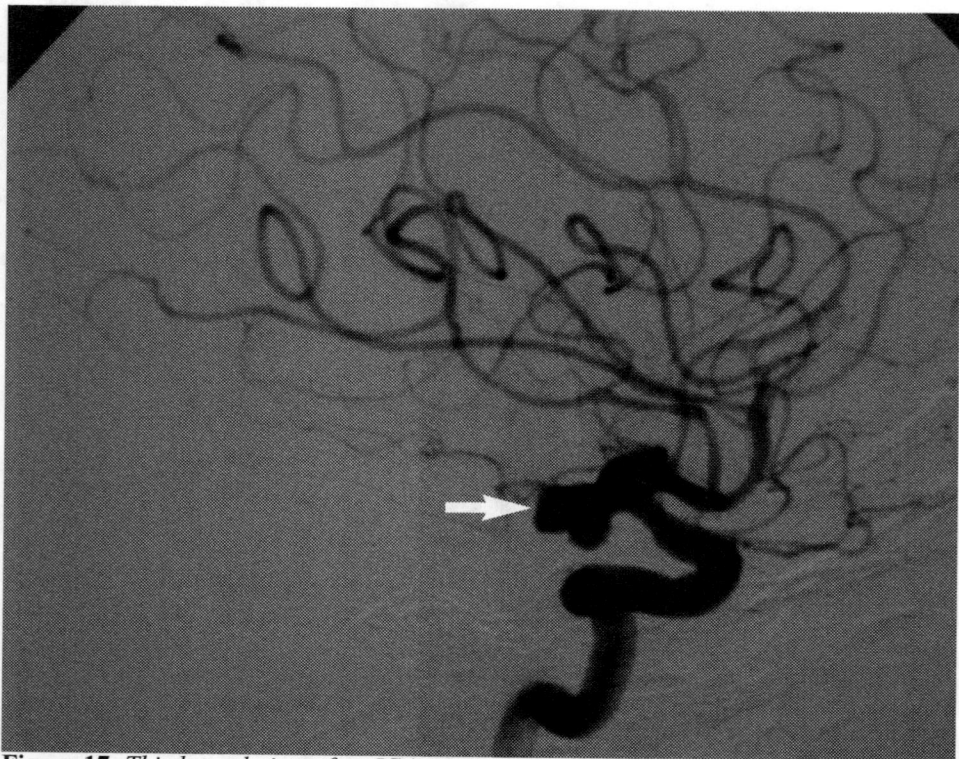

Figure 17. *This lateral view of an ICA angiogram demonstrates a posterior communicating artery aneurysm (arrow)*

How to study a cerebral angiogram

The orientation of the images is studied first whether it is in the lateral/antero-posterior or oblique plane. This could be obtained by studying the background image of the skull in the subtracted film. The injected artery should be identified. This could be the *internal carotid artery, external carotid artery, common carotid artery* or the *vertebral artery*. Identification of the vessels comes with practice and orientation of the image. Sometimes selective injection of a particular vessel could be difficult to identify. The arterial, capillary and venous phase of every angiogram should be studied in detail. The presence of vessel wall abnormalities such as aneurysms, rapid run – off of contrast in arterio-venous fistulas and presence of a nidus in an arterio-venous malformation should be identified. The presence of anomalies or variants should also be identified.

The *ophthalmic artery* is the first major supraclinoid branch of the ICA. It arises from the antero-medial surface of the ICA and courses towards the orbit. It is best seen in the lateral view, as it courses anteriorly towards the orbit.

The *posterior communicating artery* arises from the posterior surface of the ICA. It may be as large as the *posterior cerebral artery* and in this case is called the *fetal posterior cerebral artery*. On the A-P view the *posterior communicating artery* and *posterior cerebral artery* form a sigmoid curve with the *posterior communicating artery* occupying the lower, medial segment. On the lateral view, the *posterior communicating artery* has a variable course posteriorly towards the *posterior cerebral artery*.

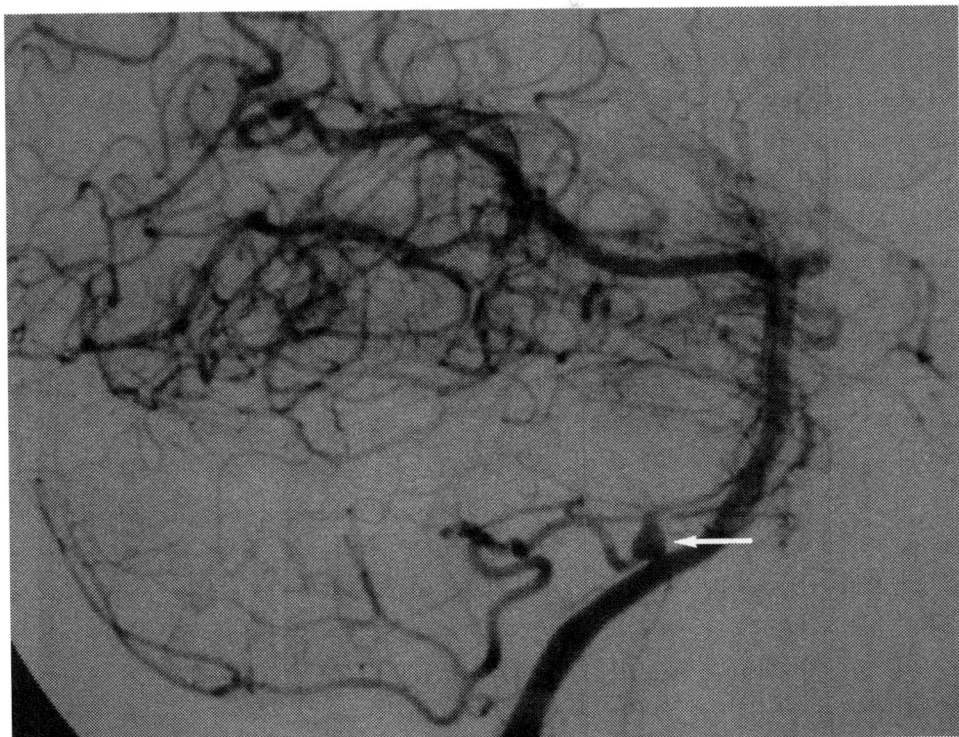

Figure 18. *This lateral view of a vertebral artery angiogram demonstrates an aneurysm (arrow) arising near the origin of the PICA.*

The *anterior choroidal artery* also arises from the posterior surface of the ICA just above the origin of the *posterior communicating artery*. It can rarely arise from the *posterior communicating artery* or the *middle cerebral artery*. It is divided into 2 segments, *cisternal* and *plexal segment*. On the A-P view the *anterior choroidal artery* is S shaped, the lower part of the S is the crural segment. On the lateral view, it courses posteriorly with the crural segment forming a superior convexity and the plexal segment forming a downward convexity.

The *anterior cerebral artery* is one of the terminal branches of the ICA bifurcation. In the antero-posterior projections, the A1 segment courses almost horisontally. The *anterior communicating artery* connects the two A1 segments in the midline and completes the anterior aspect of the circle of Willis. Visualisation of the *anterior communicating artery* requires special views such as oblique view or sub mento-vertical view and carotid cross-compression may be necessary. The A2 segment extends vertically towards the corpus callosum. In the A-P view, the A1 segments are best visualised as they approach the midline from both sides. The A2 segments lie in the inter-hemispheric fissure. In the lateral view, the A1 segment is not well visualised, but the A2 segment can be seen coursing towards the corpus callosum.

The *middle cerebral artery*

All segments of the *middle cerebral artery* are best visualised on the A-P view, while in the lateral view the M1 segment is not well visualised.

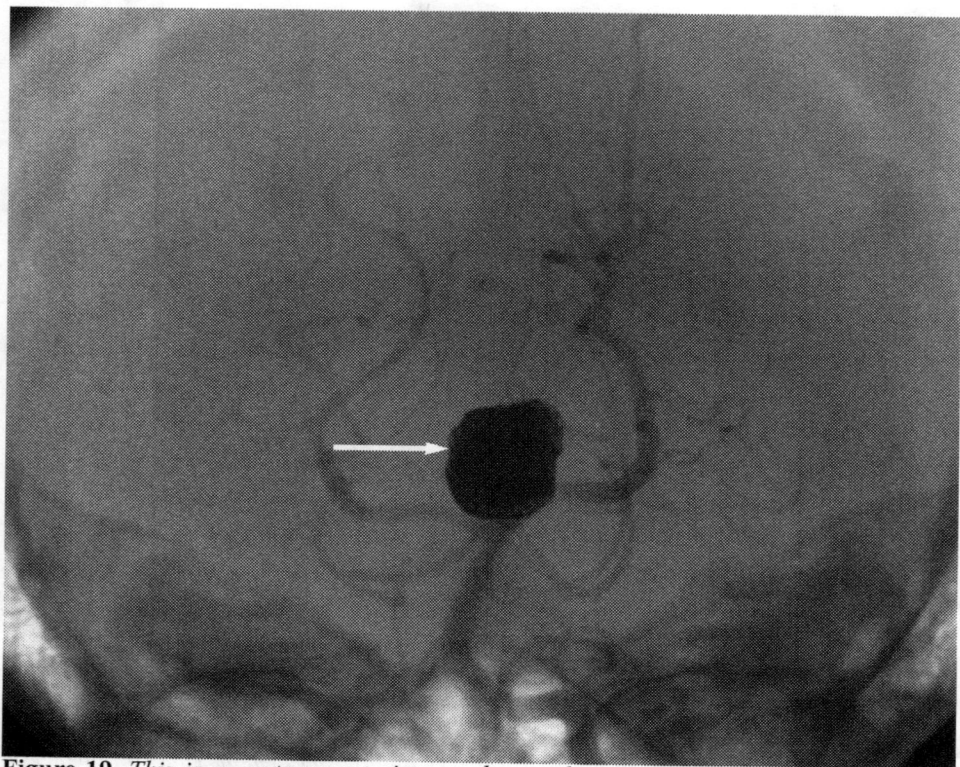

Figure 19. *This is an antero-posterior unsubtracted view of a vertebral angiogram which demonstrates a coiled basilar tip aneurysm (arrow)*

The *vertebral and basilar arteries*

The *Vertebral arteries* arise from the *subclavian arteries* on each side. The cervical and the intracranial portion are best seen on the A-P view. The *vertebral arteries* unite near the midline as an inverted Y shaped structure to form the *basilar artery*. Usually one *vertebral artery* is injected during angiography. *Vertebral artery* angiography is considered adequate if there is adequate cross flow of contrast across to the opposite *vertebral artery* up to the origin of the *posterior inferior cerebellar artery* and good visualisation of the *basilar artery* and its branches up to its bifurcation. The A-P view and the Towne's view are the best view to see the *vertebral* and *basilar arteries* with their branches.

The *posterior inferior cerebellar artery*

This is the major branch of the *vertebral artery* intracranially, and has a downward and lateral course on the A-P view and a characteristic undulant course consisting of two loops on the lateral view. It is divided into several segments such as the a*nterior medullary segment, lateral medullary segment, posterior medullary segment, supra-tonsillar segment, retro-tonsillar segment* and the *inferior vermian segment.*

The *anterior inferior cerebellar arteries*

These are two of the major branches arising from the basilar artery. They are well seen on the A-P view. They course laterally almost at right angles to the basilar artery trunk towards the internal acoustic meatus. The anterior inferior cerebellar artery size has a reciprocal relationship to the size of the posterior inferior cerebellar artery.

The *superior cerebellar artery*

This artery arises just proximal to the terminal *basilar artery* bifurcation into the *posterior cerebral arteries.* The A-P view visualises the proximal part of the vessel well while the distal part is seen best on the lateral view.

Veins

The *vein of Trolard* is the prominent superficial anastomotic vein from the *superficial middle cerebral vein* to the *superior sagittal sinus* (usually on the non-dominant side). The *vein of Labbé* is a cortical vein usually on the dominant side anastomosing the superficial *middle cerebral vein* to the *transverse sinus*. The major dural sinuses are best seen on the lateral view of the angiogram in the venous phase. The *superior sagittal sinus, inferior sagittal sinus, straight sinus, sigmoid sinus* and the *petrosal sinuses* are best seen in this view. The A-P view delineates the *transverse sinuses*, posterior aspect of the *sagittal sinus* and the *sigmoid sinuses*. The *superficial cortical* and the *deep cerebral veins* are best seen in the lateral view of the venous phase of the cerebral angiogram. The deep veins opacify late in the venous phase. The *thalamostriate vein, internal cerebral veins* and the *basal vein of Rosenthal* have characteristic configurations on the angiogram.

The lateral view of the venous phase of the vertebral angiogram show the *internal cerebral veins, vein of Galen, straight sinus, precentral cerebellar vein, superior vermian vein, inferior vermian vein* and *clival venous plexus*. The venous phase of the angiogram is essential to plan an approach that involves skeletonising or ligating a sinus such as the *sigmoid sinus*.

Evaluation of a patient with subarachnoid haemorrhage

Location of blood on a CT scan gives a clue to the site of aneurysm rupture. A complete angiographic evaluation with multiple projections of the intracranial circulation is essential starting from the region of interest based on the distribution of blood on the CT scan. Temporary cross-compression of the opposite *carotid artery* whilst injecting the ipsilateral *carotid artery* may be needed to visualise the region of the *anterior communicating artery* (the most common site of midline aneurysmal bleed). Similarly, the ipsilateral *posterior communicating artery* may be visualised with compression of the ipsilateral *carotid artery* and injecting a *vertebral artery*. *Carotid* compression should be avoided if cervical *carotid* atherosclerosis is noted. Cross-circulation should always be checked in relevant aneurysms especially in the *anterior communicating artery, posterior communicating artery* or giant aneurysms of the internal carotid artery, if temporary or permanent parent artery occlusion is necessary. The origins of both PICA's should be visualised. Multiple aneurysms should always be looked for in the angiogram. If multiple aneurysms are present, then the aneurysm that has bled must be identified. A useful clue would be the distribution of blood on the CT brain scan. Other clues would be focal vasospasm and irregular shape of the aneurysm sac with a nipple like configuration. Large aneurysms tend to bleed more and midline locations such as *anterior communicating artery* aneurysms have a high tendency to bleed. It is also usually the most proximal aneurysm that has bled. The aneurysm that had bled must be studied in detail, especially the neck, fundus, its relationship with the parent vessel and any branches arising from it. A 3-D reconstruction is helpful in difficult cases and for planning treatment. Associated vascular anomalies should also be noted, as well as presence of vasospasm, thrombus, contrast leak and mass effect. An infundibulum should be distinguished from aneurysms especially in the *posterior communicating artery*. An infundibulum is usually less than 3mm and appears rounded or conical and the vessel takes origin from the apex. Angio-negative subarachnoid haemorrhage could occur with spontaneously thrombosed small aneurysms, vascular malformations such as cavernomas, spinal vascular malformations, tumour bleeds, and non-aneurysmal perimesencephalic haemorrhage. Further radiological investigations may be needed in these cases. Dissecting aneurysms are more frequent in the vertebral circulation. The presence of a string sign, double lumen or retention of contrast in the venous phase are diagnostic. CT angiography and MR angiography have similar diagnostic accuracy of about 90% in the detection of intracranial aneurysms. Sensitivity is poorer for both in the detection of small aneurysms less than 3 mm and CT angiography is better than MR angiography.

Evaluation of a patient with an arteriovenous malformation

A complete angiographic evaluation of the intracranial circulation is essential which should include the arterial, capillary and venous phase, starting from the region of interest, since bilateral supply to the vascular malformation can occur. A super-selective study with micro-catheters of each individual feeding artery could help in planning management.

Associated aneurysms, their location, venous ectasia, stenosis and flow patterns should be analysed. The use of high-density contrast, magnification and increasing the frame rate to six per second also helps in the planning study. The nidus angio-architecture should be studied in detail to look for nature of the nidus whether it is plexiform or mixed with plexiform-fis-tulous nature. (Plexiform is a network or tangle of blood vessels whereas fistula is an abnor-mal communication between an artery and a vein).

Vascular malformations of the central nervous system

An aneurysm is an abnormal sac filled with blood in direct communication with the interi-or of a blood vessel. True aneurysms are lined by the arterial wall and false aneurysms are lined by condensed connective tissue, which communicates with the vascular compartment. True aneurysms may be saccular, fusiform or dissecting in type.

An arteriovenous malformation is a tangle of blood vessel anastomoses of varying caliber in which arteriovenous shunting occurs in a central nidus. Multiple feeding arteries converge towards this area and from this area, enlarged draining veins drain. They are usually located in the subpial space and are frequently congenital.

An arteriovenous fistula is a direct fistulous connection between an artery and a vein with-out a nidus. They could be single or multiple.

Dural arteriovenous fistulas (AVF) are abnormal direct arteriovenous shunts in the dura, between meningeal arteries of the internal carotid artery, external carotid artery, vertebro-basilar system on the one hand and the veins of the lepto-meninges, cortical veins and dural sinuses on the other hand. Sometimes pial arteries may contribute to the arterial supply. The aetiology is considered to be acquired and due to venous thrombosis. A fistula occurring between the carotid artery or its branches and the cavernous sinus directly or indirectly, is known as a **carotid cavernous fistula (CCF)**. A direct CCF arises from a defect in the cav-ernous segment of the internal carotid artery which drains directly into the cavernous sinus. This is a high flow fistula. A dural AVF of the cavernous sinus is a low flow fistulas and is supplied by dural branches of the internal carotid artery, external carotid artery or both.

Spinal dural arteriovenous fistulas are more common than arteriovenous malformations in the spine. The arterial supply may be from one or more segmental arteries. The fistula is at the level of the intervertebral foramen and venous drainage is usually through a single vein, which pierces the dura close to the segmental nerve root.

True **Vein of Galen malformations** are characterised by the presence of an aneurysmally dilated midline deep venous structure, fed by abnormal arteriovenous communications.

The dilated venous structure is the enlarged persistent median prosencephalic vein. Vein of Galen aneurysmal dilatation is caused by parenchymal arteriovenous malformations or dural arteriovenous fistulas draining into a dilated vein of Galen.

Other cerebrovascular malformations that have been described include developmental venous anomalies (venous angiomas), cavernous angiomas and capillary telangiectasias.

Type A	Direct CCF between the cavernous ICA and the cavernous sinus.
Type B	Dural AVF due to shunt between the cavernous ICA meningeal branches and the cavernous sinus.
Type C	Dural AVF due to shunt between the ECA meningeal branches and cavernous sinus.
Type D	Dural AVF due to shunt between the cavernous ICA meningeal branches and ECA meningeal branches with the cavernous sinus.

Table 1. *Barrow's classification of CCF*

Type I	DAVF draining into a sinus, with a normal antegrade flow direction
Type II	DAVF draining into a sinus. Insufficient antegrade venous drainage and reflux. The insufficiency of the venous drainage may be due to stenosis or occlusion of the sinus draining a moderate flow rate DAVF, or to a very high flow rate DAVF that cannot be drained by a normal or even enlarged sinus. Depending on the retrograde venous drainage, 3 subtypes
Type II a	Retrograde venous drainage into sinus(es) only
Type II b	Retrograde venous drainage into cortical vein(s) only
Type II a+b	Retrograde venous drainage into sinus(es) and cortical vein(s)
Type III	DAVF draining directly into a cortical vein without venous ectasia
Type IV	DAVF draining directly into a cortical vein with a venous ectasia More than 5mm in diameter and three times larger than the diameter of the draining vein.
Type V	DAVF (intracranial) draining into spinal perimedullary veins

Table 2. *Dural AVF (Revised Classification of Djindjian & Merland)*

Type I	Drainage to meningeal veins or dural sinuses
Type II	Type I as well as retrograde leptomeningeal venous drainage
Type III	Retrograde venous drainage only

Table 3. *Borden's classification of dural AVF*

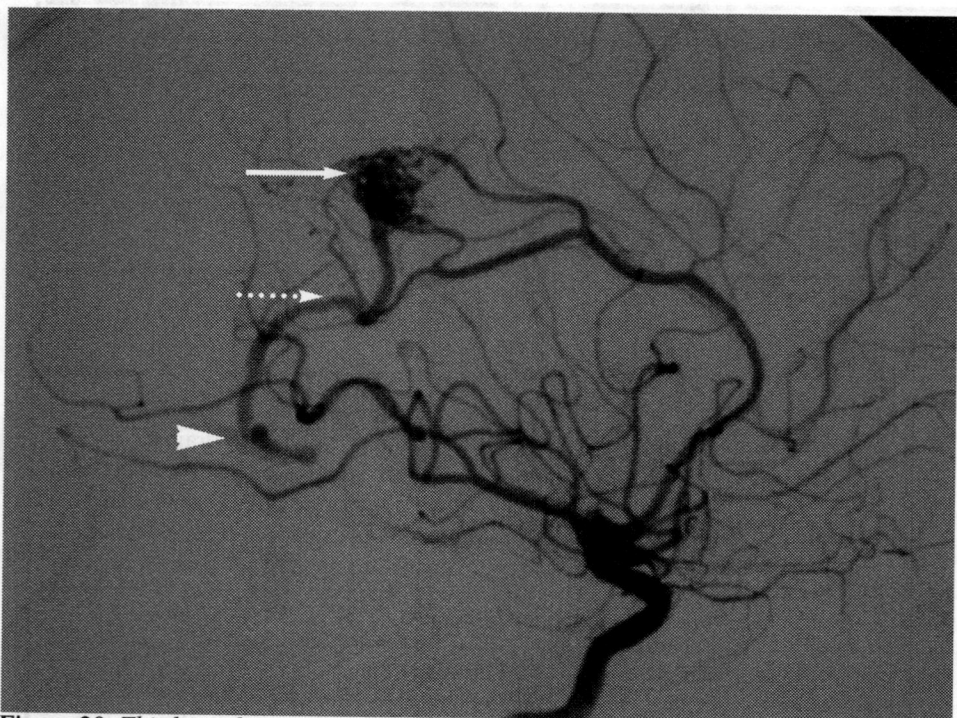

Figure 20. *This lateral view of an ICA angiogram demonstrates the nidus (arrow) of an AVM being fed by branches of the distal ACA. A large draining vein is seen draining the nidus (dashed arrow). The straight sinus (arrow head) is faintly visible.*

Preparation for cerebral angiography

Indication: The patient should fulfill the relevant clinical and morphological criteria to be investigated by cerebral angiography. The common indications are subarachnoid haemorrhage, vasospasm, intracerebral or intraventricular haemorrhage, vascular occlusive disease, vasculitis, arterio-venous malformation and evaluating the vascular supply of tumours. It is also used for physiologic testing of brain function and to outline vascular anatomy for planning and determining the effect of therapeutic measures.

Examination: The patient is assessed with a detailed history, past medical condition including allergies and the neurological state. Patients should be well hydrated before the procedure. The peripheral pulse in the legs should be examined before proceeding for a transfemoral puncture. Blood pressure should be under good control if the patient is hypertensive. Children who develop seizures and uncooperative patients may require general anaesthetic.

Investigation: The blood biochemistry, coagulation profile and the CT scan or MRI of the patient is studied to anticipate which vascular territory need to be evaluated first.

Consent: The patient is educated on the procedure and informed consent obtained which includes discussion of the indication to do cerebral angiography, nature of the procedure, the potential alternative investigations, the discomfort and risks and benefits of the procedure.

Angiography team: The angiography team should include a radiographer, scrub nurse, assistant scrub nurse and the angiographer. An anaesthetist and anaesthetic nurse are needed if general anaesthesia is required. Generally cerebral angiography is performed under local anaesthesia at the femoral arterial puncture site and without sedation.

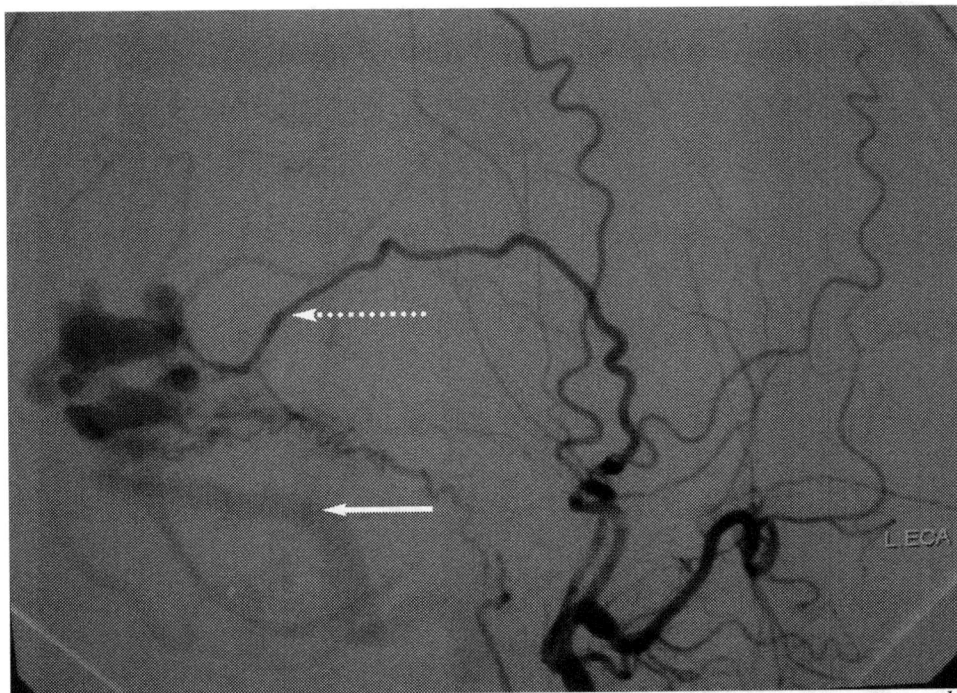

Figure 21. *This lateral view of an external carotid artery angiogram demonstrates a dural arterio-venous fistula fed by branches of the middle meningeal artery (dashed arrow) and draining into the sigmoid sinus (arrow).*

Preparation: A good intravenous access site, pulse oximetry and blood pressure monitoring is essential. The anaesthetic equipment must be in good working condition in case of an emergency conversion of a local anaesthetic procedure to a general anaesthetic procedure. The angiography tray should be checked for completeness. The arterial sheath and catheter is flushed with heparinised saline.

An algorithm should be used to study the cerebral vessels
a) First vessel to be injected should be the side of the pathology.
b) Carotid artery disease should be looked for.
c) Decide whether an external carotid artery injection is needed.
d) All cerebral vessels should be studied to look for multiple aneurysms
e) A knowledge of the collateral circulation is essential.
Temporary cross compression of the contralateral internal carotid artery may be needed to visualise the anterior communicating artery. Similarly the posterior communicating artery can be visualised by manual compression of the carotid artery during vertebral injection (Huber maneuver/Alcock's test)

To properly visualise the circle of Willis, it is essential to give up to a total of 10-12 ml contrast per second. The procedure should be of reasonably short duration. Excessive volumes of contrast agent (more than 200 ml) should be avoided.
In arteriovenous malformations larger and faster boluses of contrast is required and filming is at a minimum of 4 – 6 frames/second. Selective catheterisation and study of a feeding artery to an arteriovenous malformation or a tumour may give more detail of the pattern of blood supply.

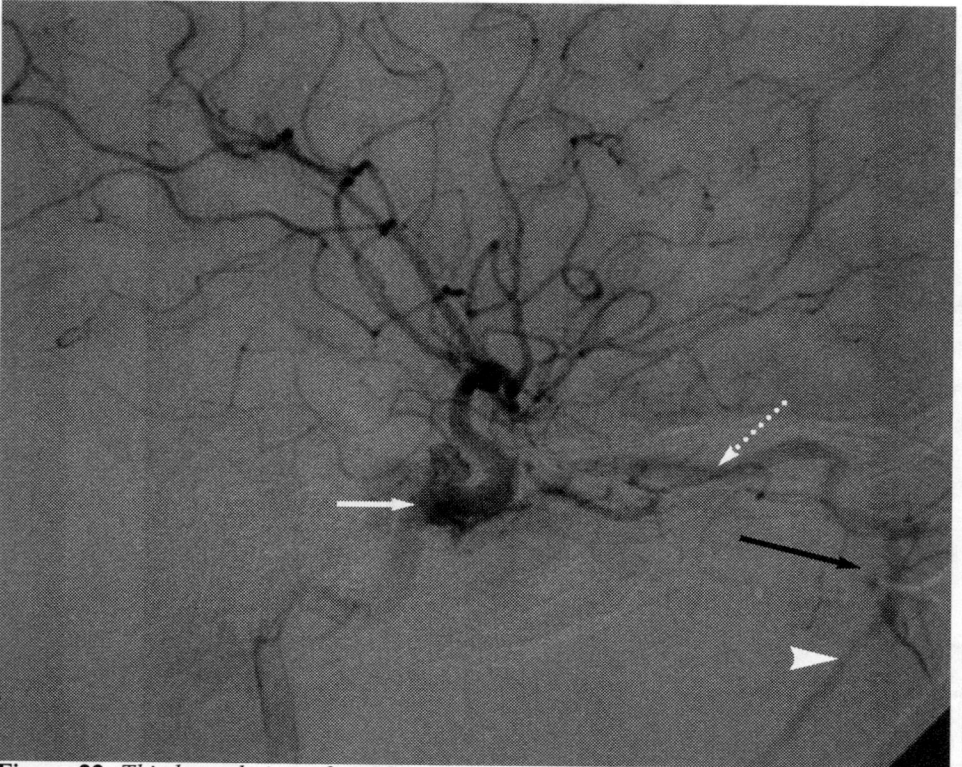

Figure 22. *This lateral view of an ICA angiogram demonstrates a carotid cavernous fistula (arrow) with anterior drainage into the superior ophthalmic vein (dotted arrow) and towards the angular vein (black arrow) and into the anterior facial vein (arrow head)*

Procedure of cerebral angiography

The access for cerebral angiography is usually through the transfemoral route, but other routes like percutaneous carotid and vertebral artery puncture, superficial temporal artery catheterisation and intravenous angiography are of historic interest. Subclavian, retrograde brachial and axillary angiography is used in selected cases. The disadvantage of the transfemoral route is the need for up to 6 hours leg immobilisation following the procedure for the fear of delayed haemorrhage, haematoma and pseudo-aneurysm formation and infection. Newer devices such as the collagen plug devices (Angio-seal, VasoSeal) and percutaneous suture devices (Perclose) are useful

Catheters

Catheters should be biocompatible, have low thrombogenicity and have a visible tip on X-ray.

Diagnostic catheters: Simmons type II (elderly patients with tortuous vessels), Mani, Headhunter, JB-II.

Guide Catheters: they are usually 5-7 French, thin walled with wide inner bore.

Microcatheters: Microcatheter technology has allowed navigation into the distal cerebral circulation. These are two types, the flow directed and the wire directed type. Some flow directed catheters can accept wires. These catheters are hydrophilic (hydrolene coating) and less thrombogenic. Catheters are made of polyethylene and polyamide. The ideal catheter for most circumstances will have low internal and external frictional resistance and low kink resistance. They are used for super selective angiography.

Micro-guidewires are used during cannulation of small caliber vessels.

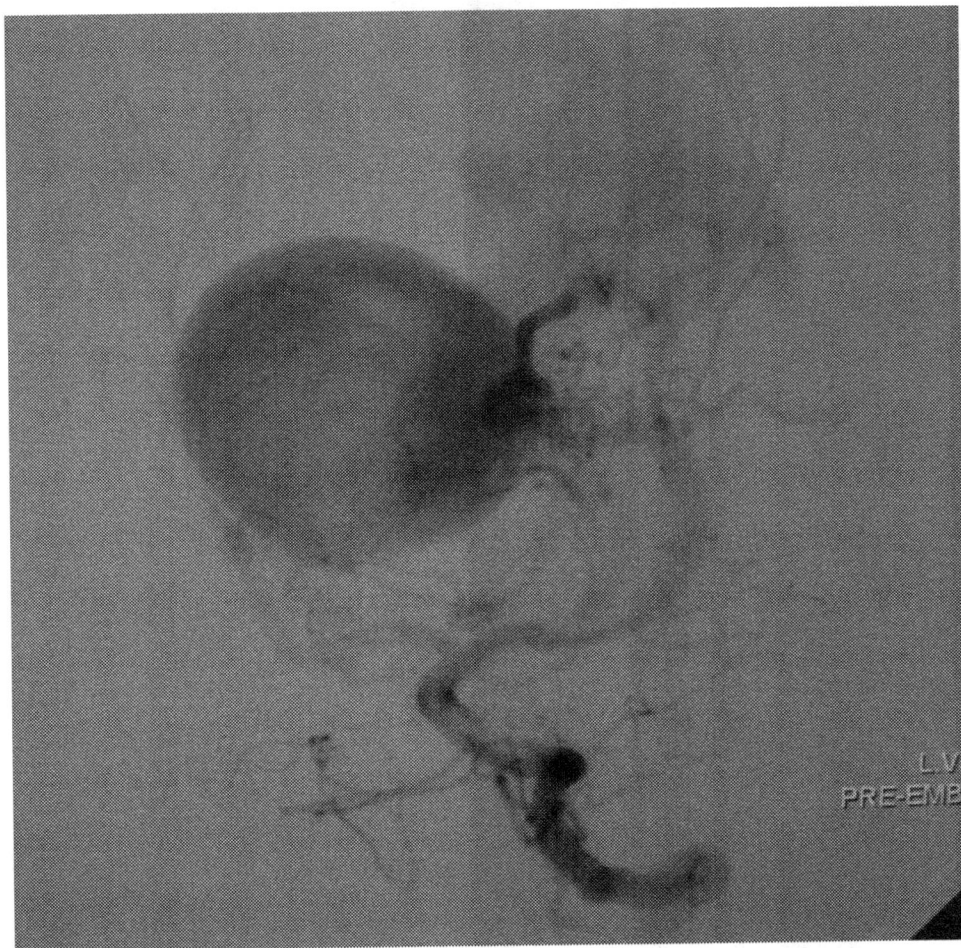

Figure 23. *This antero-posterior view of a left vertebral angiogram demonstrates the presence of a vein of Galen malformation being fed by the choroidal arteries*

The common femoral artery is palpated near the medial aspect of the femoral head. Local anaesthetic is infiltrated around the artery. The artery is punctured about 2-3 cm below the inguinal ligament. A small incision on the inguinal skin crease is made with a scalpel. The femoral artery is fixed in position and a needle is inclined to 45 degrees and with the bevel facing upwards is advanced into the femoral artery. A spurt of arterial blood should be appreciated and using the Seldinger technique, the 3mm guide wire is smoothly passed into the artery.

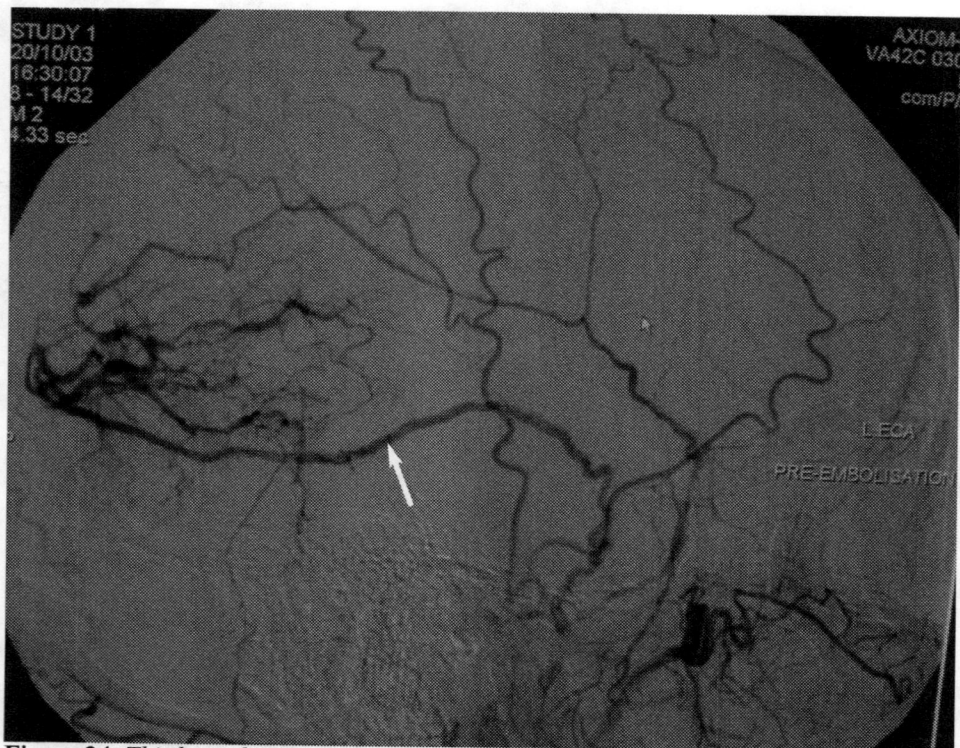

Figure 24. *This lateral view of an external carotid angiogram demonstrates a vascular blush due to a meningioma being fed by the posterior branch of the middle meningeal artery (arrow).*

Contrast agent

Any agent introduced into the tissues, globally or selectively, in order to modify contrast may be termed a contrast enhancing agent. Contrast may be changed artificially by introducing materials either with a different atomic number or by introducing materials with different density. Enhancement may be positive or negative. Iodine (mean atomic number Z = 53) is widely used as a contrast agent. Both high osmolar (ionic) and a low osmolar (non-ionic) contrast material is used in angiography. The total volume of non-ionic contrast, which could be safely used in cerebral angiography, could be roughly calculated as follows:

maximum tolerable contrast dose = Kg body weight x 5 divided by serum creatinine mg/dl. Intravascular contrast has a β half-life (elimination) of 1.5 – 2 hours in a patient with normal renal function, but this could be prolonged in renal impairment. Contrast material with concentration of more than 320mg of organic iodine per ml is generally contraindicated. In patients with renal insufficiency and those allergic to iodinated contrast agents, gadolinium could be used as an alternative. In children when the dosage of iodinated contrast approaches a toxicity level, gadolinium is an alternative.

Spinal angiography

It is the gold standard investigation for vascular lesions of the spine and spinal cord. It also helps to identify the origin of *spinal arteries* prior to spinal surgery. The angiographic study should include the pathological region of interest and the surrounding normal tissue to ensure the study to be complete. This may include study of the spinal vasculature on either side from the foramen magnum to the sacrum to look for possible dural arteriovenous malformation or fistula. It is preferable to do spinal angiograms under general anaesthesia to reduce movement artifacts with controlled respiration. Identification or marking the levels of the spine is an essential preliminary prerequisite in spinal angiography. The frontal view gives most of the information needed especially in the thoracic and lumbar spine. A lateral view may be needed if the cord appears to be rotated due to a mass lesion and a 3-D reconstruction is useful at the cervical level in difficult anatomic situations. A complete spinal angiogram should include a study of the *vertebral artery, external carotid artery, thyro-cervical trunks,* and *costo-cervical trunks* including the *superior intercostal artery, supreme intercostal arteries, segmental arteries from T4 to L3, median sacral artery* and the *lateral sacral arteries.* *Internal carotid* injections may be needed in anomalous *external carotid* branches origins. The orientation of the *segmental arteries* follows a smooth progression from cranial to caudal. The rostral (higher) vessels tend to point cephalad and the caudal (lower) vessels point inferiorly at their origin. Various catheters (such as Cobra -2, HS-1 or Mikaelsson) are used for spinal angiography based on operator preference.

Intra-operative angiography
This procedure is done in the operating room to enable the neurosurgeon to check for the adequacy of clip placement in difficult aneurysms or to look for any residual feeders after arterio-venous malformation excision. At the beginning of surgery, a sheath is placed in the *femoral artery* on a slow flowing low-dose heparinised irrigating system. The patient's head is fixed on a radiolucent head holder. When angiography is required, usually the common carotid injection with high-density contrast material (300 non-ionic) is sufficient for the anterior circulation using a mobile fluoroscopy unit.

Wada test
The Wada test is a functional test of cerebral structures. It is a useful adjunct in planning seizure surgery. It localises the dominance of the cerebral hemisphere with relation to language and whether the cerebral hemisphere contralateral to the epileptogenic focus is capable of supporting memory after cortical resection of the epileptogenic focus. A base-line assessment of neurological function and EEG is performed followed by a cerebral angiogram to evaluate the distribution of the *internal carotid artery*, to check for cross-flow, *carotid-basilar* anastomosis and arterio-venous malformation. Each cerebral hemisphere is then anaesthetised with selective injection of sodium Amytal into the *internal carotid artery*. Simultaneous EEG monitoring is done. A neurologist and a neuro-psychologist do a battery of tests to check for cerebral dominance and memory function. The test is contra-indicated if a carotid-basilar anastomosis is present, which could lead to anaesthesia of the brain stem due to direct supply from the carotid artery to the basilar artery.

Inferior petrosal sinus sampling
Plasma adrenocorticotropic hormone (ACTH) levels are determined by radioimmunoassay, which is elevated in patients with Cushing's disease and in patients with an ectopic source of adrenocorticotropic hormone. The assay is more definitive, if the venous blood is obtained from the organ suspected of being the site of abnormal secretion. This assay is best used by selective sampling for adrenocorticotropic hormone in blood from the *petrosal sinus*, which contains the venous effluent from the pituitary gland. Furthermore, it also helps to localise the side of the pituitary gland harbouring the tumour secreting abnormal levels of the hormone by measuring the differences in the levels of the ACTH between the two petrosal sinuses.

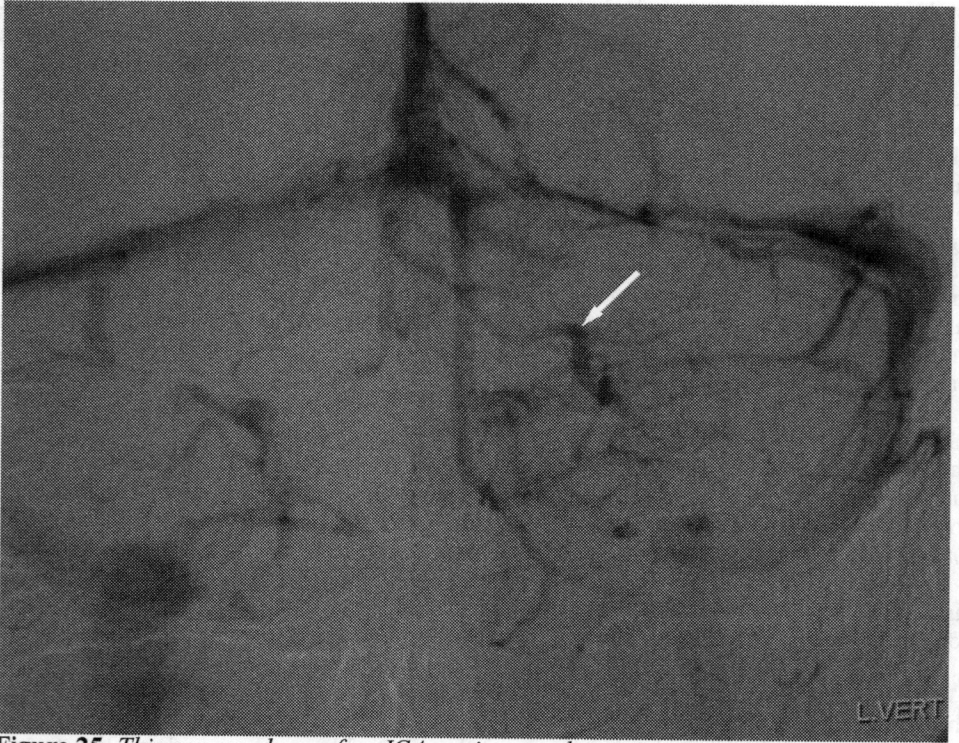

Figure 25. *This venous phase of an ICA angiogram demonstrates a caput medusae appearance with a draining vein (arrow) which is typical of a developmental venous anomaly.*

Complications of cerebral angiography

Angiography is an invasive procedure, hence it should be used judiciously by trained operators who are sufficiently skilled with neuro angiography techniques and are knowledgeable with neurovascular anatomy and pathology to avoid and deal with any complications, which may arise. Every cerebral angiogram carries a potential risk of stroke. Knowledge of radiation physics and radiation biology is also essential for patient and the angiography team safety.

Local complications related to the puncture site include haematoma formation at the femoral puncture site in about 6.9 - 10.7%, retroperitoneal haematoma, femoral nerve damage, sepsis, deep venous thrombosis, pseudoaneurysm formation, dissection and arterio-venous fistula. Avascular necrosis of femoral head and leg length discrepancies due to vascular stenosis in children has also been described. Airway compromise in carotid punctures has also been reported.

Contrast material related complications include non-allergic complications like renal impairment in patients who were dehydrated or had previous renal disease, and patients with multiple myeloma. Patients with diabetes mellitus who are on metformin therapy could develop lactic acidosis.

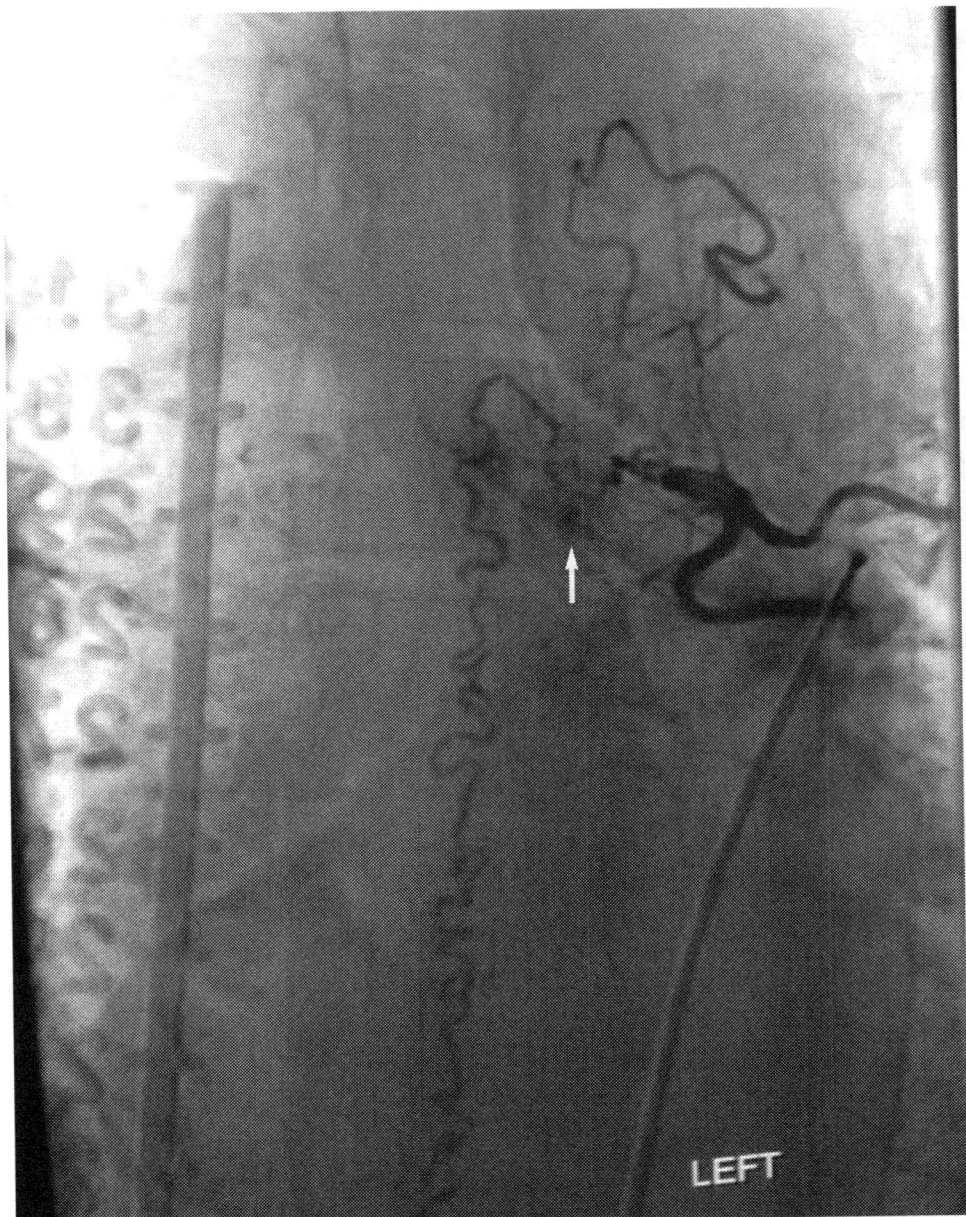

Figure 26. *This spinal angiogram in the antero-posterior plane demonstrates a spinal dural arteriovenous fistula (arrow). The tortuous vessels in the midline are dilated veins. Note the markings of the levels of the spine which is essential for localising the correct level.*

Contrast related neurotoxicity is usually self-limiting and include cortical blindness, tinnitus, amnesia and mono ballismus. Myocardial infarction, cardiac arrest, nausea and vomiting, cardiac arrhythmias, paresthesia in the lower limbs are other reported complications. Allergic reaction to contrast is uncommon with non-ionic contrast media.

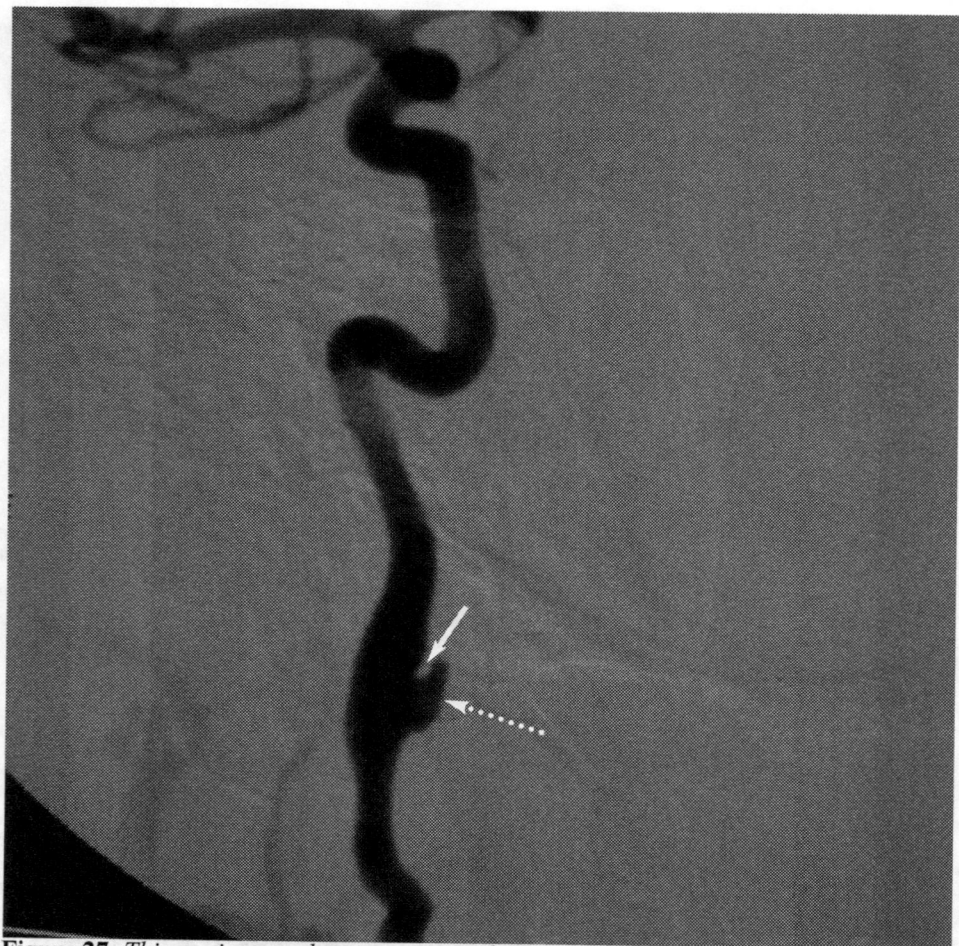

Figure 27. *This angiogram demonstrates evidence of intimal dissection (arrow) as a double lumen (dotted arrow) which arose during vessel catheterisation.*

The incidence is about one in 2500 patients. Patients with known allergic history could be premedicated with steroids and anti-histamines or an alternative contrast agent such as gadolinium could be used.

Neurologic complications within 24-72 hours of cerebral angiography occurs in 0.5 – 4%. These are transient deficits with permanent deficits occurring in 0.1-0.5%. Compromise of cerebral blood flow is the commonest event.

Thromboembolic complications due to clots, air, foreign bodies or plaques can occur which could be avoided with meticulous technique.

Non-embolic vascular complications such as vessel rupture, aneurysm rupture, and vasospasm can occur.

The risk of neuroangiography is higher in older patients with advanced age with atherosclerosis, acute subarachnoid haemorrhage, certain vascular dysplasia such as Ehler Danlos syndrome and in migraine patients. The risks are also related to the length of the procedure, number of catheter exchanges, catheter size and manipulation and the amount of contrast medium used. Non-ionic low osmolarity contrast media are safer than ionic, high osmolarity contrast media among in patients with previous history of contrast medium hypersensitivity or nephropathy. The risk of contrast medium induced nephropathy is greater in patients with diabetes mellitus with pre-existing azotemia.

Conclusion

The introduction of less invasive imaging techniques such as magnetic resonance angiography and computed tomographic angiography have been complimentary to the diagnostic evaluation of neurovascular pathology by digital subtraction angiography (DSA). DSA still plays a significant role because of its superior spatial resolution and the flow information obtained. Moreover, the advances in interventional neuroradiology have further highlighted the importance of neuro angiography in neurovascular pathology.

8

BRAIN TUMOURS

W Adriaan Liebenberg

Contents

Epidemiology
Genetics factors in brain tumours
Environmental factors in brain tumours
Neuropathology
Tumours according to anatomical distribution
Tumours according to the WHO classification
Neuroepithelial tumours of the CNS
Other CNS neoplasms

Adjuvant therapies
Radiotherapy
Chemotherapy

Neurofibromatosis and other phakomatoses
Von Hippel – Lindau (VHL) syndrome
WHO classification of CNS tumours

Epidemiology

The annual incidence of primary brain tumours is about 10-20 per 100,000 person years. Brain tumours are either primary or secondary. Primary brain tumours can be divided according to their histology. The most prevalent primary brain tumours are meningiomas which occur in about 25% of all primary brain tumours, followed by glioblastomas which occur in about 23%. Astrocytomas occur in around 11% and nerve sheath tumours follow at 8%. Ependymomas, oligodendrogliomas, medulloblastomas, craniopharyngiomas, pituitary tumours and lymphomas all individually constitute less than 5% each of all primary brain tumours.

Genetic factors in brain tumours

Brain tumours are caused by a combination of unchecked proliferation of a cell line as well as decreased apoptosis. This occurs when there is loss of control of the cell cycle and of programmed cell death (apoptosis). The cell cycle and cell death are normally well controlled and is disrupted by a combination of a suppression or inactivation of tumour suppression genes and an over expression and amplification of oncogenes. This occurs due to the accumulation of a series of genetic mutations.

221

Tumour suppressor genes - In brain tumours, the most frequently found genetic aberration is that of the tumour suppressor gene *p53* located on chromosome 17p. The *p53* gene is a transcription factor that induces and suppresses several genes that have influences on the cell cycle, genomic stability and programmed cell death. This mutation of the *p53* gene happens early in the series of genetic alterations that occur and is present in more than 50% of all gliomas. The *p53* protein up regulates the transcription of the *p21* gene that blocks the cell in the G_1 phase. Another effect of the *p53* protein is to up regulate BAX (BAX proteins regulate apoptosis in cellular pathways), which promotes apoptosis. The absence of this protein (and resultant decrease in *p21* and BAX) leads to uncontrolled cell proliferation. Other important suppressor genes are located on chromosome 9p (gene *16p*), chromosome 22q and chromosome 10.

Oncogenes – Gene amplification is a common activation pathway for oncogenes which leads to an overstimulation of growth. There are three sets of growth factors implicated in the formation of glial tumours. These growth factors all have tyrosine receptors and are epidermal growth factor (chromosome 7), platelet derived growth factor (chromosome 17p) and basic fibroblast growth factor. Another group of oncogenes on chromosome 12q inactivate the gene products of tumour suppression genes.

Environmental factors in brain tumours

There are several risk factors that may play a role such as exposure to ionising radiation, non-ionising radiation (electro magnetic field radiation), maternal alcohol consumption, chronic aspartame ingestion, exposure to vinyl chloride, infections like tuberculosis and HIV and previous cranial trauma.

Neuropathology

Most histological specimens are interpreted with hematoxylin and eosin staining. There are other stains to assist the pathologist in differentiating tissues. Reticulin is useful in differentiating meningiomas and pericytomas, and trichrome is useful in differentiating collagen and glial tissue.

Immunohistochemistry is probably the most useful adjunct in neuropathology:

Glial fibrillary acidic protein (GFAP) is a filamentous protein that is specifically expressed by astrocytes and therefore astrocytic tumours or tumours that are mixed and contain astrocytes express it. Up to 50% of ependymomas also express it.
Neuron specific enolase (NSE), synaptophysin and neurofilament, as their names suggest, are expressed by neuronal tumours as well as medulloblastomas.
Meningiomas and choroid plexus tumours express *epithelial membrane antigen (EMA)*.
Leucocyte common antigen as well as B and T-cell markers are expressed by lymphomas.

Markers of cell proliferation help to build up a biological profile of a tumour. Bromodeoxyuridine, Ki-67 and MIB-1 are markers that are frequently used. Bromodeoxyuridine is a thymidine analogue that is taken up by cells in the S-phase of the cell cycle and Ki-67 and MIB-1 is expressed by cells in all phases of the cell cycle except for G_0

Tumours according to anatomical distribution
Tumours of the skull base
Skull base tumours are difficult to treat since they abut critical neurological and vascular

structures and complete resection is difficult if not impossible. A clue to the possible diagnosis might be gained from the anatomical location of the tumour. The anterior cranial fossa contains meningiomas, esthesioneuroblastomas and sometimes nasopharyngeal carcinomas; the posterior cranial fossa contains tumours of the CPA and on the floor of the posterior cranial base; chordomas, chondrosarcomas and paragangliomas. The middle cranial fossa may contain chordomas, craniopharyngiomas, pituitary adenomas, metastases and meningiomas.

Suprasellar tumours
This area may contain arachnoid cysts, Rathke's cleft cysts, pituitary adenomas, craniopharyngiomas, giant aneurysms, meningiomas and metastases. Approaches are transsphenoidal and transcranially. Transcranial approaches are via subfrontal or pterional approaches.

Tumours of the CPA (cerebellopontine angle)
This area may contain epidermoid cysts, dermoid cysts, arachnoid cysts, choroid plexus tumours, schwannomas, metastases and meningiomas. Access to it is via a retromastoid, middle fossa or translabyrinthine approach.

Tumours of the posterior fossa
Posterior fossa astrocytomas are no different in character to the supratentorial variant. The main differential diagnosis for a tumour in the posterior fossa in children is that of medulloblastoma, ependymoma and astrocytoma. Medulloblastomas usually are in the midline with astrocytomas and ependymomas being off-centre. Astrocytomas (especially pilocytic astrocytomas) are more frequently cystic than ependymomas.

Intraventricular tumours
These can be ependymomas, subependymomas, choroid plexus tumours, meningiomas, subependymal giant cell astrocytomas or central neurocytomas.

Pineal region tumours
These tumours most commonly cause obstructive hydrocephalus, Parinaud's syndrome (paresis of upward gaze) and nystagmus. The differential diagnosis for tumours in this region include germ cell tumours, pineal parenchymal tumours, pineal cysts, meningiomas, dermoids and epidermoids, gliomas and vascular abnormalities like aneurysms.

Tumours according to the WHO classification

Neuroepithelial tumours of the CNS

Gliomas
Gliomas are primary brain tumours that are made up of the three basic glial cells; namely astrocytes, oligodendrocytes and ependymal cells. Astrocytic gliomas are more common than oligodendroglial tumours or ependymal tumours. Astrocytic tumours can be divided into the following groups; low grade astrocytoma (grade 2), anaplastic astrocytoma (grade 3) and glioblastoma multiforme (grade 4, WHO grading scheme) and three more tumours that are not included in the above but are denoted grade 1. These tumours are the juvenile pilocytic astrocytomas, pleomorphic xanthoastrocytoma and subependymal giant cell astrocytomas. All three these tumours have vascular proliferation and nuclear atypia that would in the normal grading scheme place them in the anaplastic group, yet they continue to grow slowly with mostly an indolent course.

Astrocytic tumours
(Low grade) Astrocytoma (WHO grade II)
This accounts for about 10% of all gliomas. The differentiation between the four grades of

gliomas is made on the presence or absence of mitotic figures, nuclear polymorphism, neo-vascularity and the presence of necrotic areas. Low-grade astrocytomas have only one of these histo-pathological features and are non-enhancing, hypodense lesions on T1 WI with minimal or no surrounding oedema on T2 WI. Median survival time is approximately 5 years although survival rates in excess of 10 years are known. Low-grade astrocytomas unfortunately have the propensity to change into more malignant astrocytomas.

Anaplastic (malignant) astrocytoma (WHO grade III)

Up to 30% of gliomas are anaplastic and defined histologically by having more than one histo-pathological feature and usually includes neovascularity. They may enhance following contrast enhancement on MRI and CT scanning and they have a median survival rate in the range of 5 years with maximal surgical, radio- and chemotherapy.

Glioblastoma multiforme (WHO grade IV)

This is the most common of the glial tumours and accounts for about half of all glial tumours. These tumours enhance on MRI scanning, usually in a heterogeneous fashion and frequently have a necrotic core (outstanding feature). Glioblastomas usually have the histological criteria of mitosis, nuclear polymorphism, neovascularity and necrosis. Median survival with aggressive treatment is in the order of about 1 year. The main prognostic factors for survival are the Karnofsky score (measures the patient's pre-morbid functional level) as well as the age at presentation.

Score	Description
100	Normal
90	Able to perform normal activity; minor signs and symptoms of disease
80	Able to perform normal activity with effort; some signs and symptoms of disease
70	Cares for self, unable to perform normal activity or to do active work
60	Requires occasional assistance but is able to care for most of own needs
50	Requires considerable assistance and frequent medical care
40	Requires special care and assistance; disabled
30	Hospitalisation indicated, although death not imminent; severely disabled
20	Hospitalisation necessary; active supportive treatment required, very sick
10	Fatal processes progressing rapidly; moribund
0	Dead

Table 1. *Karnofsky score*

Pilocytic astrocytoma (non-invasive, WHO grade I)

These tumours are prevalent in the paediatric population although a quarter of them occur in adults. It is a relatively rare astrocytic tumour accounting for less than 5% of astrocytic tumours. They are usually slow growing and relatively benign tumours and grow slowly despite having nuclear atypia and mitosis. These are the only astrocytic tumours with a defined margin histologically and on imaging they enhance vividly with contrast. Due to their defined margins, they can be excised and 10-year survival rates of 80-100% have been reported following surgery.

Subependymal giant cell astrocytoma (non-invasive, WHO grade I)

These intraventricular tumours are associated with tuberous sclerosis and occur in children and young adults. They usually arise from the head of the caudate nucleus. On imaging, they are calcified, intraventricular lesions that enhance strongly with contrast. Surgical excision is the treatment of choice and long-term survival is possible.

Pleomorphic xanthoastrocytoma (non-invasive, WHO grade I)

This tumour presents in children and young adults with seizures. On imaging they are large, superficial cortical hemispheric masses with heterogeneous appearance (solid and cystic components mixed) and calcification and enhances with contrast. Treatment is complete macroscopical removal and this is often curative.

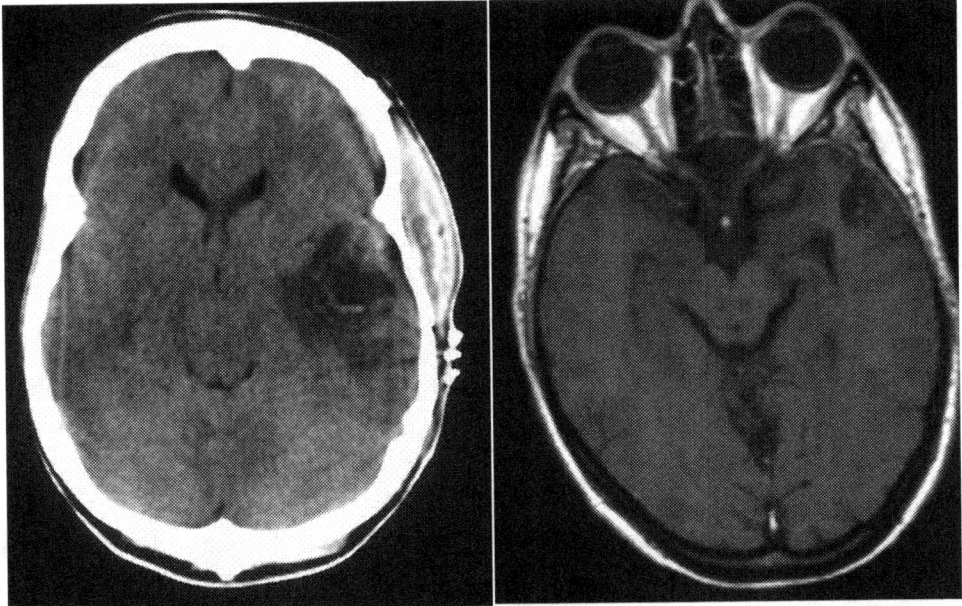

Figure 1. *Pleomorphic xanthoastrocytoma. The image on the left is a contrast enhanced axial CT scan and the image on the right is a contrast enhanced axial T1 WI. The lesion is hypodense on the CT scan and hypointense on the T1 WI.*

Oligodendroglial tumours

Oligodendroglioma (WHO grade II)

Arise from oligodendrocytes, are sensitive to both radiotherapy and chemotherapy, and have longer survival rates than astrocytomas. They usually present with seizures in the fifth and sixth decades of life and comprise as much as 20% of gliomas. They may be difficult to diagnose since there is no specific immunohistochemistry marker for them.

Anaplastic (malignant) oligodendroglioma (WHO grade III)

These are even more susceptible to chemotherapy and respond well to PCV (procarbazine, carmustine, and vincristine) chemotherapy as well as temozolomide. Median survival is 4 years compared to 15 years for oligodendrogliomas.

Ependymal cell tumours

Ependymoma (WHO grade II)

These are tumours found in the paediatric population and young adulthood. They can arise anywhere in the central nervous system but arise mostly in the ventricular system of the posterior fossa (children) and cerebrum (adults). They are relatively uncommon brain tumours and have a definite margin, so resection can be curative. They may seed throughout the CNS and the whole neuraxis should be screened for drop metastasis. Incomplete resection should be followed by radiotherapy as these tumours are very radiosensitive. The 5-year survival is in the order of 50%.

Anaplastic ependymoma (WHO grade III)
Malignant transformation warrants the use of radiotherapy and chemotherapy, although chemotherapy has limited success.

Myxopapillary ependymoma
Although they behave unpredictably, myxopapillary ependymomas in the filum terminale are less malignant than ependymomas in the spinal cord and, in turn ependymomas of the spinal cord, are less malignant than those in the posterior fossa or the cerebrum.

Subependymoma (WHO grade I)
These rare, slow growing masses arise in the ventricular system. They usually have a lobulated appearance and resection is curative.

Mixed gliomas
Mixed oligoastrocytoma (WHO grade II)
Anaplastic (malignant) oligoastrocytoma (WHO grade III)

Neuroepithelial tumours of uncertain origin
Polar spongioblastoma (WHO grade IV)
Astroblastoma (WHO grade IV)
Gliomatosis cerebri (WHO grade IV)

Tumours of the choroid plexus
Choroid plexus papilloma
These tumours are mostly found in children and arise throughout the ventricular system but are found mostly in the lateral ventricles. In adults they are found mostly in the fourth ventricle. Patients usually present with hydrocephalus and like all tumours of the ventricular system, may seed. Treatment is complete macroscopic excision and care should be exercised in these vascular tumours to isolate the blood supply early in the procedure. Gross macroscopic excision has a survival rate approaching 100%

Choroid plexus carcinoma (anaplastic choroid plexus papilloma)
Adjuvant chemotherapy and radiotherapy should be considered for these.

Neuronal and mixed neuronal-glial tumours
These are rare tumours of children and young people and arise from the neurones and neuronal elements of the CNS.

Gangliocytoma
Consist of ganglion cells and variable deposits of neoplastic glial cells. In most cases gross total macroscopic removal of these tumours leads to resolution or improvement of the seizures that are their presenting feature. Both this tumour and gangliogliomas occur mostly in the temporal lobe. These are benign tumours with a good prognosis.

Dysplastic gangliocytoma of the cerebellum (also called Lhermitte-Duclos disease)
This is a rare disease of young adults and presents with a slow growing unilateral cerebellar mass with probable hamartomatous origin. The mass frequently causes obstructive hydrocephalus. It is hypointense on T1 WI, hyperintense on T2 WI and does not enhance with contrast. It is graded as WHO I and is cured with complete resection.

Ganglioglioma

Gangliogliomas consist of purely ganglion cells. In most cases gross total macroscopic removal of these tumours leads to resolution or improvement of the seizures which, like gangliocytomas, are their presenting feature. These are benign tumours, but the glial component may undergo malignant transformation.

Anaplastic (malignant) ganglioglioma

Desmoplastic infantile ganglioglioma

These tumours present with large heterogeneous hemispheric masses in infancy. The solid component enhances intensely. These tumours are completely resectable and have a good prognosis.

Central neurocytoma

These tumours are found in the ventricular system and are histologically quite similar to oligodendrogliomas. Usually they attach to the septum pellucidum or the wall of the lateral ventricle and frequently cause obstructive hydrocephalus. On imaging, they are typically calcified with some cystic components and have variable contrast enhancement. Treatment of choice is complete surgical resection with favourable prognosis.

Dysembryoplastic neuroepithelial tumor

This is a rare condition made up of dysplastic axons, oligodendrocytes and neurons intermixed with oligodendrocytes and astrocytes. Clinical presentation is with epilepsy. They are hypointense on T1 WI and hyperintense on T2 WI. They do not commonly enhance with contrast and surgical resection is the treatment of choice with uniformly good prognosis.

Olfactory neuroblastoma (esthesioneuroblastoma)

These tumours arise from the olfactory epithelium. They involve the sinuses, anterior skull base and leptomeninges. On imaging they are heterogenous lesions with hypointensity on T1 WI, enhancement with contrast and hyperintense on T2 WI. Complete surgical resection is the aim but late recurrences are well known and lifelong follow up of the patient is necessary. This lesion metastasises in up to 30% of cases. The 5 year survival rate is in the order of 70%.

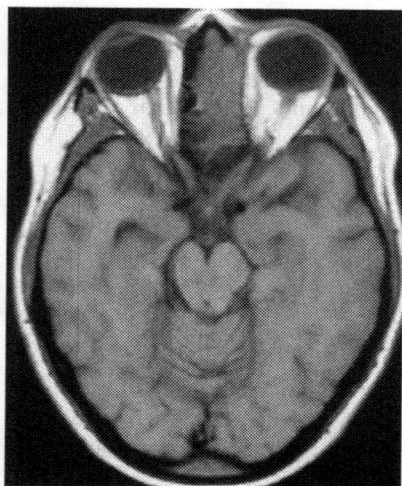

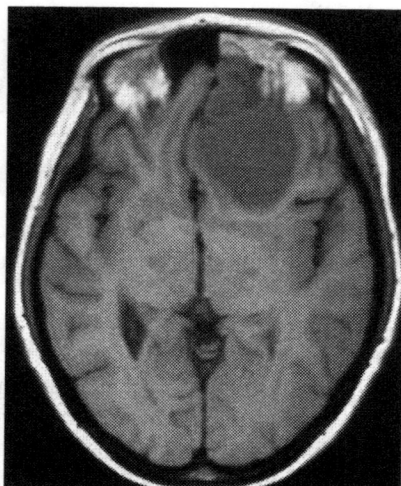

Figure 2. *Olfactory neuroblastoma (esthesioneuroblastoma). These images are uncontrasted axial T1 WI. The lesion arises in the nasal sinuses in the image on the left and extends intracranially on the image on the right.*

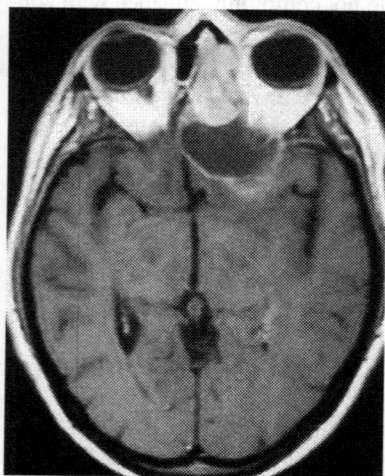

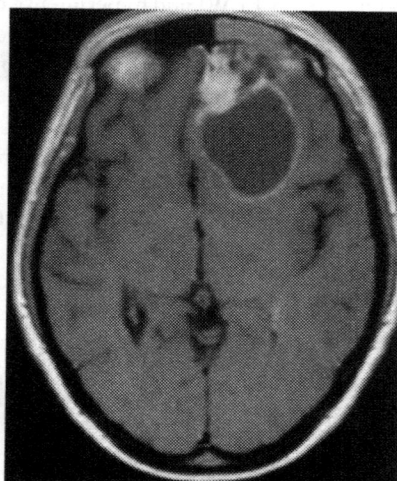

Figure 3. *Olfactory neuroblastoma (esthesioneuroblastoma). These images are contrast enhanced axial T1 WI. Note the enhancement of both the solid component and the cyst wall.*

Pineal parenchymal tumours

Pineal cysts

These are asymptomatic, incidental lesions found on MRI scanning but should be differentiated from epidermoid and dermoid cysts.

Pineocytoma

Pineocytomas are low grade tumours and pineoblastomas high grade. Pineocytomas occur in adults and can be cured with resection. They may seed throughout the CSF.

Pineoblastoma

Pineoblastomas are seen more frequently in children and are highly malignant, unresectable tumours. They are true primitive neuroectodermal tumours (PNET's) and replace the tissue of the pineal gland. Resection plus adjuvant chemotherapy is the treatment of choice. They may seed throughout the CSF.

Mixed pineocytoma/pineoblastoma

Tumours with neuroblastic or glioblast elements (embryonal tumours)

Medulloepithelioma

Primitive neuroectodermal tumours with multipotent differentiation

a) Medulloblastomas are primitive neuroectodermal tumours (PNET) found mostly in the midline in the posterior fossa and mostly in children. They frequently infiltrate and obstruct the fourth ventricle, causing hydrocephalus. These tumours are associated with CSF seeding and drop metastasis of the spine and the initial work up should include full craniospinal imaging. The treatment of choice is surgical debulking with craniospinal radiotherapy and chemotherapy. Five year event free survival rates of up to 80% have been reported following multimodal therapy (female patients do better).

b) Cerebral PNET's are supratentorial primitive neuroectodermal tumours. The may seed via the CSF throughout the neural axis and resection plus radiotherapy and chemotherapy are used in their management.

Neuroblastoma

Retinoblastoma

Ependymoblastoma

Other CNS neoplasms

Tumours of the sellar region

Pituitary adenoma

These are the third most common type of primary intracranial tumour after meningiomas and glial tumours. Pituitary adenomas may be either non-functioning or functioning. The functioning adenomas are frequently small and excert a clinical effect due to their hormone secretion. Non-functioning adenomas are usually macro adenomas, and exhibit their symptoms due to compression of the optic tracts or obstructive hydrocephalus. Pituitary apoplexy is a medical emergency during which bleeding into a pituitary adenoma can cause ophthalmoplegia, visual loss and acute hypopituitarism. Cardiovascular depression secondary to adrenal failure occurs and emergency treatment with steroids is imperative. Adenomas can be divided into micro adenomas (less than 1cm) and macro adenomas (greater than 1 cm). There is a wide differential diagnosis for tumours in the sellar area including pituitary adenoma, carotid aneurysm, metastasis, germ cell tumour, craniopharyngioma, Rathke's cleft cyst, optic glioma, meningioma, abscess, sarcoidosis and lymphocytic hypophysitis.

Hormone secreting adenomas

Prolactinomas

These are the most common, accounting for about one third of these tumours. Symptoms are caused by hormone secretion with amenorrhea and galactorrhoea in women and associated decreased libido, headache and dyspareunia. In men it can be associated with hypogonadism. In some cases of prolactinoma, the prolactin level is only mildly elevated and this can be due to the stalk effect where the adenoma is not prolactin secreting but, because of compression of the pituitary stalk, the prolactin levels rise. Prolactinomas are treated with a dopamine agonist, which patients need to take for the rest of their lives. Surgery is reserved for cases where there is compression of the optic complex or failed medical therapy.

Growth hormone secreting pituitary adenomas

These tumours are usually slightly larger than prolactinomas and are diagnosed with elevated levels of growth hormone and IgF1. They exert their effects via the hormones and the hallmarks of this disease are acromegaly in adults and gigantism in children. Surgery is the main treatment but adjunctive therapy with Octreotide (somatostatin analogue) is also useful.

ACTH secreting pituitary adenomas

Women are more affected than men by this disease and the pituitary adenomas are usually very small. It is important in cases with Cushing's syndrome to exclude exogenous (outside of the pituitary) production of ACTH and to confirm that the high levels of ACTH with resultant Cushingoid features are due primarily to a pituitary adenoma (Cushing's disease). Several tests including the Dexamethasone suppression test are used for this. The main treatment for this is surgery. The patients should receive exogenous corticosteroids following surgery and this should commence after surgery as soon as a cortisol level has been sent to the lab. Resection of the adenoma is immediately proven with this cortisol level and is taken as proof of cure.

TSH secreting pituitary adenomas

These are relatively rare and a combination of surgery and radiotherapy is usually required to control them.

Gonadotrophin secreting pituitary adenomas

Despite secreting FSH or LSH, these usually cause symptoms due to compressive effects and are treated surgically.

Non-functional macroadenomas

These exert their symptoms due to compressive effects and surgery is the treatment of choice.

Pituitary carcinoma
Craniopharyngioma

These derive from Rathke's pouch remnants. They arise in the suprasellar region and can be divided into adamantimatous, which usually occur in children, and squamous papillary lesions that usually occur in adults. On imaging, these tumours frequently have calcification (more than 70%) and frequently have the features of a lipid filled sac. In children these tumours can lead to growth failure or obstructive hydrocephalus and in adults they frequently cause visual failure and hormonal deficiencies. Surgery is the treatment of choice but total macroscopic removal is difficult. Although these tumours are benign, they recur in 25% of patients following total resection.

Hematopoietic tumours

Primary malignant lymphomas

This is a form of non-Hodgkin lymphoma that is confined to the CNS. The incidence of these tumours is increased in immuno-incompetent patients but they do also occur in immuno-competent patients. They are mostly B-cell lymphomas and demonstrate widespread infiltration of the normal parenchyma. B-cell lymphomas usually also have reactive but benign T-lymphocytes that infiltrate between the B-lymphocytes. These tumours are usually hyperdense before contrast on CT scanning and isointense on T1- and T2 WI and enhance uniformly with contrast. They are mostly found in a periventricular location but can be found at other locations too and may have variable imaging characteristics. Nearly half of patients will have leptomeningeal dissemination and 10-15% of patients will have ocular involvement. It is interesting to know that, conversely, patients with isolated ocular lymphoma disseminate to the brain in up to 75% of cases. These tumours are exquisitely radiosensitive and the current recommendation is not to debulk these tumours but obtain a stereotactically guided tissue biopsy. It is unusual for these tumours to be secondary to systemic lymphoma but systemic screening tests like CT scans of the abdomen and chest may be performed to exclude systemic lymphoma. Treating these patients with steroids frequently leads to involution of the tumour cells and negative biopsies. If clinical circumstances permit, steroids should be witheld until the biopsy has been performed in cases of suspected lymphoma. Whole brain radiotherapy is the treatment of choice and the current life expectancy is about 18 months. This can be extended to about 5 years with the concomitant use of Methotrexate. In patients with HIV, primary central nervous system lymphoma is the second most common intracranial mass lesion after toxoplasmosis.

Plasmacytoma
Granulocytic sarcoma

Germ cell tumours

Germ cell tumours arise from pluripotential germinal cells with a germinoma being the most common and accounting for about half of all cases. Other germ cell tumours include teratomas, choriocarcinomas, endodermal sinus tumours and embryonal carcinoma. These are tumours of children and young adults and germ cell tumours can be diagnosed according to their tumour marker that includes alpha-fetoprotein, beta HCG and placental alkaline phosphatase (see table 2). These tumours can be diagnosed with serum and CSF levels of tumour markers as well as stereotactic biopsies. Pure germinomas should be treated with radiotherapy whereas other germ cell tumours benefit from radical resection and mature teratomas can be cured with complete resection.

Germinoma
Embryonal carcinoma
Yolk sac tumor (endodermal sinus tumor)
Choriocarcinoma
Teratoma
Mixed germ cell tumours

Type of tumour	ß-HCG	Alpha-FP	PLAP
Teratoma			±
Germinoma	+		±
Choriocarcinoma	++		±
Mixed germ cell tumour	++	++	±
Endodermal sinus tumour	±	++	±
Embryonal carcinoma	±	±	±

Table 2. *Tumour markers in germ cell tumours.*

Tumours of the meninges
Meningiomas
Meningiomas arise from the arachnoid cap cells in the dura and are benign in at least 90% of cases. The malignant meningiomas are invasive. Meningiomas are diagnosed on imaging by their typical appearance of having a dural attachment (dural tail), the fact that they are homogeneous and that they enhance vividly with contrast. They may be associated with oedema and because they are slow growing they are sometimes found as incidental lesions. These tumours should be completely resected with a normal rim of dura wherever possible and the extent of resection is the basis for the Simpson grading (see table 3). Meningiomas may be highly vascular lesions and are frequently embolised prior to the surgery. Skull base meningiomas can usually not be completely removed and stereotactic radiosurgery or radiotherapy is used as an adjunct in residual tumours.

Grade	Tumour resection	Recurrence
I	Macroscopically complete removal including dura and bone	9%
II	Macroscopically complete removal, dural coagulation	19%
III	Complete tumour resection, dura not coagulated	29%
IV	Partial removal	44%
V	Simple decompression	

Table 3. *Simpson grading.*

Atypical meningioma
Anaplastic (malignant) meningioma
Non-meningothelial tumours of the meninges

Benign Mesenchymal tumours
Osteocartilaginous tumours
Lipoma
Fibrous histiocytoma

Malignant mesenchymal tumours
Chondrosarcoma
Chondrosarcomas typically arise from the middle cranial fossa and are frequently large at the time of diagnosis. Tumours should be maximally surgically resected but only about half are resectable due to their location at the skull base. Concurrent radiotherapy is usually administered and more than 80% local control and more than 80% five year survival rates are reported with combination proton and photon therapy.
Haemangiopericytoma
These tumours arise from pericytes and are sometimes difficult to distinguish from meningiomas. They also have a dural attachment and are vascular tumours but unlike meningiomas usually have lytic destruction of the adjacent skull on X-rays and CT scans. They can be distinguished from meningiomas by immunohistochemistry as they are negative for epithelial membrane antigen. There is a greater than 50% local recurrence rate and postoperative radiotherapy is mandatory. In about 25% of cases, there are extracranial metastasis.
Rhabdomyosarcoma
Meningeal sarcomatosis

Primary melanocytic lesions
Diffuse melanosis
Melanocytoma
Malignant melanoma

Tumours of uncertain histogenesis
Hemangioblastoma
These are mostly cystic (may be solid) tumours of the posterior fossa in adults and usually appear as a large non-enhancing cyst with an enhancing mural nodule. These may be sporadic or be part of the Von Hippel – Lindau (VHL) syndrome that is an autosomal dominant inherited condition. Resection of the mural nodule is the therapy of choice and results are generally favourable with recurrence less than 25%.

Tumours of cranial and spinal nerves
Schwannoma (neurinoma, neurilemoma)
These arise from Schwann cells and most commonly arise from the vestibular nerve (vestibular schwannoma - previously called acoustic neuroma) but can also arise from the trigeminal nerve or other lower cranial nerve. These tumours arise eccentrically from the nerve. The aim of surgery is to completely resect the tumour without damage to the associated nerves. These are relatively slow growing tumours and in vestibular schwannomas the aim of treatment is facial nerve preservation.
Neurofibroma
Neurofibromas and schwannomas are derived from a common Schwann cell origin. Neurofibromas are made up of fibrous tissues as well as nerve fibres. There is a fusiform enlargement of the nerve and it is not possible to distinguish between the nerve tissue and the fibrous tissue.
Malignant peripheral nerve sheath tumor (malignant schwannoma)

Local extensions from regional tumours
Paraganglioma (chemodectoma)
These arise from the paraganglionic tissue and can arise from the glomus tympanicum in the middle ear or the glomus jugulare at the jugular base. They present with lower cranial nerve deficits and complete surgical resection and radiotherapy for residual tumour is the treatment of choice.
Chordoma
Chordomas are rare tumours that arise from bone, typically the clivus. Tumours should be maximally surgically resected. Concurrent radiotherapy is usually administered with a 10-year local control rate of approximately 40% to 50%.
Chondrosarcoma
Carcinoma

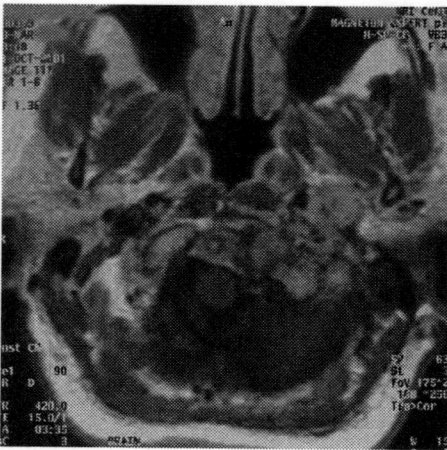

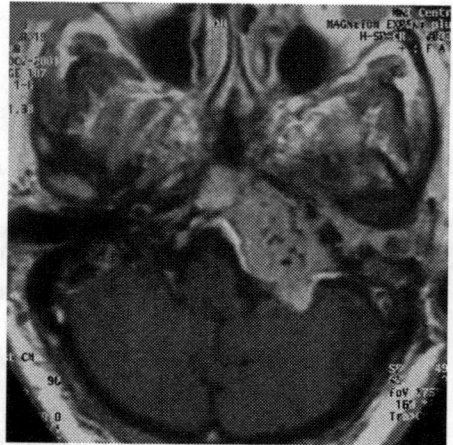

Figure 3. *Glomus jugulare tumour. The image on the left is an uncontrasted axial T1 WI and the image on the right is a contrast enhanced T1 WI. This paraganglioma is hyperintense on these images, heterogeneous and enhances with contrast.*

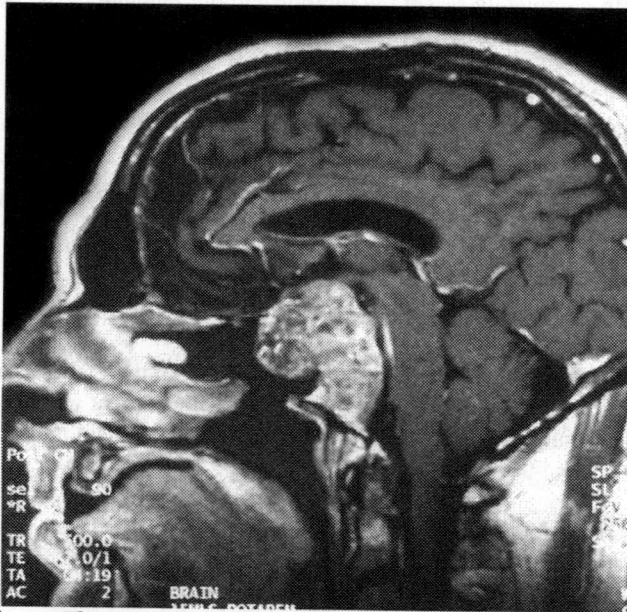

Figure 4. *Chordoma. This image is a contrast enhanced sagittal T1 WI and demonstrates a chordoma infiltrating and destroying the clivus.*

Metastatic tumours

Unclassified tumours

Cysts and tumor-like lesions
Rathke cleft cyst
These are usually found in the sellar region and can be difficult to distinguish from cranio-pharyngiomas. However, they usually have less calcification than craniopharyngiomas and

craniopharyngiomas have the tendency to erode the posterior clinoids.

Epidermoid and Dermoid Cysts
These are midline tumours found in the suprasellar area, the area of the fourth ventricle and the spine. Epidermoids can also be found off the midline in the CP angle and the ear (cholesteatoma). They are mostly made up of inclusion squamous keratinised epithelium and dermoids in addition, are characterised by dermal appendages. Dermoids are more common in childhood whereas epidermoids are more common in adulthood. In children, epidermoids can frequently be associated with a dermal sinus and can be a cause of repeated CNS infections.

Colloid cyst of the third ventricle
These are usually attached to the choroid plexus of the foramen of Monroe. They cause obstructive hydrocephalus that may cause sudden death. Treatment is with bilateral ventriculoperitoneal shunting, open surgical removal or endoscopic marsupialisation.

Arachnoid cysts
These are duplications of arachnoid membrane that are thought to fill up with a ball valve mechanism or osmotic diffusion and can typically be found in the Sylvian fissure, CPA and suprasellar area. The have a similar appearance to epidermoid cysts on CT and MR scanning and can only be distinguished with FLAIR images (fluid attenuation inversion recovery) which suppresses the CSF in an arachnoid cyst and epidermoid cysts appear hyperintense demonstrating abnormal fluid. Treatment is resection and is reserved for symptomatic cases.

Neurenteric cysts
These are found either in the posterior fossa or in the spinal canal and give local compressive symptoms. They are formed secondary to epithelial inclusions during the embryonic period.

Enterogenous cyst
Neuroglial cyst
Granular cell tumor (choristoma, pituicytoma)
Hypothalamic neuronal hamartoma
Nasal glial heterotopia
Plasma cell granuloma

Adjuvant therapies

Radiotherapy
The aim of radiotherapy is to damage the DNA of rapidly dividing cancer cells so that they die with little or no associated damage to surrounding normal brain.

External beam radiotherapy is delivered via intersecting beams in a three dimensional space with the patient fixed in a face mask.

Stereotactic radiosurgery is a more precise means of delivering radiotherapy to a very small target. The radiotherapy beams can be either from a cobalt unit (Gamma knife) or from a linear accelerator.

Particle beam radiotherapy administers heavy particles such as neutrons and protons. This is used for skull base tumours such as chordomas, chondrosarcomas and pituitary adenomas

Interstitial radiotherapy (brachytherapy) is the implantation of radiation sources within the tumour bed and many oncologists currently use Gliadel wafers (carmustine).

There are complications of radiation therapy such as increased brain swelling. Complications up to 6 months may be due to reversible demyelinisation that is usually responsive to steroid treatment. Complications after 6 months and up to several years later include irreversible radionecrosis that is unresponsive to steroid administration. It can be difficult to differentiate between this, tumour progression and abscess formation. Single photon emission computed tomography (SPECT) scanning, which demonstrates biologically active tissue, is useful to distinguish between these. Another late complication is that of malignancy. Irradiation can cause intracranial malignancies. This usually happens when a slow growing tumour is irradiated and years later a new tumour develops in the area where the radiation was administered.

Chemotherapy

Used mostly in children because many childhood tumours are chemosensitive and radiation is toxic to the developing brain. Therefore chemotherapy is used as a first line treatment (neoadjuvant chemotherapy). These agents can only kill cells that are in the active phase of the cell cycle and dividing.

Procarbazine is an alkylating agent and it acts against synthesis of DNA, RNA and proteins. It is used against gliomas, medulloblastomas, PNET's and lymphomas.

Nitrosoureas (carmustine and lomustine) are the most commonly used agents and exert their effects via DNA alkylation and are used against glioblastomas, anaplastic astrocytomas, low-grade gliomas, oligodendrogliomas, medulloblastomas and PNET's.

Vincristine inhibits mitosis and is active against gliomas, medulloblastomas, PNET's and lymphoma.

PCV (procarbazine, carmustine, and vincristine) is a frequently used combination.

Temozolomide is a DNA alkylating agent now commonly used against glioblastoma and anaplastic gliomas

Cisplatin and carboplatin are platinum analogues used against gliomas, medulloblastomas, ependymomas, PNET's and germ cell tumours.

Neurofibromatosis and other phakomatoses

Neurofibromatosis

Neurofibromatosis (NF) is an autosomal dominant neurocutaneous disorder that can involve almost any organ system. Neurofibromatosis Type 1 (most common) is referred to as peripheral NF and is associated with a defect on chromosome 17q and NF type 2 is referred to as central NF with an associated abnormality of chromosome22q.

The criteria for the diagnosis of NF are as follows:

NF 1: (Two or more of the following)
Six or more cafe au lait spots (more than 5 mm before puberty and more than 15mm post puberty)
Axillary or inguinal freckling
Two or more neurofibromas or one plexiform neurofibroma
Optic glioma
Two or more Lisch nodules (hamartomas of the iris)
Sphenoid bone dysplasia, atrophic long bone cortexes or other bony lesions
A first-degree relative with NF-1
NF2
Bilateral vestibular schwannomas

Or
Unilateral vestibular schwannoma (or intracranial meningioma or glioma) and a first-degree relative with NF 2

Tuberous sclerosis (TS)

Tuberous sclerosis (TS) is an autosomal dominant genetic disorder (chromosome 9, 16) which results in hamartoma formation in multiple organs (brain, eyes, dermal, renal, and cardiac).

Criteria for diagnosing TS - There are major and minor features and the diagnosis is made if there are two major features or one major feature plus two minor features.

Major features

Dermal:
Facial angiofibromas
Ungual fibromas (finger or toenail)
Hypomelanotic macules ($\geq$3)
Shagreen patch (connective tissue nevus)

CNS:
Subependymal giant cell astrocytoma
Cortical tuber
Subependymal nodule
Multiple retinal nodular hamartomas

Systemic:
Cardiac rhabdomyoma
Lymphangiomyomatosis
Renal angiomyolipoma

Minor features

Multiple random pits in dental enamel
Bone cysts
Cerebral white matter radial migration lines
Gingival fibromas
Hamartomatous rectal polyps
Confetti skin lesions (reticulated hypomelanotic lesions)
Multiple renal cysts
Retinal achromic patch (round or oval gray-yellow flat spots)
Nonrenal hamartoma

Von Hippel – Lindau (VHL) syndrome

This is an autosomal dominant, inherited, neurocutaneous dysplasia complex with an 80-100% penetrance and variable delayed expression. The gene has been located on chromosome bands 3p25-26

Haemangioblastomas are typical for this syndrome and other manifestations of VHL are:

Retinal angiomas
Renal cysts and renal cell carcinoma
Pancreatic cysts and islet cell carcinoma
Hepatic cysts
Splenic cysts
Epididymis cysts, testicular germ cell tumours

Pheochromocytoma
Cafe au lait spots and skin nevi

Criteria for the diagnosis of VHL:
More than one CNS hemangioblastoma
One CNS hemangioblastoma and one systemic manifestation
One manifestation and known family history

Patients with known hemangioblastomas and at risk family members can be screened using several established protocols - a standard approach is:
Yearly
Clinical examination
Direct and indirect ophthalmoscopy
Fluorescein angiography
Twenty-four hour urine collection for vanilmandelic acid (VMA) levels
Three yearly
MRI or CT scan of the brain to age 50 years then every five yearly
Abdominal CT scanning

WHO classification of CNS tumours

Neuroepithelial tumours of the CNS

Gliomas
Astrocytic tumours
(Low grade) Astrocytoma (WHO grade II)
Anaplastic (malignant) astrocytoma (WHO grade III)
Glioblastoma multiforme (WHO grade IV)
Pilocytic astrocytoma [non-invasive, WHO grade I]
Subependymal giant cell astrocytoma (non-invasive, WHO grade I)
Pleomorphic xanthoastrocytoma (non-invasive, WHO grade I)

Oligodendroglial tumours
Oligodendroglioma (WHO grade II)
Anaplastic (malignant) oligodendroglioma (WHO grade III)

Ependymal cell tumours
Ependymoma (WHO grade II)
Anaplastic ependymoma (WHO grade III)
Myxopapillary ependymoma
Subependymoma (WHO grade I)

Mixed gliomas
Mixed oligoastrocytoma (WHO grade II)
Anaplastic (malignant) oligoastrocytoma (WHO grade III)

Neuroepithelial tumours of uncertain origin
Polar spongioblastoma (WHO grade IV)
Astroblastoma (WHO grade IV)
Gliomatosis cerebri (WHO grade IV)

tumours of the choroid plexus
Choroid plexus papilloma
Choroid plexus carcinoma (anaplastic choroid plexus papilloma)

Neuronal and mixed neuronal-glial tumours
Gangliocytoma
Dysplastic gangliocytoma of cerebellum (Lhermitte-Duclos)
Ganglioglioma
Anaplastic (malignant) ganglioglioma
Desmoplastic infantile ganglioglioma
Central neurocytoma
Dysembryoplastic neuroepithelial tumor
Olfactory neuroblastoma (esthesioneuroblastoma)

Pineal parenchymal tumours
Pineocytoma

Pineoblastoma
Mixed pineocytoma/pineoblastoma

Tumours with neuroblastic or glioblast elements (embryonal tumours)
Medulloepithelioma
Primitive neuroectodermal tumours with multipotent differentiation
Medulloblastoma
Cerebral primitive neuroectodermal tumor
Neuroblastoma
Retinoblastoma
Ependymoblastoma

Other CNS Neoplasms

Tumours of the sellar region
Pituitary adenoma
Pituitary carcinoma
Craniopharyngioma

Hematopoietic tumours
Primary malignant lymphomas
Plasmacytoma
Granulocytic sarcoma

Germ cell tumours
Germinoma
Embryonal carcinoma
Yolk sac tumor (endodermal sinus tumor)
Choriocarcinoma
Teratoma
Mixed germ cell tumours

Tumours of the meninges
Meningioma
Atypical meningioma
Anaplastic (malignant) meningioma
Non-meningothelial tumours of the meninges

Benign mesenchymal tumours
Osteocartilaginous tumours
Lipoma
Fibrous histiocytoma

Malignant mesenchymal tumours
Chondrosarcoma
Haemangiopericytoma
Rhabdomyosarcoma
Meningeal sarcomatosis

Primary melanocytic lesions
Diffuse melanosis
Melanocytoma
Malignant melanoma

Tumours of uncertain histogenesis
Hemangioblastoma

Tumours of cranial and spinal nerves
Schwannoma (neurinoma, neurilemoma)
Neurofibroma
Malignant peripheral nerve sheath tumor (Malignant schwannoma)

Local extensions from regional tumours
Paraganglioma (chemodectoma)
Chordoma
Chondrosarcoma
Carcinoma

Metastatic tumours

Unclassified tumours

Cysts and tumour-like lesions
Rathke cleft cyst
Epidermoid
Dermoid
Colloid cyst of the third ventricle
Enterogenous cyst
Neuroglial cyst
Granular cell tumour (choristoma, pituicytoma)
Hypothalamic neuronal hamartoma
Nasal glial herterotopia
Plasma cell granuloma

9

SPINAL TUMOURS

W Adriaan Liebenberg

Contents

Extradural compartment

Primary tumours
Bony tumours
Cartilaginous tumours of the spine
Lymphoproliferative tumours
Tumour of notochordal origin
Round cell tumours

Metastatic tumours

Intradural, extramedullary compartment
Nerve sheath tumours

Intramedullary compartment
Ependymoma
Astrocytoma
Others

Spinal Tumours

Tumours of the spine are located in one of three anatomical compartments, the extradural compartment, the intradural, extramedullary compartment or the intramedullary compartment.

Extradural compartment

Primary tumours

Bony tumours
Osteoid osteoma
This is a benign skeletal neoplasm presenting in young people but rarely in children younger than five. The salient clinical feature is pain that is worse at night and is relieved by small doses of salicylates. On imaging, the lesion presents as a small island of sclerotic bone with a radiolucent centre that is usually less than 1.5 cm in diameter. Radionuclide scans are a

243

good way to locate the tumours. The tumour sometimes involutes spontaneously. Treatment is with surgical excision or radiofrequency ablation and the aim is complete ablation or resection of the tumour, which is curative.

Osteoblastoma

This is a benign tumour that is closely related to the osteoid osteoma and is differentiated by the ability of the nidus to grow larger than two centimeters. Patients usually present in the first three decades of life. It has to be differentiated from the aggressive osteosarcoma. On imaging, the lesion usually presents as a well-circumscribed radiolucent lesion with a thin rim of new bone that separates it from the surrounding soft tissues. Osteoblastomas that are more aggressive display local resorption of the cortex, destruction of bone, and extension into surrounding soft tissues. For tumours that remain subcapsular local resection is acceptable. More aggressive types with extracapsular extension require resection with a wide margin, which is usually curative.

Osteosarcoma

This malignant tumour usually presents in the lumbosacral spine in the fourth decade of life and has a male preponderance. These tumours present with pain and local mass effects. On imaging, this is usually a tumour of the vertebral body that extends into the soft tissues and may incorporate the posterior elements. The tumour is usually intensely hyperdense and the vertebrae have been called ivory vertebrae. There is frequently a loss of height of the vertebrae. Despite wide surgical resection and adjuvant chemotherapy and radiotherapy, the diagnosis is poor with life expectancy usually less than two years.

Cartilaginous tumours of the spine

Osteochondroma

These are benign tumours presenting in the third and fourth decades of life. They involve the cervical spine mostly (especially C2) and are usually located in the posterior elements. On imaging the lesion presents as an exostosis with a cartilaginous cap. In adults this cap should be less than 2 cm, if not; malignant transformation to chondrosarcoma should be suspected. Complete surgical resection is usually curative.

Chondrosarcoma

These are malignant tumours presenting mostly in men in the fifth decade of life and most commonly in the thoracic spine. They present on imaging with a characteristic matrix arranged in the form of rings and arcs and in approximately 30% extend through the disc spaces into adjacent levels. Complete cure can be achieved with total excision and a wide margin. Adjuvant chemotherapy may be used to reduced tumour mass. These lesions have the potential to metastasise (mostly to the lungs) and lesions that are not resected with a wide margin mostly recur.

Lymphoproliferative tumours

Multiple myeloma

This is a systemic disease of middle-aged people caused by malignant plasma cells that produce elevated levels of immunoglobulins. This is the most common primary bone tumour and presents with local bone destruction. Diagnosis is confirmed by detecting immunoglobulins with protein electrophoresis in the patient's serum and urine. The mainstay of treatment is radiation therapy and chemotherapy with surgical stabilisation of destructed and unstable levels.

Solitary plasmacytoma

These are also caused by malignant plasma cells, but are solitary lesions that occur in younger people and have a better prognosis. Radiation therapy and surgical stabilisation as above are the mainstay of treatment. These lesions can transform into multiple myeloma and it is important to follow patients up life long.

Lymphoma

This can either be primary lymphoma of the bone or secondary deposits of both Hodgkin and non-Hodgkin lymphomas (cranial lymphoma is Non-Hodgkin). These patients present with local compressive effects due to tumour growth. On imaging lymphoma appears as a large soft tissue mass extending from the bone and is homogenous and hypointense on T1 WI images and enhances strongly with contrast. Technetium bone scans are very sensitive in detecting these lesions. The mainstay of treatment is radiotherapy with surgery reserved for cases requiring decompression and stabilisation.

Tumours of notochordal origin

Chordoma

These tumours arise from a notochord remnant (the notochord evolves into the nucleus pulposus of the intervertebral discs). These are large soft tissue masses and have associated vertebral destruction. More than half demonstrate calcification on imaging and they are hypointense on T1 WI and hyperintense on T2 WI since they have high water content and enhance with contrast administration. Surgical resection with adjuvant chemotherapy and radiotherapy is the treatment of choice. Sacrococcygeal tumours have 8-10 year survival and tumours at other sites have 4-5 year survival. These lesions may metastasise but death is usually due to the local effects of the tumour.

Round cell tumours

Ewing sarcoma

These malignant tumours occur in children and mostly in the sacrococcygeal region. Diffuse sclerosis is usually evident on imaging and these lesions are usually located in the vertebral bodies with soft tissue extension. Treatment consists of radiotherapy and chemotherapy and this achieves nearly 100% local control with nearly 90% long-term survival. This is less true for sacral tumours since they are usually larger at presentation.

Metastatic tumours

The tumours that most commonly metastasise to the spine are carcinoma of the prostate, breast adenocarcinoma, lung adenocarcinoma, renal cell carcinoma and gastric carcinoma. Treatment is based on several factors including the general status of the patient, status of the systemic disease, amount of neural compression and the presence of intractable pain. Metastatic tumours cannot be cured by local excision of the metastasis and the treatment is aimed at local decompression of the tumour. Concurrent stability procedures are aimed at preserving anatomical integrity and for pain relief. The mainstay of treatment for metastatic tumours of the spine is radiotherapy.

Intradural, extramedullary compartment

Nerve sheath tumours

Neurofibromas and schwannomas are derived from a common Schwann cell origin. Neurofibromas are made up of fibrous tissues as well as nerve fibres. In neurofibromas there is a fusiform enlargement of the nerve and it is not possible to distinguish between the nerve tissue and the fibrous tissue. Schwannomas are round or ovoid masses that are suspended from the nerve and are made up of bipolar cells that are either arranged in a palisade formation, called Antoni – A or are loosely arranged, called Antoni – B. The latter is less common.

These tumours occur between the fourth and the sixth decade, arise mostly from a dorsal nerve root, and are mostly intradural. Some extend through a neural foramen as the classical dumbbell tumours and rarely they are entirely extradural. These are benign tumours and the treatment is excision with excellent prognosis.

Meningiomas

Both these and the nerve sheath tumours make up 25% each of intradural tumours. They arise from the arachnoid cap cells on the dura at the edge of the root sleeve and are therefore found mostly in a lateral position. There is a female preponderance and they arise mostly in the thoracic spine. These are also mostly benign lesions, just like their cranial counterparts and treatment is complete excision with excellent prognosis.

Filum terminale ependymomas

Nearly half of spinal canal ependymomas arise in the filum terminale. There is a slight male preponderance and these tumours tend to occur in the third to fifth decade of life. The histological arrangement is myxopapillary and consists of tumour cells surrounding a core of hyalinised and poorly differentiated connective tissue. These are benign tumours for the most part and the treatment is excision.

Intramedullary compartment

Ependymoma (55% of intramedullary tumours)

These benign tumours occur mostly in men in the fourth decade. They can occur throughout out the spine but a specific type, the myxopapillary ependymoma arises in the conus and filum terminale. These tumours are homogenous and well circumscribed, discrete and cause their symptoms by intrinsic compression of the spinal cord rather than infiltration. They are hypointense on T1 WI, enhance strongly with contrast and are hyperintense on T2 WI. Resection results in prolonged survival. Some lesions may undergo malignant transformation, infiltrate, and metastasise within the CNS.

Astrocytoma (30% of intramedullary tumours)

Low-grade astrocytomas and pilocytic astrocytomas are slow growing, usually have cleavage planes and may be totally or nearly totally excised. Residual tumours may be treated expectantly although the treatment of these residual tumours is controversial. Anaplastic glioma and glioblastoma multiforme are rare but lethal. Resection of these malignant tumours is not possible and life expectancy is generally less than 2 years.

Other tumours

Generally these tumours have the same imaging characteristics of their cranial counter parts. Intramedullary oligodendrogliomas are rare, the optimal management is not yet known and chemotherapy sensitivity, unlike the cranial type, is unproven. Dermoid cysts, epidermoid cysts and lipomas are inclusion tumours that are slow growing. The aim of treatment is total resection with prolonged survival in dermoids and epidermoids but lipomas are frequently difficult to excise completely. Hemangioblastomas can be cured by complete removal. They are vascular and piecemeal removal is risky. Gangliogliomas are more common in childhood, are benign and the aim of treatment is total resection with prolonged survival. Subependymoma are rare lesions and experience with their management is limited but total resection is the main aim of treatment.

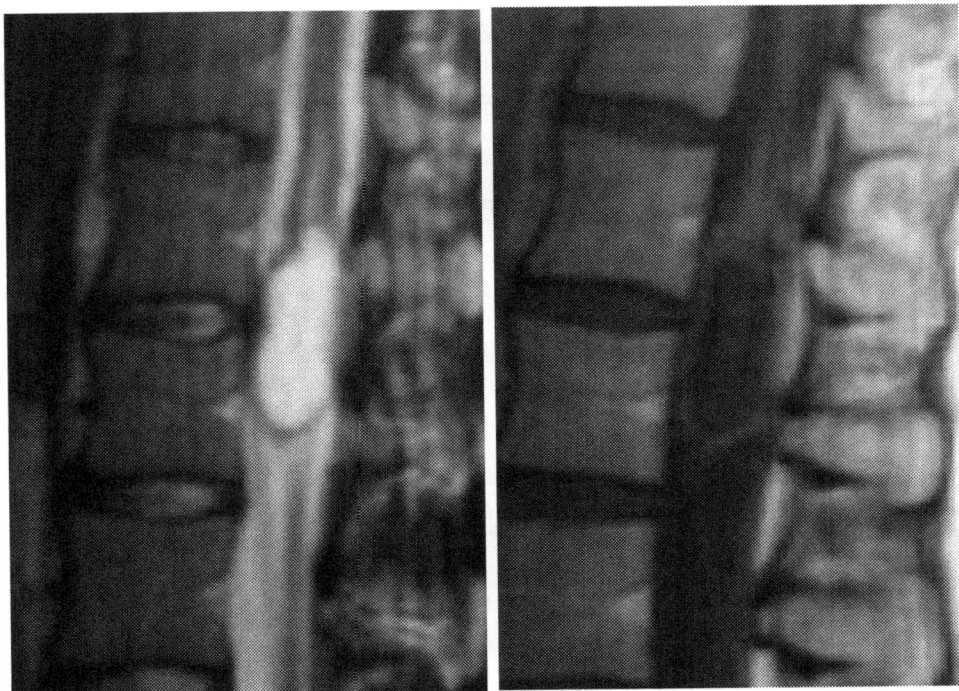

Figure 1. *Hemangioblastoma. The image on the left is a sagittal T2 WI and the image on the right is a contrast enhanced sagittal T1 WI. Note how this lesion is mostly composed of cyst material and has a peripherally placed nodule that usually enhances with contrast*

10

VASCULAR ABNORMALITIES

W Adriaan Liebenberg

Contents

Intracranial vascular abnormalities
Arteriovenous malformations
Cavernous angiomas
Venous angiomas
Cerebral aneurysms
Treatment of incidental and unruptured aneurysms
Aneurysmal subarachnoid haemorrhage (SAH)
General effects of SAH
Specific effects of SAH
Vasospasm
Definitive treatment of the aneurysm

Intracranial vascular abnormalities

The intracranial vasculature develops pathology in several ways. There may be occlusion of arteries or venous structures or haemorrhage can occur into the parenchyma, the intraventricular system, the subdural space or subarachnoid space.

Occlusion of cerebral blood vessels is usually due to embolic phenomena and these can be secondary to atherosclerotic plaques, infected emboli or foreign material. Occlusion of the arterial side of the circulation leads to ischaemia and, if the blood flow is not restored instantly, it will lead to cell death and infarction. Occlusion of the venous part of the circulation will lead to venous hypertension, intraparenchymal bleeds and infarction. Hypertensive spontaneous intraparenchymal bleeds are secondary to the rupture of friable blood vessels. Spontaneous haemorrhages can also be secondary to vascular anomalies and/or aneurysms.

Arteriovenous malformations (AVM) are lesions in which the arterial system short-circuits directly into the venous system without the intervening capillary bed. The venous circulation is not designed to function under such high pressure and this leads to tortuous vessels and associated flow aneurysms may also develop. AVM's recruit additional blood vessels and may grow quite large. They are graded according to the Spetzler-Martin grading scale based on three factors, namely the size of the lesion, its location and the type of venous drainage. AVM's either cause effects secondarily to brain irritation (seizures) or may present with spontaneous intraparenchymal bleeds.

Size	Score	Eloquent brain	Score	Deep draining vein	Score
more than 6cm	3	Yes	1	Yes	1
3-6cm	2	No	0	No	0
less than 3cm	1				

Table 1. *The Spetzler-Martin grading scale. The size of the lesion is divided into categories of less than 3cms (1 point), 3-6cms (2 points) and greater than 6cms (3 points). If the AVM is located in an eloquent area of the brain such as the speech area, motor area, visual cortex or brain stem then another point is added. If the venous draining system is deep and if the lesion, for instance, drains directly into the vein of Galen or the straight sinus, then another point is added. The maximum score therefore is five.*

Cavernous angiomas (cavernomas, cavernous malformations) do not fill from the systemic circulation and do not drain via veins but rather are abnormal thin-walled vascular channels (caverns). They can present with spontaneous haemorrhage or seizures and are more prevalent in the paediatric population. Cavernous angiomas are sometimes found in the spinal cord and can cause potentially devastating neurological sequelae secondary to haemorrhage. Since cavernomas do not fill or drain from the systemic circulation, they are diagnosed on MRI scanning and are non-detectable on angiography. Lesions can be watched expectantly if they are discovered incidentally. Symptomatic lesions with multiple haemorrhagic events, can be treated surgically if accessible, or with radio surgery if surgically inaccessible.

Venous angiomas are most likely to have formed during the embryonic period due to an arrest of venous development. They are composed of dilated venous channels that drain normal brain and converge into medullary veins which are enlarged and these in turn drain into normal cortical veins. They may sometimes be found in association with cavernous angiomas. The majority of these lesions are discovered incidentally and present only infrequently with haemorrhage. These lesions can be diagnosed on MRI scanning as well as angiography. On contrasted MRI scanning they form a characteristic 'caput medusa lesion' where dilated capillary veins drain centrally towards a main draining vein. They can be diagnosed on angiography when, in the venous phase, a persistent pattern of dilated medullary veins is seen that drains towards a single draining vein. They are usually managed expectantly.

Cerebral aneurysms are usually found amongst the medium sized arteries of the circle of Willis and can be fusiform dilatations or saccular berry aneurysms. Saccular aneurysms form due to weakness of the interna and media of the artery wall resulting in outpouching. These are true aneurysms. False aneurysms can be found secondary to trauma or infection and are not contained by the vessel wall but rather by the surrounding tissues. Aneurysms are thought to be flow related in their mechanism of origin and are usually found at vessel bifurcation on the side of the greatest flow.

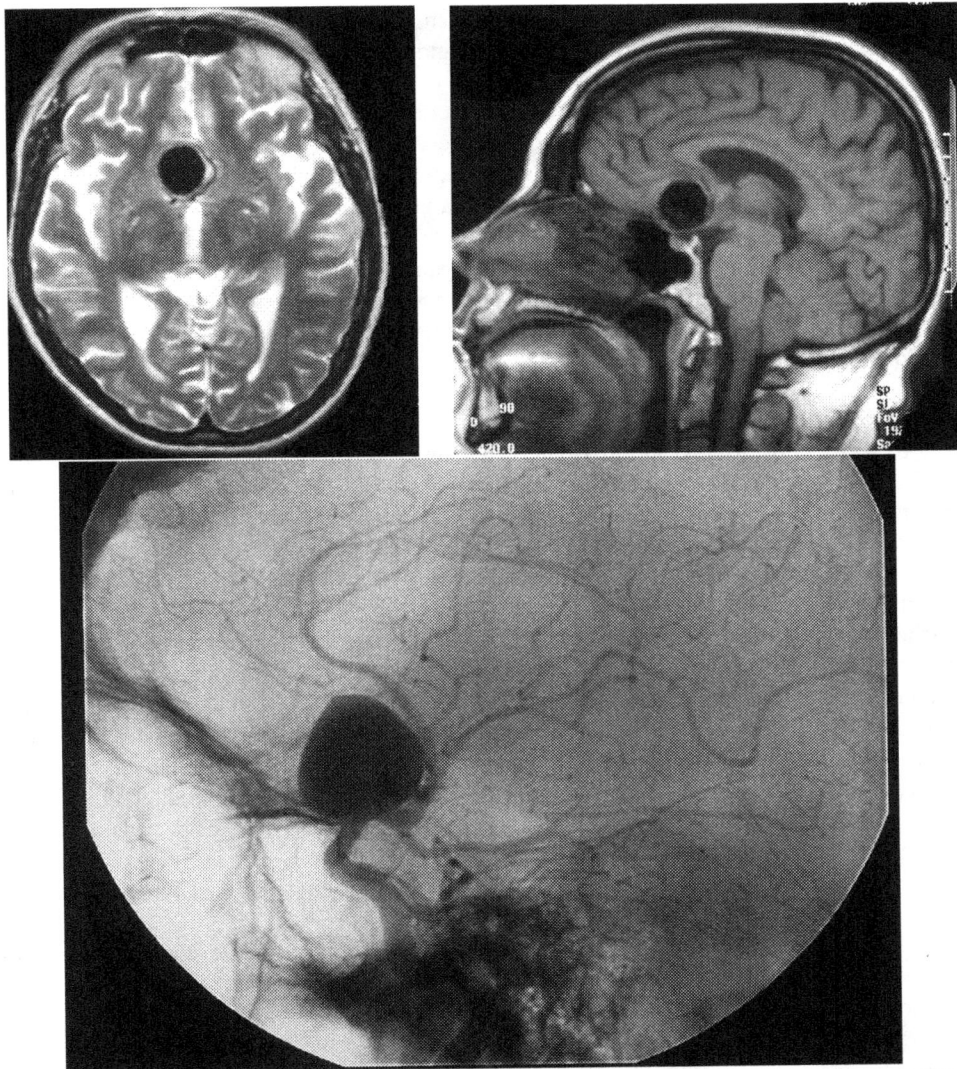

Figure 1. *The image top left is an axial T2 WI, the image top right is a sagittal T1 WI and the image directly above is that of a cerebral digital subtraction angiogram. The hypointensity seen on both top images represents flowing blood and the angiogram demonstrates a giant aneurysm.*

Some inherited conditions are associated with the formation of cerebral aneurysms, including polycystic kidney disease, Ehlers-Danlos syndrome, Marfan syndrome and neurofibromatosis type 1. Aneurysms, unlike the other malformations noted above, usually present with subarachnoid haemorrhage as they are located in the subarachnoid space. The other lesions usually cause intraparenchymal haemorrhage. In cases of intraparenchymal haemorrhage, the clinical effects are due to direct destruction of brain and to secondary pressure effects of the intraparenchymal clot. In the case of aneurysms that have previously leaked, the dome of the aneurysm can become adherent to brain and subsequent bleeds can also have an intraparenchymal component. Saccular (berry) aneurysms are classified according to size into small (less than 10mm), large (more than 10mm) and giant (greater than 25mm); their location in the anterior or posterior circulation of the circle of Willis and which blood vessel they originate from. The risk of rupture grows with increase in size and rupture usually occurs when the aneurysm reaches 5-10mm. Rupture commonly occurs during activities that increase blood pressure and a constant environmental factor that has been associated with increased risk of subarachnoid haemorrhage is cigarette smoking.

Treatment of incidental and unruptured aneurysms

This can sometimes be a difficult situation. Patients should be advised that these rupture at an average rate of 1 – 1.4% per year. The risk for rupture in a patient, who is less than 59 years old, is enough to negate the risks of treatment.

Aneurysmal subarachnoid haemorrhage (SAH)

This is a devastating disease and 10-30% of patients die before reaching hospital and for those that do reach the hospital, another 30-60% pass away. Survival does not equate with normality and only 30% of all patients with non-traumatic SAH survive without major disability. Patients who suffer SAH associated with AVM and those associated with perimesencephalic SAH carry a good prognosis. The sudden onset of an excruciating headache, usually reported as the worst ever in the patient's life is the hallmark of SAH. Unfortunately headache is a frequent presenting complaint to primary care physicians and it is frequently misdiagnosed. SAH is frequently associated with nausea, vomiting, meningism, photophobia, retinal haemorrhages on fundoscopy and decreased level of consciousness. A specific type of pre-retinal haemorrhage, called a subhyaloid haemorrhage is associated with SAH. Another ocular complication is haemorrhage into the vitreous, called Terson's syndrome. This may require elective surgery by an ophthalmic surgeon. There are 2 clinical grading systems in use, the Hunt and Hess grading scale (table 2) and the World Federation of Neurological Surgeons (WFNS) grading scale (table 3). Both have been correlated with outcome, but the WFNS grading scale is less likely to have inter-observer variations.

CT scanning is 98% sensitive for SAH in the first 12 hours after the haemorrhage but decreases over time and is only about 70% sensitive on day three following the ictus. The Fisher grading scale is used to predict the likelihood of vasospasm based on CT scan appearances (see chapter 5). In cases where there is a good history but negative CT scan, lumbar puncture and spectroscopy is invaluable. Following SAH, the red blood cells that entered the CSF undergo lysis and it takes several hours for the liberated oxyhaemoglobin to be converted via deoxyhaemoglobin to bilirubin. The enzyme, haem-oxygenase, which is responsible for the process is only found in the CNS. If a period of 12 hours is allowed following a suspected SAH, CSF obtained with a lumbar puncture can be spun down and spectroscopy performed on it. The presence of bilirubin is diagnostic for SAH. This is a very sensitive test for the first 14 days following SAH. The test should be delayed for 12 hours to allow the break down process into bilirubin to be completed, if not, a traumatic tap will be too early to pick up bilirubin and may contaminate the CSF sufficiently to make future test unreliable. The presence of high systemic levels of bilirubin and high levels of CNS protein may give false positive results but there are formulae to compensate for this.

Sudden severe headache, 'worst headache ever'
+/-
meningism, photophobia, nausea and vomiting, decreased consciousness,
retinal haemorrhages, cranial nerve pa lsy

Uncontrasted CT scan of the brain

positive for SAH

SAH CONFIRMED

LP > 12 hours after SAH
by experienced clinician

bilirubin peak +/ -
oxyhaemoglobin peak

oxyhaemoglobin peak alone

no peaks

SAH CONFIRMED **PROBABLY A TRAUMATIC TAP** **NO SAH**

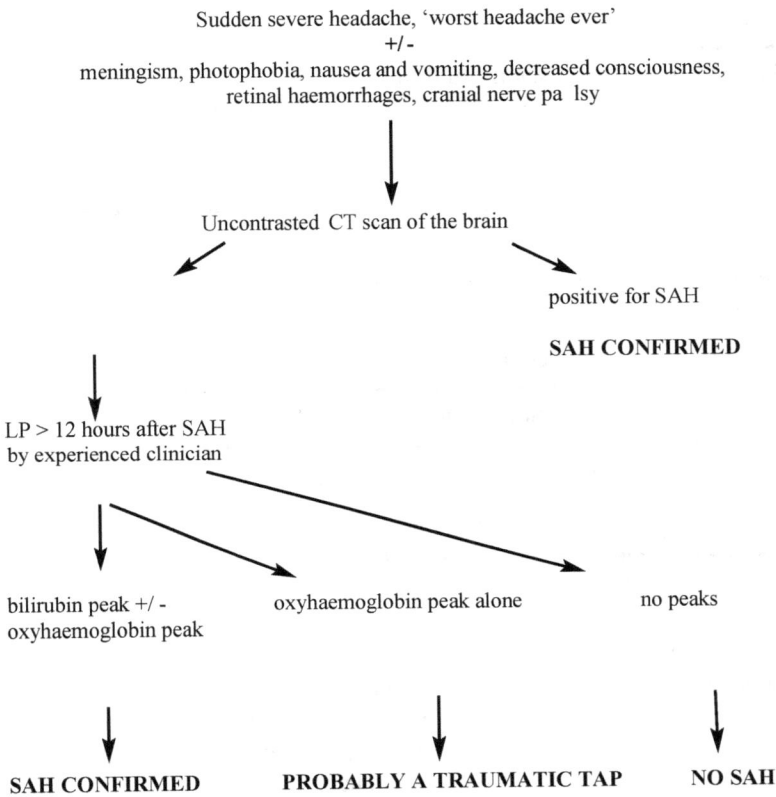

Figure 2. *Suggested scheme for diagnosing subarachnoid haemorrhage. (Aneurysmal sub-arachnoid haemorrhage: guidance in making the correct diagnosis, W A Liebenberg, R Worth, G B Firth, J Olney, and J S Norris, Postgrad Med J 2005; 81: 470-473).*

The definitive diagnosis of an underlying vascular abnormality is made with conventional digital subtraction cerebral angiography, which is the gold standard, but non invasive angiography (CT and MR) is approaching the same sensitivities. The most common sites of aneurysm ruptures are the internal carotid artery, anterior communicating artery/anterior cerebral artery and the middle cerebral artery. Approximately 85% of berry aneurysms occur in the anterior circulation of the circle of Willis.

Grade 1	Asymptomatic, mild headache, slight nuchal rigidity
Grade 2	Moderate to severe headache, nuchal rigidity, no neurological deficit other than cranial nerve palsy
Grade 3	Mild alteration in mental status, mild focal neurological deficit
Grade 4	Stupor and/or mild to moderate hemiparesis
Grade 5	Comatose and/or decerebrate rigidity

Table 2. *Hunt and Hess grading scale.*

Grade 1	Glasgow Coma Score (GCS) of 15, motor deficit absent
Grade 2	GCS of 13-14, motor deficit absent
Grade 3	GCS of 13-14, motor deficit present
Grade 4	GCS of 7-12, motor deficit absent or present
Grade 5	GCS of 3-6, motor deficit absent or present

Table 3. *The WFNS grading system*

General effects of SAH

Hyponatremia is common in SAH. It is usually due to the syndrome of cerebral salt wasting (CSW) or less often due to the syndrome of inappropriate secretion of antidiuretic hormone (SIADH) - see chapter 16. These syndromes can be difficult to tell apart. A reduced intravascular volume is the hallmark of CSW and is the best way to differentiate between the conditions. It is important to avoid fluid restriction in patients with SAH (especially in cases with CSW) and should be reserved for severe cases of SIADH where there is water intoxication.

Neurogenic pulmonary oedema is associated with advanced age and poor grades of SAH. It may occur in the first two weeks after SAH but most commonly occurs on day three. It is thought to be due to the catecholamine surge that occurs in SAH. Diuretics and positive end-expiratory pressure (PEEP) ventilation are the mainstays of treatment.

Neurogenic sympathetic hyperactivity with increased levels of systemic catecholamines leads to a whole host of different cardiac abnormalities. Arrhythmias are very common in the first 48 hours following SAH. ECG changes are also very common and cardiac enzymes are useful to diagnose true cardiac infarction from the benign ECG changes caused by the catecholamine shower.

Hydrocephalus - Acute obstructive hydrocephalus occurs in roughly 20% of SAH patients and is managed with external ventricular drainage. Late onset (after one week) communicating hydrocephalus caused by blockage of the CSF pathways occurs in approximately 10-15% of patients with SAH. There may be a general deterioration of patients and it can be difficult to distinguish it from symptomatic vasospasm. These patients can be managed by external lumbar CSF drainage, serial lumbar punctures or in persistent cases, ventriculoperitoneal shunting.

Specific effects of SAH

The medical management of SAH is extremely important and is based on the prevention of rebleeding and symptomatic vasospasm. The greatest risk of rebleeding is on the first day (4.1%) and the cumulative risk in the first two weeks is 19%. Rebleeding is associated with a 78% mortality rate and strict bed rest, restriction of visitors, quiet surroundings, adequate analgesia, stool softeners and antihypertensive agents when the mean arterial pressure (MAP) exceeds 130 mm Hg are measures used to try to prevent this catastrophe. Intravenous beta-blockers are popular for blood pressure control since they have a relatively short half-life, can be titrated easily and do not increase ICP. Seizures occur in as many as 25% of patients following SAH (most common in middle cerebral artery aneurysms) and increase the risk of rebleeding. Two anticonvulsants that allow for rapid IV loading, Phenytoin and Phenobarbital, are both used for prophylaxis. Patients in a poor grade and with increased ICP should be intubated and ventilated and care taken to keep the pCO_2 between 30-35 mm Hg (4-4.6 kPa), avoiding excessive hyperventilation which may cause vasospasm and brain ischaemia/infarction. The cerebral perfusion pressure (CPP) should be kept above 60-70 mm Hg (see chapter 16 for the management of ICP and CPP).

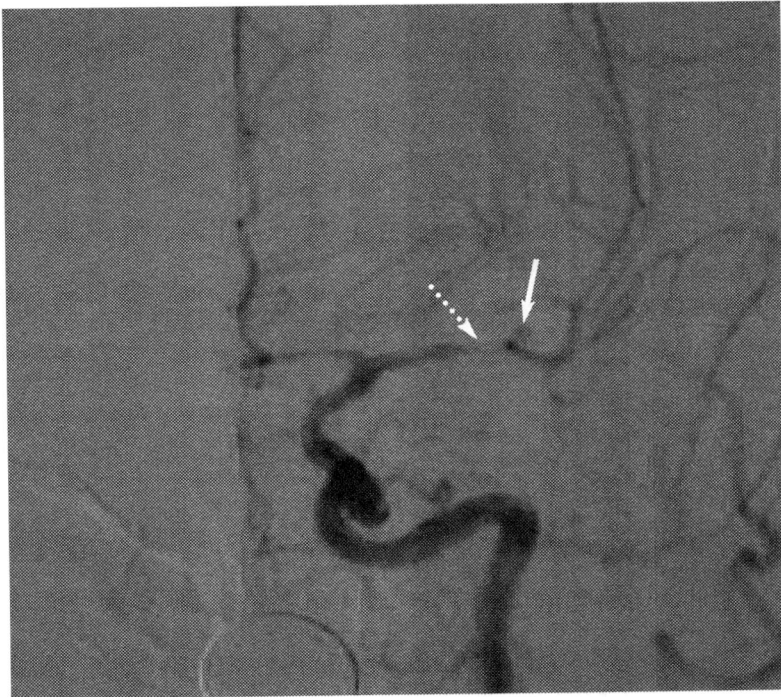

Figure 3. *This antero-posterior view of a left ICA angiogram demonstrates diffuse vasospasm (dashed arrow) following subarachnoid haemorrhage. A left MCA bifurcation aneurysm is also visible (arrow).*

Vasospasm

Vasospasm mostly occurs 4-14 days after the haemorrhage and is present in up to 70% of patients. Clinically symptomatic vasospasm is present in up to 30% of patients, may lead to cerebral ischaemia and infarction, and is more common in females, young patients, those who smoke, patients who presents in a poor clinical grade and those with large volumes of blood in the subarachnoid space. Patients present with a new onset decrease in consciousness or focal neurological deficit. Conventional angiography is the gold standard for diagnosing vasospasm but the diagnosis can be made reliably as a bedside test with transcranial Doppler. Other imaging modalities including single photon emission computed tomography (SPECT) and perfusion imaging (Xenon CT, dynamic perfusion CT and MRI), have been used successfully.

Prophylaxis for vasospasm:

Prophylaxis with Nimodipine is now standard practice and it improves overall outcome within 3 months of aneurysmal SAH. It appears that Nimodipine may have a neuroprotective effect by blocking calcium influx into damaged brain cells. Current practice is to maintain normovolemia to slight hypervolemia to prevent hypoperfusion. Results suggest that subarachnoid blood removal with intracisternal injections of recombinant tissue plasminogen activator (rTPA) during surgery for aneurysm clipping may carry some benefit.

Treatment for proven vasospasm:

Hypertensive, hypervolemic, and haemodilution therapy (HHH therapy, triple H), the standard of treatment for proven vasospasm, should be reserved for patients with secured aneurysms to reduce the risk of rebleeding.

Hypervolemia - The central venous pressure (CVP) should be maintained at 10-12 mm Hg. The pulmonary artery wedge pressure (PAWP) should be maintained at 19-20 mm Hg.

Haemodilution - The hematocrit should be maintained at 30-35% with dilution or packed cell transfusion to optimise blood viscosity and oxygen delivery.

Hypertensive therapy - Inotropic support and vasopressors may be needed to keep the mean arterial pressure (MAP) between 90 and 110 mm Hg.

Cerebral angiography with transluminal balloon angioplasty has been reported to lead to improved neurologic outcome in 70% of patients with symptomatic vasospasm. It is effective in treatment of large proximal vessels and is not effective in treatment of smaller distal vessels. Cerebral angiography with intra-arterial injection of Papaverine and nimodipine is also effective. Approximately 15-20% of patients with symptomatic vasospasm will have a poor outcome despite maximal therapy.

Definitive treatment of the aneurysm

Both surgical clipping and endovascular obliteration are highly successful treatments modalities. The international subarachnoid aneurysm trial (ISAT) which included mostly patients with small anterior circulation aneurysms showed a 22.5% relative and 6.9% absolute risk reduction at one year in the disability outcome of patients who were treated with coiling compared to those treated with surgery. There are many caveats to the interpretation of this study and the results cannot be extrapolated to all aneurysms. It has however fixed endovascular management firmly in the mind of physicians and the lay public alike. The main concern of endovascular treatment is the paucity of data on the longevity of this form of treatment. The following are broad guidelines:

Indications for surgical clipping include
Presence of a large parenchymal haematoma that requires evacuation
Young, fit patients with a good clinical grade (WFNS or Hunt and Hess grades 1-3)
Giant aneurysms
Complicated vascular anatomy with arteries originating from the aneurysmal dome
Wide-necked aneurysms (the coils escape from the aneurysm and block distal vessels)
Recurrent aneurysm after endovascular treatment with coil embolisation
Patient's wishes

Indications for endovascular treatment include
Patients who are medically unfit for a long general anaesthetic
Patients presenting with a poor clinical grade
Aneurysms located in the cavernous sinus and basilar tip aneurysm
Patients with symptomatic vasospasm who may benefit from endovascular treatment of their vasospasm
Multiple aneurysms not located close together anatomically
Patient's wishes

Timing of intervention
Early surgery within the first 3 days allows for the prevention of rebleeding, the removal of blood clots that may reduce vasospasm and for the use of maximal HHH therapy since transluminal pressure fluctuations are negated by clipping. However surgery is technically more difficult due to brain swelling and fragility of the aneurysm dome with increased surgical morbidity. Delayed surgery removes most of the technical difficulties except for very late surgery that brings the complication of adhesions. However, the aneurysm remains unprotected for this period and rebleeding carries a high mortality rate. It has been found that patients with good grades (grade 1 and 2) fare better with early treatment. This is less conclusive for grade 3 patients and grade 4 and 5 patients should be managed on a case per case basis. Patients with significant hydrocephalus may sometimes improve significantly on their clinical grading with the simple act of placing an external ventricular drain (EVD). Many centres employ endovascular treatment as a first line of management for patients in a poor clinical grade and some centres are using endovascular treatment as the mainstay of treatment.

11

HYDROCEPHALUS

W Adriaan Liebenberg

Contents

Hydrocephalus
Childhood hydrocephalus
Adult hydrocephalus
Normal pressure hydrocephalus
Benign intracranial hypertension (pseudotumour cerebri/ idiopathic intracranial hypertension)
Shunt complications

Hydrocephalus

CSF is produced in the brain through an active process by the choroid plexus and ependyma and is passively reabsorbed by the arachnoid villi. An adult produces about 20mls of CSF every hour (0.5L per day) and the adult ventricular system contains approximately 150mls CSF. There is a very fine balance between production and absorption of CSF and, with the large volume of CSF produced every day, obstruction in the pathway of CSF flow or decreased reabsorption will lead to a build up of fluid and increase in the size of the ventricles (ventriculomegaly). Ventriculomegaly is called hydrocephalus if the ventricles are enlarged because of fluid build up. In older people, the reduced size of the brain might lead to the ventricular spaces and subarachnoid spaces enlarging due to shrinkage of the brain, and this is not called hydrocephalus but purely brain atrophy with secondary ventriculomegaly (hydrocephalus ex vacuo).

Childhood hydrocephalus

This can be either congenital or acquired. A large proportion of childhood hydrocephalus is congenital and nearly half of those cases are due to aqueduct stenosis of which there are several anatomical variants which include small multi-channels and membranes across the lumen of the aqueduct. These children frequently become hydrocephalic in utero and this can be diagnosed in perinatal ultrasonic screening. Another cause of congenital childhood hydrocephalus is Chiari malformations. Chiari 2 malformation found in children is frequently associated with myelomeningocele. Up to 90% of patients with myelomeningocele will have associated Chiari 2 malformations and up to 80% of these children will also have associated hydrocephalus. This is particularly true for lesions higher up in the spinal cord. Chiari 2 malformation consists of downwards displacement of the vermis of the cerebellum and the fourth ventricle into the cervical spinal canal. The displaced tissue is fused to the underlying brain stem and this causes hydrocephalus by blocking the foramen of Magendie. These children need combination therapy of closure of the myelomeningocele and VP shunting.

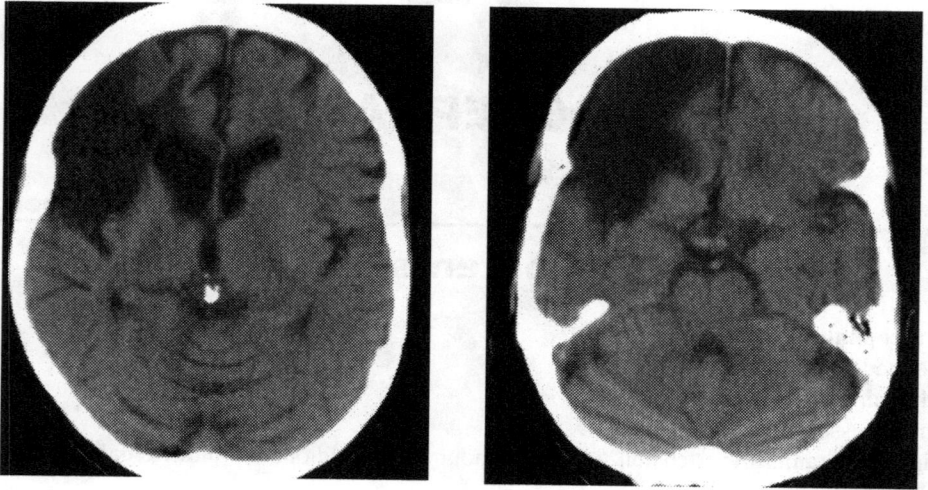

Figure 4. *Porencephalic cyst. These images are axial T1 WI and demonstrates a poren-cephalic cyst. A porencephalic cyst is a cavity within the cerebral hemisphere, filled with cerebrospinal fluid, that communicates directly with the ventricular system. The image on the right demonstrates the communication with the ventricle.*

Cysts are other causes of congenital hydrocephalus. Porencephalic cysts (cysts within the brain parenchyma), arachnoid cysts (cysts within the subarachnoid space) and Dandy-Walker cysts can cause hydrocephalus by compression of the ventricular system or of its outlet foramina. A Dandy-Walker cyst is a posterior fossa cyst that is in communication with the enlarged fourth ventricle with associated aplasia of the vermis of the cerebellum.
This has to be distinguished from a mega cisterna magna (large cisterna magna without hypoplasia of the vermis). Hydrocephalus is caused due to atresia of the foramina of Magendie and hydrocephalus with associated Dandy-Walker cyst is seen. The main differ-ential diagnosis of a Dandy-Walker cyst is an arachnoid cyst of the posterior fossa and a mega cisterna magna. Another congenital form of hydrocephalus is caused by aneurysms of the vein of Galen that causes obstruction of the CSF pathway.

Acquired hydrocephalus can be obstructive due to childhood tumours or can be communicat-ing due to post-inflammatory hydrocephalus and obstruction of the basal cisterns. Tuberculous meningitis, *Escherichia Coli* meningitis and *Haemophilus Influenza* meningitis are all well known to cause this. Premature infants weighing less than 0.5kg at birth, fre-quently develop intraventricular haemorrhage which can lead to obstruction of the CSF path-ways. The incidence of these bleeds can be reduced with phenobarbital. Repeated CSF tap-ping and treatment with Diamox (acetazolamide), which reduces the production of CSF, can frequently treat communicating hydrocephalus. Persistent cases, however, need shunting. Patients with obstructive hydrocephalus may be treated by removal of the obstruction and opening of the CSF pathways but in some cases temporary CSF diversion with ventriculosto-my is required or permanent diversion with third ventriculostomy or ventriculoperitoneal shunting (VPS).

Adult hydrocephalus

In adults, obstructive hydrocephalus, which is characterised by dilatation of only a part of the ventricular system, is caused by external compression of the ventricular system as in aqueduct stenosis or intraventricular obstruction by masses or bleeds. Obstructive hydrocephalus is usually treated by ventriculoperitoneal shunting. Obstructive hydrocephalus caused by aqueduct stenosis, either congenital or due to external compression, can also be treated by endoscopic third ventriculostomy. Communicating hydrocephalus (non obstructive) is due to dysfunctional absorption of CSF.

Normal pressure hydrocephalus (NPH) is a condition that occurs mostly in people older than 60. NPH is a misnomer however since it has been found that in these individuals the intracranial pressures, although mostly normal, are periodically transiently high. The condition is characterised by enlarged ventricles on imaging and a clinical triad of dementia, ataxia and incontinence. This supports dysfunction in the region of the medial frontal lobes. In about half the patients with NPH, there is a defined cause such as trauma, meningitis or subarachnoid haemorrhage which can be held accountable for the reduced absorption of CSF. The mechanism is thought to be blockage of the subarachnoid fluid pathways and blockage of some of the arachnoid villi which reabsorb CSF passively. The term idiopathic NPH is reserved for cases where there is no known cause for the hydrocephalus. Investigating NPH includes monitoring the intracranial pressure with pressure monitors, measuring the CSF pressure with a lumbar puncture (patient in decubitus position), infusing CSF through a lumbar puncture whilst measuring intracranial pressure and therapeutic drainage of CSF through either a lumbar puncture or an indwelling lumbar drain and measuring improvement in walking and mental function by the neuropsychologist. Treatment is with permanent CSF diversion via either a Lumboperitoneal or VP shunt.

Benign intracranial hypertension (BIH) also called pseudotumour cerebri or idiopathic intracranial hypertension is a disorder of unknown aetiology which affects predominantly obese women of childbearing age. The condition is characterised by raised intracranial pressure, headaches and visual disturbances secondary to papilloedema and optic nerve damage. There is thought to be either abnormalities of the arachnoid granulations or some form of venous outflow obstruction that accounts for the condition. On imaging the ventricles are usually slit-like and compressed by a generally 'tight' and swollen brain. The management is based on careful ophthalmological follow up since blindness is the major complication of this condition. Medical treatment is based on weight loss, diuretic treatment and acetazolamide (Diamox) administration. Diamox is a carbonic anhydrase inhibitor and decreases CSF production. When medical therapy fails optic nerve fenestrations are an option as well as CSF diversion with lumboperitoneal shunting. Some surgeons employ subtemporal decompression.

Shunt complications

Presentation

Beyond the age of 2 years shunt underdrainage presents with signs and symptoms of raised intracranial pressure. Up to the age of 2 years, the pliant skull and open cranial sutures allow for some compensation and resultant macrocephaly. Headaches that are worse in the recumbent position, nausea, vomiting and photophobia are typical symptoms. Patients that are completely shunt dependant and have complete occlusions typically become unwell very quickly. Considering that we produce nearly 500ml of CSF every day,   this is not entirely surprising.

About 50% of shunt complications are due to malfunction of the shunt unit, approximately 20% are due to symptoms related to pressure changes or overdrainage and about 10% are due to infection.

Infection

An infection rate of 5 – 10% is the accepted norm. Most infections are usually diagnosed within two months. *Staphylococcus Epidermidis* (40%) and *Staphylococcus Aureus* (20%) are the most frequently diagnosed organisms. Most of these infections have their origin in the perioperative period. Late infections after 2 months are usually due to bowel organisms (Gram negative Bacilli). Immediately after shunt placement a glycoprotein layer forms over the shunt. There are receptors on this glycoprotein layer that present for bacterial adhesion, but if normal body cells bind on these before bacteria can, this gives a barrier against infection. It is during this period of adhesion that a sterile enviroment needs to be insured. If there is bacterial adhesion, then bacterial multiplication follows with formation of a biofilm containing bacteria, polymers and caught up cells. Clinical infection is the last stage. The biofilm gives very good protection against anti bacterial agents such as antibiotics, white cells, surfactants and antibodies. *Staphylococcus Epidermidis* is much better at producing a biofilm than *Staphylococcus Aureus.* There are three main ways that the shunt can become colonised: the first is primary colonisation at the time of surgery, the second mechanism is haematogenous spread of infection and the third is transmission of an intra-abdominal infection.

The clinical effects of infection can be local infection around the shunt, meningitis, peritonitis, obstruction or cor pulmonale and nephritis in the case of ventriculoatrial shunts. Useful adjuncts in making the diagnosis are a blood white cell count, C-reactive protein, erythrocyte sedimentation rate and blood cultures. CSF sampling is 95% accurate and can be done from the shunt reservoir or LP. A CT scan is mandatory for comparison of ventricular size.

Risks for shunt infection are young patient age, poor skin condition, concomitant systemic infections at the time of shunt placement, postoperative wound dehiscence, prolonged operation time, limited surgeon experience, shunt revision rather than primary procedure, surgery done after hours, cases where the indication for shunt placement is myelomeningocele and importantly, an increased number of people in the operating room.
Some units have reported shunt infection rates of less than 2% by aggressively focusing on these factors and trying to eliminate them.
Management of the infected shunt is aimed at maintaining continued CSF drainage and eradication of the infection. In managing an infected shunt there are basically three options. The first and least successful option is to leave the shunt in position and to administer IV antibiotics. The second option is to externalise the distal end of the shunt, administer IV antibiotics

and, if the CSF obtained from the distal end is clear, then to replace the shunt. The third option is to completely remove the shunt and place an external ventricular drain, monitor the CSF drainage and, as soon as this is clear following antibiotic treatment, replace the whole shunt. The last option is the most successful and should be the aim in all cases. It is usual practice to give prophylactic antibiotics at the time of shunt placement and there is good evidence for this in the literature.

Mechanichal failure
In 20- 40% failures present within one year. After one year the incidence is 5% per year. The mean time until revision for a standard valve is 5 yrs. It is imperative that all valves are tested at surgery for failure.

Occlusions - cause up to 50% of shunt dysfunction in pediatric population. The risk is highest immediately post operatively secondary to debris or improper ventricular catheter placement Late occlusions can be due to choroid plexus, ependymal reactions or immune reactions. Ventricular catheter occlusion can be due to debris in the CSF, improper location of the ventricular catheter point and slit ventricles (up to 40% incidence of proximal obstruction). Valve occlusions can be due to a factory fault, accumulation of debris with insertion, bacterial proliferation or immune reaction. There may be relative obstruction to flow from ascites or a pseudocyst in a ventriculo peritoneal shunt or thrombi in the lumen of a ventriculoatrial shunt. Suggestions to reduce occlusions are to make sure that the shunt inserted is clean, to place the ventricular catheter in area of most ventricular dilatation, to check patency of the valve before insertion and to choose the appropriate shunt and shunt setting to avoid over drainage and slit ventricles.

Disconnection or fracture - this is the second most frequent reason for dysfunction in the pediatric population. Reasons are improper selection of shunts, loose ties, the use of absorbable sutures, multiple connections and a rough technique during insertion.

Migration - very low profile and streamlined valves and reservoirs may be prone to migration and occlusion. Improper fixation of the shunt and excess tubing is another reason for migration and subsequent kinking and occlusion.

Improper placement of the ventricular catheter - usually directly related to the surgeon's experience.

Skin complications and subcutaneous CSF accumulations
Skin complications are seen in patients with open wounds, septic and potentially septic areas adjacent to the shunt or its tract. Poor host immune system, poor placement of the valve and large valves with sharp edges are also potentially dangerous. CSF fluid collections are seen when shunt is non functioning or when functioning but under the following conditions: loose skin, valves with high pressure, large ventricles with relatively small area of cortex or large dural openings

Overdrainage
Overdrainage occurs in up to 10% of children and 30% of adults. A standard low resistance, medium pressure valve can allow drainage of 200ml/hr in a 25cm water differential pressure. The production of CSF is only 21ml/hr. There are large variations in pressure gradients during different physiological conditions such as postural changes, REM sleep and physical

exertion. The risk of overdrainage can be decreased by: increasing the opening pressure of the valve, adding an anti siphoning device or adding a flow regulatory device. The complications of overdrainage are subdural fluid collections, slit ventricles, craniostenosis, loculation of ventricles and orthostatic hypotension

12

CRANIOSPINAL TRAUMA

W Adriaan Liebenberg

Contents

Traumatic brain injury (TBI)
Focal injury
Diffuse brain injury
Secondary brain injury

Spinal Trauma
Cervical spine
Thoracic spine
Lumbar spine

Spinal dysfunction syndromes
Grading scales for spinal injury

Traumatic brain injury (TBI)

Approximately 52,000 people die in the United States every year from TBI.
TBI is divided into primary and secondary injury. Primary injury can either be focal injury or diffuse injury. The severity of TBI is classified according to the GCS as follows:

Severe	3-8
Moderate	9-12
Mild	13-15

Focal injury
Soft tissue injury
Trauma can lead to severe soft tissue injuries with degloving, tissue loss and macerated tissue depending on the nature of the force brought to bear on the cranium. The scalp is vascular and patients may suffer significant blood loss from lacerations.

Skull fractures
Linear fractures
A linear fracture is when the opposing edges of the skull defect are directly opposing each other. These can be difficult to tell apart from suture lines on CT scans and X-rays. They differ from sutures in that they are wider at the centre and narrower at the points, run in a straight line and have angular turns. Sutures on the other hand are the same width throughout and run in gentle curves. When these fractures cross dural arteries like the middle meningeal artery or cross dural venous sinuses, they may lead to epidural (extradural) haematomas.

Depressed fractures

When the two edges of a fracture do not directly oppose each other, a fracture is depressed or indriven. They are only of clinical significance if the one edge is depressed as least as much as the thickness of the opposing edge. These may require elevation if they are cosmetically unacceptable or if there is dural penetration. Closed fractures may be treated non-surgically but open fractures should be explored and débrided.

Comminuted fractures

A fracture that contains more than two fragments is deemed to be comminuted. These are usually associated with a direct blow to the head.

Open (Compound)

A skull fracture where the overlying skin is lacerated is called an open fracture and these may lead to infection and therefore should be properly debrided, and the scalp closed without tension.

Base of skull fractures (BOS fracture)

These linear fractures run through the skull base and are produced by considerable force. There are two types:

Longitudinal BOS fracture (to the axis of the petrous bone)

These fractures of the petrous portion of temporal bone lead to ossicular chain disruption and conductive deafness and need urgent ENT consultation.

Transverse BOS fracture (to the axis of the petrous bone)

These fractures of the petrous portion of temporal bone lead to damage of the VIIth cranial nerve and damage to the labyrinth leading to facial weakness, ataxia and permanent sensorineural hearing loss.

Ping pong fractures

In babies where the bone is still very pliable, a specific type of depressed fracture occurs. Just like a ping-pong ball may be dented, the baby's skull may be dented and may require surgical correction. They are easily corrected with an elevator due to the softness of the bone.

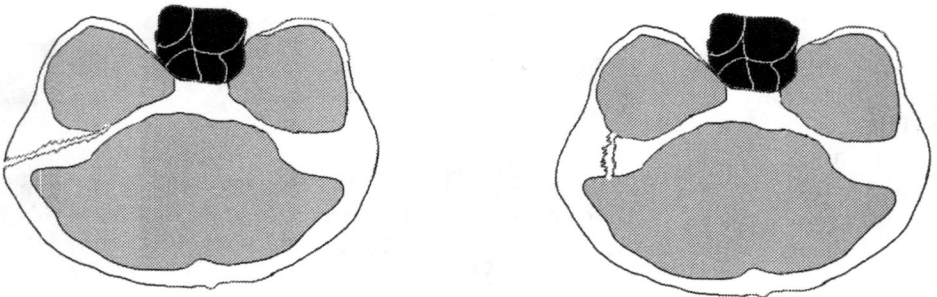

Figure 1. *The image on the left is a diagrammatic representation of a longitudinal BOS fracture and the image on the right, that of a transverse BOS fracture through the petrous bone.*

Extra-axial haemorrhages

These haemorrhages are outside the parenchyma of the brain.

Epidural haematomas

These form between the bone and the dura and occur when dural arteries or venous sinuses are damaged. They are frequently associated with minor or no underlying damage to the brain itself and carry a favourable prognosis if evacuated promptly. It may however be part of a generalised diffuse brain injury with associated subdural haematoma and diffuse brain damage. This is frequently seen where there is a focal injury as well as rotational and acceleration/deceleration forces in motor vehicle accidents. In these cases the focal injury frequently occurs when the patient's head comes into contact with the windscreen or dashboard. Seldom are lesions treated conservatively, since they have the propensity to continue enlarging.

Subdural haematomas

These can either be caused by focal damage or by diffuse brain injury. In contrast, the epidural haematomas are nearly always caused by a focal injury, which may be on a background of a diffuse injury, as described above. Direct focal forces that penetrate the dura can lead to haematomas. In diffuse brain injuries, the rotational and deceleration/acceleration forces tear the fragile veins that drain from the cortex to the overlying dural sinus and leads to haemorrhage. Subdural haematomas are a marker of severe injury and usually associated with a less favourable prognosis. In the elderly and patients with atrophic brains, frequently only minor trauma is needed to cause a subdural haematoma. This is because of the increased distance between the dura and the shrunken atrophic cortex, allowing veins to tear easily. Since there is a large CSF space and fluid around the atrophic brain, these haemorrhages frequently need to be quite extensive before they compress the brain and cause symptoms. Therefore there may be a delay in diagnosis of these haematomas. As the red blood cells lyse, the haemoglobin denaturises into bilirubin and the density of these haematomas reduce on CT scanning and they become first isodense to brain and then hypodense. In the acute stage, when the subdural consists mostly of clots, it can only be removed with a craniotomy but in the chronic phase, the more liquid chronic subdural is usually drained with burr holes. The decision to drain a subdural is based on the patient's status as well as the findings on CT scan. The most important findings on CT scan are the size of the lesion, the amount of shift and whether there is any herniation of brain tissue.

Penetrating head injuries

These can be missile or non missile injuries and can be devastating injuries. In the case of missile injuries, the velocity of the missile is the main determinant of the resultant damage ($E=mv^2$). The tumble and yaw of the projectile as it passes through tissue is incredibly destructive locally and the passage of the projectile leads to a temporary cavity that explodes outwards and then collapses again, causing damage in a wide area. A secondary effect is the generation of distant shockwaves that race through the brain causing a severe, global cerebral dysfunctional state. Admission GCS predicts outcome and mortality has been reported to be wide ranging from about 45% in more recent series to 80% in older series. Suicidal gunshot wounds carry a poorer prognosis. Non penetrating injuries have the best prognosis. There are three types of penetrating injuries. The first type is a tangential injury where the projectile glances of the skull and only bone fragments penetrate the dura. The second type is simply called a penetrating gunshot wound and per definition the projectile passes through the dura into the brain parenchyma. The third type is called a perforating gunshot wound and in this case the projectile passes through the cranium. Treatment includes debridement, broad spectrum antibiotics, anticonvulsants and ICU care to limit secondary brain injury. The prognosis is poor in bihemispheric injuries and especially in transventricular injuries.

Coup and contrecoup lesions

We frequently see coup and contrecoup injuries where the impact side (coup side) has underlying pathology as well as the contrecoup side. This may be seen when patients fall from standing or from a height onto their heads. They have focal soft tissue swelling over the site of impact with some focus of pathology there, frequently an intracerebral haemorrhage with some associated subarachnoid haemorrhage. As the brain then moves forward and rubs over the surface of the orbital roof and reaches the anterior cranial fossa, this then leads to bifrontal contusions. There are frequently associated bitemporal contusions as the anterior poles of the temporal lobes collide with the sphenoid ridge which forms the anterior border of the middle cranial fossa. These can frequently be devastating injuries and can have longterm sequelae. These contusions quite often blossom as they enlarge and have associated oedema, usually about a week after the injury. Other intracerebral haemorrhages, called haemorrhagic contusions, can be larger versions of the pinpoint bleeds in diffuse brain injury and is caused by the same mechanism. It is frequently seen at the white matter/grey matter interface but the term is also used to refer to coup and contrecoup lesions.

Diffuse brain injury

Diffuse brain injury (DBI) is part of a wide spectrum ranging from concussion to severe diffuse axonal injury. The hallmark of diffuse brain injury on imaging is pinpoint bleeds. These occur due to acceleration, deceleration and rotational forces placed on the brain with subsequent tears in the white matter tracts, leading to pin point haemorrhages. A frequent accompaniment of diffuse brain injury is the presence of intraventricular or subarachnoid blood, denoting a serious injury.

On imaging there are three grades of DBI.

Grade 1 – diffuse point bleeds throughout the brain
Grade 2 – as above with point bleeds in the corpus callosum
Grade 3 – as grade 2 with point bleeds in the dorsal mid-brain

These three grades correlate well with prognosis and mid-brain haemorrhages are usually associated with a poor prognosis. Histopathologicaly the injury is the greatest at the grey-white matter interface and the basis for the clinical syndrome of diffuse brain injury is the histological condition of diffuse axonal injury (DAI). The axons are damaged by shear forces. Some are torn and some sustain damage and are not completely torn, but due to damage in the membrane, there is disruption in the axoplasmic flow, which causes the axon to swell up and ultimately split up. A retraction ball forms, which is a pathologic hallmark of shearing injury. The axon then undergoes Wallerian degeneration. DAI was always believed to represent a primary injury. However, it has become apparent that the axoplasmic membrane damage and retraction ball formation represents a secondary set of events.

Secondary brain injury
Local factors

Traumatic brain injury (TBI) leads to mechanical cell membrane deformation with subsequent depolarisation and activation of ligand-gated ion channels which allow ions to move down their electrochemical gradients. Membrane depolarisation from this ionic flux trigger voltage-sensitive ion channels that open even more routes for ionic movement. The ionic movement leads to an increase in extracellular potassium and an increase in intracellular sodium, calcium and chloride that is followed passively by water, leading to cellular oedema and in turn brain oedema and raised ICP. Normally membrane ionic pumps would rectify this imbalance, but in brain swelling and hypoperfusion states, the available ATP is reduced to supply these energy dependant pumps. The final pathway of cell death is calcium influx and a lot of research efforts are aimed at trying to combat this. Secondary brain injury is controlled and initiated through mediators released following TBI. The excitatory amino acids (EAA) glutamate and aspartate are released in significant amounts following TBI. They are responsible for an excitotoxic cascade that ultimately leads to cell damage and cell death. They cause an influx of chloride and sodium, leading to acute neuronal swelling which may lead to cell death. EAAs also can cause delayed damage secondary to an influx of calcium. EAAs in association with N-methyl-D-aspartate receptor agonists, which also contribute to increased calcium influx, may decrease high-energy phosphate stores (ATP). Another effect of both is an increase in free radical production.

Systemic factors

Hypoxemia (SaO_2< 90%) or hypotension (Systolic BP< 90 mm Hg) are significant parameters associated with a poor outcome in patients with severe head injury. After TBI, reduced levels of vasodilators (nitric oxide, cGMP and cAMP) contribute to decreased intracranial blood flow and conversely increased levels of vasoconstrictors, such as endothelin -1, also contribute to vascular dysregulation. Hypotension has been said to be the sine qua non of secondary brain injury.

Spinal Trauma
Cervical spine

This highly mobile and relatively weak part of the human body is the conduit for the spinal cord that carries all nerve impulses between the brain and the body. The normal biomechanics of the cervical spine allow for ample flexion and lateral flexion since these are anatomically limited. Forward flexion is limited by the chin striking the chest wall and lateral flexion is limited by the head striking the shoulders. However extension is only limited by the head striking the patient's back and this is significantly outside the limit of the normal biomechanical range. A high proportion of cervical trauma is sustained in motor vehicle accidents (MVA), and 20% of all MVA deaths include fatal or severe cervical spine injuries. The level most often involved in cervical fractures or fracture dislocations is C2 followed by C5 and then C6.

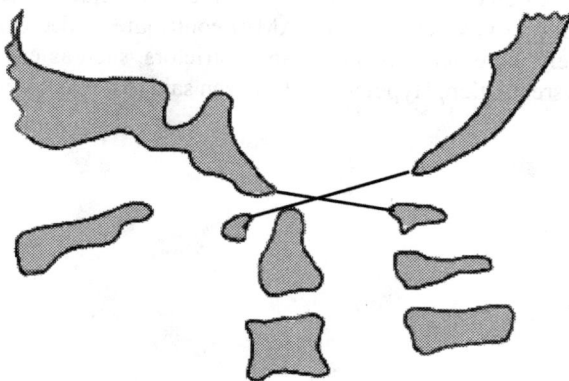

Figure 2. *The Power's ratio is calculated by dividing the distance between the edge of the clivus and the posterior arch of the atlas by the distance between the anterior arch of the atlas and the posterior edge of the foramen magnum*

Specific fractures and dislocations:
Occipital condyle fractures

Type 1 – axial loading mechanism with comminution of the condyle but no displacement (stable)

Type 2 – part of a base of skull fracture (stable)

Type 3 – avulsion fracture of the condyle, due to lateral flexion forces (potentially unstable)

Atlanto-occipital dislocation

These are produced by distraction forces, are usually unstable, and must not be treated by traction. External immobilisation such as halo vest followed by internal fixation is the treatment of choice. The injury is diagnosed by demonstrating an increased distance between the base of the skull and the tip of the dens. A Power's ratio (see fig 2) of greater than one suggests the diagnosis. The Power's ratio is calculated by dividing the distance between the edge of the clivus and the posterior arch of the atlas by the distance between the anterior arch of the atlas and the posterior edge of the foramen magnum.

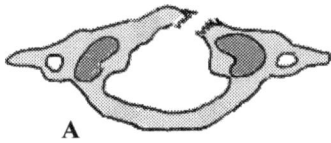

A

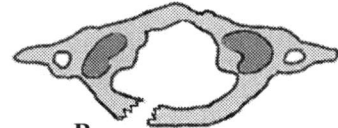

B

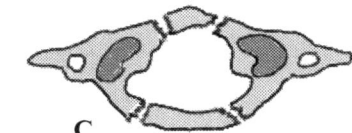

C

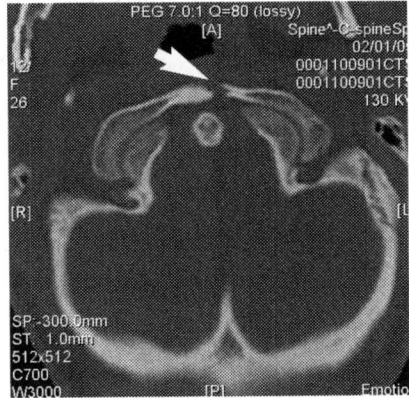

Figure 3a. *This axial CT scan demonstrates a fracture of the anterior arch of the atlas*

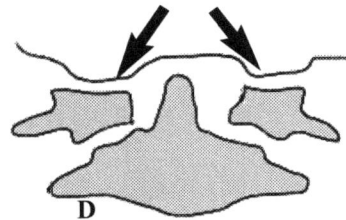

D

Figure 3. *Fractures of the atlas. A: demonstrates a fracture of the anterior arch; B: demonstrates a fracture of the posterior arch; C: demonstrates a Jefferson's fracture and D: demonstrates the force vectors when the skull base is forced downward onto the atlas that leads to a Jefferson's fracture.*

Fractures of the atlas
Posterior arch fractures
These are stable fractures that can be treated in a hard collar or halo vest.
Anterior arch fractures
These are stable fractures that can be treated in a hard collar or halo vest.
Jefferson fracture (burst fracture of the ring of C1)
This is caused by axial compression and is manifested by fractures of both the anterior and posterior arches. The lateral masses are displaced laterally and if they are displaced more than 7mm from their normal position, this signifies rupture of the transverse ligament. A halo vest is adequate for cases where the transverse ligament is intact. Rupture of the transverse

271

ligament usually necessitates recumbent traction.

Lateral mass fracture

These can generally be treated in a hard collar or a halo vest

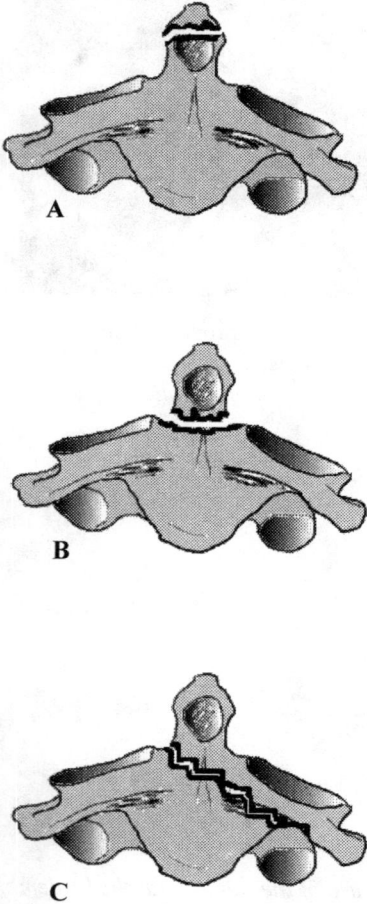

Figure 4. *Fractures of the dens (odontoid peg). A: demonstrates a type 1 fracture; B: demonstrates a type 2 fracture and C: demonstrates a type 3 fracture.*

Fractures of the axis
Odontoid
Type 1 – avulsion of the tip, treated with cervical collar.
Type 2 – fracture through the base, most common type, treatment in halo vest leads to union in about half. Otherwise posterior C1-C2 fusion required.
Type 3 – fracture through the base and extends into the body of the axis. These heal well in a halo vest.
Fractures of the lateral mass

These occur secondary to an axial loading mechanism, usually heals well in hard collar or halo vest.

Hangman's fracture (traumatic spondylolisthesis of C2)

These fractures are caused by bilateral pars interartricularis (pedicle) fractures

Type 1 – no angulation of C2 relative to C3 and less than 3mm spondylolisthesis, treat in hard collar

Type 2 – both greater than 11 degree angulation and more than 3mm spondylolisthesis, reduce and treat in halo vest

Type 3 – the above plus either unilateral or bilateral facet dislocation, reduce and treat in halo vest

Type 4 (Type 2 A) – no spondylolisthesis but significant angulation, reduce and treat in halo vest

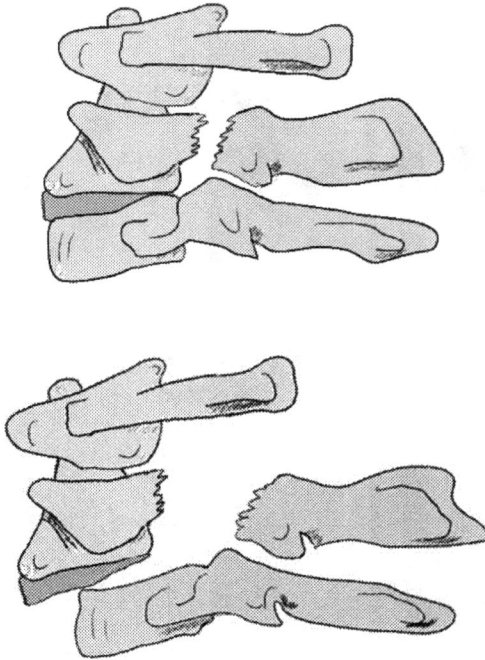

Figure 5. *Hangman's fracture. The top image demonstrates a type 1 fracture and the bottom image demonstrates a type 2 fracture.*

Fractures and dislocations of the subaxial cervical spine

Unilateral facet dislocations

These are typified by a spondylolisthesis of 25% or less at the affected level and rotation of the spinous process on the anterior-posterior view. Treatment is based on reduction with spinal traction followed by halo vest immobilisation or open reduction and fixation in cases where closed reduction is not possible.

Bilateral facet dislocations

This is a hyperflexion injury leading to rupture of the posterior ligaments. There is usually a spondylolisthesis of 50% or more and these are highly unstable fractures associated with neurological deficit. They may be reduced with spinal traction but universally require open fixation.

273

Subaxial fractures

Panjabi and White suggest that the sub axial cervical spine is unstable or on the brink of instability when any of the following conditions are present:

All the anterior or all the posterior elements have been destroyed

More than 3.5 mm spondylolisthesis is present

More than 11 degrees angulation is present.

Compression fractures – flexion injuries, usually failure of the anterior column

Burst fractures – axial loading injuries may have neurological compromise, they are mostly treated with surgery.

Tear drop fractures – flexion injuries, small chip of bone breaks off on anterior aspect of the vertebral body. May have neurological compromise, may require surgery.

Clay shoveller's fracture – hyperflexion, avulsion fracture of the spinous process of C7, occasionally caused by a direct blow, painful but stable.

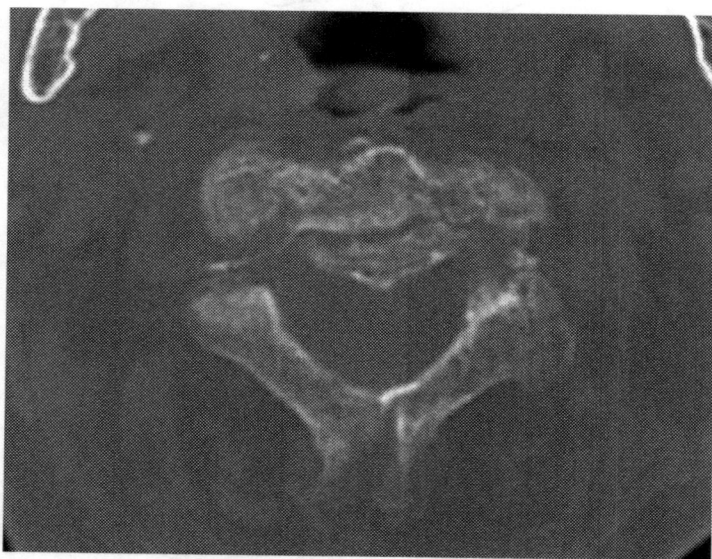

Figure 6. *This axial CT scan demonstrates a burst fracture of C2 with a segment of bone slightly retropulsed..*

Spinal cord injury without radiological abnormality (SCIWORA)

These patients present with neurological compromise following trauma with no radiologically identifiable fracture. In adults, it is due to hyperextension on the background of pre-existing cervical spondylosis and critical cervical canal stenosis. It is common in paediatric patients for the following reasons: the articulating facets are arranged more horisontally, there is forward wedging of the anterior portion of the vertebral bodies, the ligaments of the spine are more lax and the muscles of the neck are relatively underdeveloped for the relatively large size of the paediatric cranium.

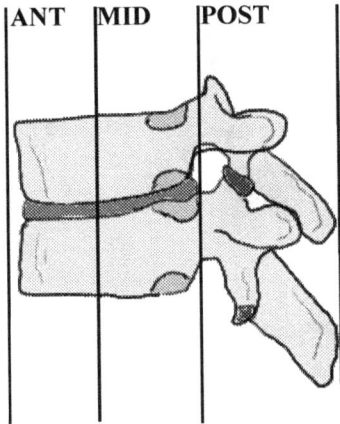

Figure 5. *Denis's three column theory*

Thoracic spine

Spinal instability in the thoracic spine is based on Denis's three column model which is an adaptation of Holdsworth's two column theory. The three columns are divided as follows:

Anterior column – anterior half of the vertebral body and the anterior longitudinal ligament
Middle column – posterior half of the vertebral column and the posterior longitudinal ligament
Posterior column – Posterior bony elements (pedicles, lateral masses, laminas and spinous processes) and the posterior ligaments (interspinous and supraspinous ligaments and ligamentum flavum)

Injury to two columns causes instability, therefore involvement of the middle column along with the posterior or the anterior column equates to instability and requires internal fixation.

Lumbar spine

Denis's model for spinal instability is used in the lumbar spine as well. However for both the thoracic and the lumbar spine there are other classification systems. The AO classification is widely used.

The four major spine injuries as per Denis:

Wedge compression fractures

Most common type of fracture, stable as middle column not involved
Type A: fracture of both superior and inferior endplates with avulsion of segment of bone on anterior aspect
Type B: fracture of the superior endplate
Type C: fracture of the inferior endplate
Type D: Fracture of anterior aspect of vertebral body, endplates unaffected

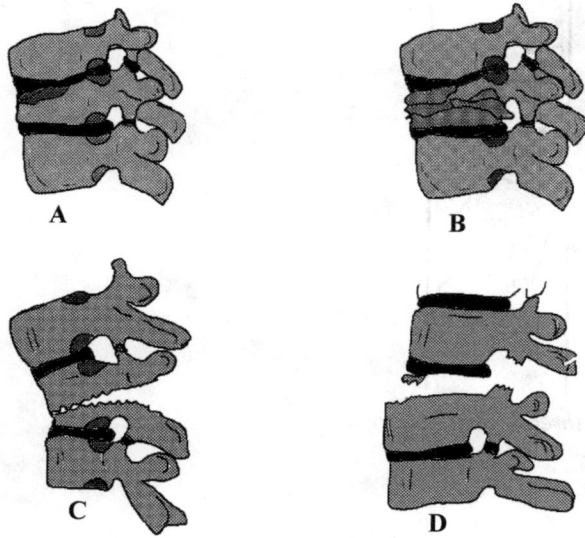

Figure 6. *The 4 major spine injuries as per Denis; A: Wedge compression fracture; B: Burst fracture; C: Chance fracture; D:Fracture-dislocation.*

Burst fractures

In theory unstable as anterior and middle columns involved and sometimes the posterior elements as well. It has been suggested by McAfee that these fractures are only truly unstable if all three columns are involved. These fractures are also in some instances associated with retropulsed segments that compress the conus/cauda equina.

Type A: fracture of both superior and inferior endplates
Type B: fracture of the superior endplate
Type C: fracture of the inferior endplate
Type D: rotational component
Type E: lateral flexion component

Seat belt-type injuries

These are distraction and hyper flexion injuries. The classic description of this was done by Chance in 1948. He described a fracture through the posterior arch and pedicles of the vertebral body with extension into the posterior aspect of the vertebral body. There are 4 types
Type A: the classic Chance fracture
Type B: rupture of the posterior ligamentous complex, no bony fracture
Type C: the same as Type A, only over 2 levels
Type D: the same as Type B, only over 2 levels.

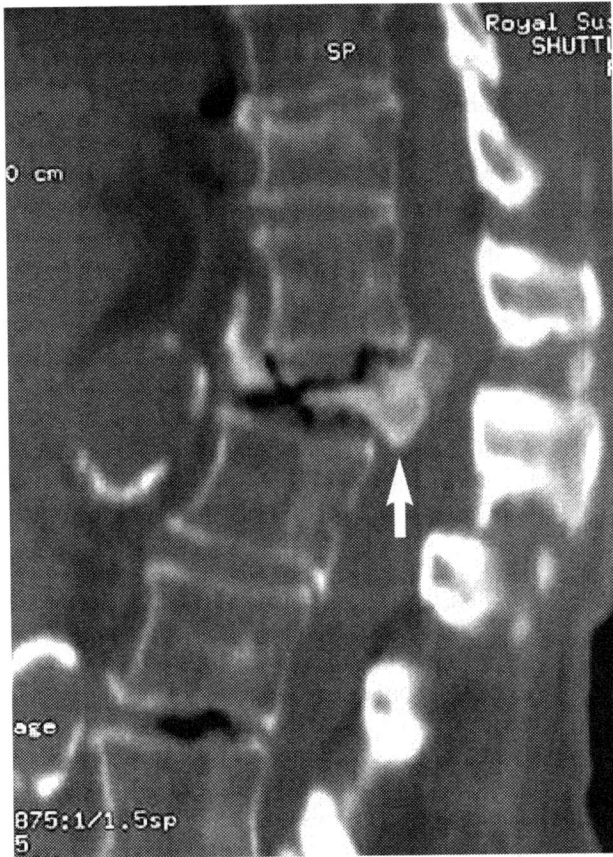

Figure 7. *This CT scan of the thoracic spine demonstrates a burst fracture with retropulsed fragment of bone (arrow).*

Fracture-dislocations

These are when the superior vertebral body undergoes both a traumatic spondylolisthesis and rostral displacement secondary to failure of all three columns either by a fracture extending through the whole of the vertebra or as a result of a separation of the intervertebral disc. There are 3 mechanisms that can lead to these injuries: flexion-rotation, flexion-distraction and shear injuries. There are 2 types

Type A: lesions associated with bony fracture and ligamentous disruption

Type B: lesions with ligamentous disruption and the separation of the vertebrae occurring through the disc.

Spinal dysfunction syndromes

The management of spinal trauma is based on reduction of anatomical abnormalities, decompression of neural elements and fixation to re-establish the integrity and stability of the spinal column. Closed reduction in cases of cervical trauma can be performed with spinal traction. Open reduction and fixation are used for cases of failed closed reduction. Operative approaches are tailored according to the elements damaged and whether there is canal compromise. Anterior as well as posterior approaches and fixation are used, sometimes in combination.

Brown Séquard syndrome

This syndrome results from damage to the one half of the cord. The clinical manifestations are the loss of power, proprioception and light touch on one side and pain and temperature on the other side of the body distal to the level of the injury. Thinking back to the anatomy of the cord, it would mean that the one side's anterior elements (motor – corticospinal, light touch – anterior spinothalamic), posterior elements (proprioception) and in the cases of the lateral elements (pain and temperature – lateral spinothalamic), the opposite side's pain sensation will be affected. This is because the pain fibres cross over in the spine and not at the medulla like other fibres. Pain fibres enter the cord and run in the lateral spinothalamic tract for a few segments and then cross over. The prognosis for these injuries is moderately good.

Anterior spinal cord syndrome

This is due to occlusion of the anterior spinal artery or anterior cord compression and leads to complete motor and sensory loss with some sparing of proprioception. These injuries have a poor prognosis.

Central cord syndrome

This frequently occurs in the elderly with pre-existing cervical canal stenosis, who suffer hyperextension injury, frequently with a simple fall. Due to the arrangement of the motor fibres in the spinal cord, with the arm fibres being more centrally located than the leg fibres, the patients present with motor symptoms which are more severe in the upper limbs than the lower limbs. These patients also present with a variety of sensory deficits.

Conus medullaris syndrome

When the conus and the origin of the cauda equina are compressed, there is both cord and radicular compromise. This leads to mixed upper and lower motor neurone signs with motor weakness, bowel and bladder dysfunction and sensory deficit.

Cauda equina syndrome

Compression of the cauda equina at a level below that of L1/2 produces lower motor neurone signs and symptoms in the lower limbs and bowel and bladder dysfunction. Lesions above L1 compress the conus as well and patients will have a conus medullaris syndrome.

Grading scales for spinal injury

The Frankel grading system is used for gross neurological impairment grading and correlates with prognosis:
Frankel A: complete deficit
Frankel B: sparing of some sensory function
Frankel C: sparing of non useful motor function
Frankel D: sparing of useful motor function
Frankel E: recovery

American Spinal Injury Association (ASIA) Impairment Scale

The Asia Impairment Scale is a finer scale:
ASIA A: **Complete** - No motor or sensory function down to the level of S4 and S5
ASIA B: **Incomplete** – Sensory but not motor function is preserved below the neurological level and extend through the sacral levels of S4 and S5.

ASIA C: **Incomplete** – Motor function is preserved below the neurological level and the majority of the key muscles below the neurological level have a muscle grade less than 3.

ASIA D: **Incomplete** – Motor function is preserved below the neurological level and the majority of the key muscles below the neurological level have a muscle grade greater than or equal to 3.

ASIA E: **Normal** – Motor and sensory function is normal

13

CRANIOSPINAL INFECTION

W Adriaan Liebenberg

Contents

Cranial infection

Extra-axial infection
Osteomyelitis
Epidural abscess (empyema)

Intra-axial infection
Bacterial meningitis
Subdural empyema
Cerebritis and brain abscess
Ventriculitis
Viral infections
Parasitic diseases

Spinal infection
Osteomyelitis
Epidural empyema (abscess)
Subdural abscess (empyema)
Intramedullary abscess
Discitis
Tuberculosis of the spine

Cranial infection
Extra-axial infection
This includes infection of the scalp, the skull (osteomyelitis) and the epidural (extradural) compartment.
Osteomyelitis
Osteomyelitis is relatively rare and usually follows either penetrating trauma or neurosurgical intervention but may also be spontaneous. *Staphylococcus Aureus* most commonly causes the infection and the treatment includes complete debridement and long-term antibiotic cover.
Epidural abscess (empyema)
Epidural and subdural empyema have the same pathogenesis. The most common causes are penetrating trauma, neurosurgical procedures and infection of nearby anatomical spaces

(facial air sinuses, the mastoid and middle ear sinuses) and haematogenous spread is less likely. Epidural empyema is usually associated with osteomyelitis and the main complications of epidural abscess are thrombosis of nearby vascular structures and intracranial spread. In extradural empyema without any subdural spread, CSF studies are usually normal. The peripheral white blood cell count and inflammatory markers are usually elevated and the patient might be pyrexial with signs of increased intracranial pressure. Management is complete surgical evacuation and long-term antibiotic cover.

Intra-axial infection
Intra-axial cranial infection includes meningitis, subdural empyema, cerebritis, brain abscess and ventriculitis.

Bacterial meningitis
Meningitis is either aseptic or septic. Septic meningitis can be acute (within hours or days) or chronic (for at least 4 weeks) and can be iatrogenic or spontaneous. Clinically patients present with symptoms and signs that include the following: lethargy or confusion, fever, neck stiffness and Kernig's sign (meningeal irritation), photophobia, nausea and vomiting. CSF analysis shows increased white cells (leucocytosis). In bacterial or septic meningitis, there is a polymorphonuclear pleocytosis and in aseptic meningitis, a predominant lymphocytosis. Certain patient factors (age and immune status) and iatrogenic factors play a role in the type of organism involved (see table 1.) In septic meningitis CSF must be obtained emergently and the patient placed on a broad spectrum antibiotic regime (see table 2). There is usually a polymorphonuclear leukocytosis, low CSF glucose and, the gram stain will be positive in 80% of patients that have not had any antibiotic therapy. The yield drops to 50-60% in patients who have had antibiotic treatment. Aseptic meningitis, which is much more common than septic meningitis, is frequently due to a non-bacterial infective agent and less often to partially treated septic meningitis. Basic supportive and symptomatic treatment is usually all that is required in aseptic meningitis if it is of viral origin or if the cause cannot be found. If it is due to fungal or other infection, the treatment is based on the organism isolated.

Subdural empyema
This accounts for between 5 – 25% of intracranial infections. It is associated with nearby pyogenic infections (sinusitis and mastoiditis) or overlying osteomyelitis and extradural empyema. There is a classical triad - namely sinusitis, fever and neurological deficit. When the empyema progresses it acts like an intracranial mass lesion causing raised intracranial pressure. Subdural empyema leads to an intense reaction in the underlying brain causing oedema and, in cases of cortical vessel thrombosis, to infarction. A hallmark of subdural empyema, which should raise a definite suspicion of infection, is that of seizures and thus all patients should be treated with prophylactic anticonvulsants. The microbiology of the infection is related to the source of infection and sinusitis causes empyema by anaerobic organisms and less commonly by aerobic *Streptococci and Staphylococci*. In iatrogenic infections or post-traumatic infections *Staphylococcus Aureus* is the predominant organism. In children there is a pattern of subdural empyema that follows infection with *Haemophilus Influenza* and *Streptococcus Pneumonia* meningitis. Both extradural and subdural empyema are diagnosed on CT scanning with the administration of intravenous iodine contrast which demonstrates enhancement of the collection, the overlying dura and the underlying cortex. MRI scanning, however, is much more sensitive for diagnosing empyema, especially in subtemporal collections or collections that are located on the tentorium cerebelli. Coronal cuts are especially useful. Treatment is complete surgical evacuation and long-term intravenous antibiotics. These cases should be treated as an emergency as the spread of the organism and subsequent cortical thrombosis can lead to cerebral infarction and malignant brain swelling.

Age/predisposing factors	Bacteria implicated
< 3months	*Listeria Monocytogenes* *Group B Streptococci* *Eschericia Coli* *Haemophilus Influenzae* *Streptococcus Pneumoniae* *Neisseria Meningitidis*
3 months to 50 years	*Haemophilus Influenzae* *Streptococcus Pneumoniae* *Neisseria Meningitidis*
Older than 50 years or immunocompromised state	*Streptococcus Pneumoniae* *Neisseria Meningitidis* *Listeria Monocytogenes* *Aerobic gram-negative bacilli*
Iatrogenic Introduction (surgery)	*Staphylococcus Aureus* *Coagulase-negative Staphylococci* *Aerobic gram-negative bacilli*
Fractures extending into sinuses (base of skull)	*Streptococcus Pneumoniae* *Haemophilus Influenzae* *Group A Streptococci*

Table 1. *The Most Common Bacteria implicated in different age groups and different clinical scenarios.*

Age/predisposing factors	Antibiotic regime
Neonates	Ampicillin plus third generation cephalosporin
Older than 1 month	Ampicillin plus third generation cephalosporin plus vancomycin
Immunocompromised state	Ampicillin plus ceftazidime plus vancomycin
Iatrogenic Introduction (surgery) and trauma	Vancomycin plus ceftazidime

Table 2. *The suggested antibiotic regime for different age groups and different clinical scenarios.*

Cerebritis and brain abscess

Infection of the brain parenchyma leading to cerebritis and brain abscess is mostly, but not exclusively, due to pyogenic bacteria. The foci that seed the parenchyma vary and bacteria can enter the CNS via several mechanisms including spread from infection in adjacent structures such as dental infection, infection of the cranial and facial sinuses, middle ear infection and from mastoiditis. The location of the intracranial infection is usually adjacent to the extra cranial infection, giving a clue as to the cause (middle and posterior fossa in mastoiditis and anterior fossa in frontal sinusitis). It may also occur as haematogenous spread from local (retrograde thrombophlebitis) or distant sites of infection. Another mechanism is direct innoculation at the time of surgery, penetrating trauma or base of skull fractures. In children, patent dermal tracts (lumbar lipomyelomeningocele, dermal sinus etc) are a congenital cause of CNS infection. The most common organisms are the *Streptococci and Staphylococci*. When infection has spread from nearby sinuses, gram-negative bacteria are prevalent.

There are 4 stages in the evolution of cerebritis into a brain abscess.
Early Cerebritis: In the first 5 days, there is a localised but non-capsulated area of oedema, pin point haemorrhage and small areas of necrosis.
Late Cerebritis: For the next week to two weeks, the infection attains a core of central necrosis. Neovascularity in the periphery leads to contrast enhancement.
Early capsule formation: Collagen and reticulin is laid down, the surrounding oedema starts to subside and there is early gliosis around the abscess.
Late capsule formation: This may go on for months and ends up with the capsule consisting of an outer gliotic layer, a middle collagenous layer and an inner inflammatory layer.
Patients may present with seizures or symptoms due to mass effect. Treatment is that of drainage, long term antibiotic treatment and treatment with prophylactic anticonvulsants.

Ventriculitis
Ventriculitis is infection of the CSF contained in the ventricles, and this can be due to the spread of infection in other anatomical compartments, but is mostly due to infection of ventricular shunts or external ventricular drains. In cases where intraparenchymal abscesses break through into the ventricular space by rupturing through the ependyma, there is a high associated morbidity and mortality. These cases are treated aggressively by external ventricular drainage, washout of the pus from the ventricular space and systemic antibiotics.

Viral infections
Human immunodeficiency virus infection
The spectrum of neurological disorders caused by this virus is large and is a direct effect either of the infection or because of the associated immunosuppression. The direct effects are those of meningitis, encephalopathy and myelopathy. Secondary or opportunistic infections are those of other viral infections such as progressive multifocal encephalopathy (PML), which is a result of a papovavirus infection with the JC virus and fungal infections.

JC virus (PML)
This virus infects oligodendrocytes and astrocytes and is characterised pathologically by demyelination and adjoined astrocytes with abnormal oligodendrocytes. Clinically these patients usually present with limb weakness followed by cognitive dysfunction, gait disturbance, visual loss, speech and language disorder and headache. On CT scanning patients usually have hypodense white matter lesions in the centrum semi-ovale and the cerebellum. This is a very aggressive condition and the mean survival time is reported to be 2-4 months.

Cryptococcus meningitis
This is an encapsulated fungus with yeast-like properties found mainly in dirt and bird droppings. About half of the cases of *C. Neoformans* meningitis occur in immunocompromised patients, and the rest occur in patients with normal cellular immunity. This is a chronic basilar meningitis and appears to be a result of activation of primary disease with cystic lesions, containing clusters of yeast surrounded by inflammatory and reactive gliosis, throughout the cerebral cortex. Clinical presentation includes signs of increased intracranial pressure and focal neurological signs. CSF examination shows a mononuclear pleocytosis and depressed

glucose with elevated protein. The CSF streptococcal antigen and serum streptococcal antigen latex agglutination tests have a high degree of sensitivity and the definitive diagnosis is made on culture of the CSF. CT scan findings are usually normal. A mortality of 30% is reported. Treatment is with systemic intravenous amphoteracin B for a minimum of 6 weeks, followed by fluconazole to prevent remission.

Toxoplasma gondii

This is a protozoal infection and is one of the most common complications associated with HIV infection. It accounts for up to half of identified neurological illnesses in patients with HIV. Approximately 25-50% of patients who are serum positive for *T Gondii* develop toxoplasma encephalopathy. *T Gondii* is an intracerebral parasite that is found in mammals, and people are usually infected by eating raw or undercooked meat that contains cysts. The house cat is the normal host of this parasite. The usual presenting neurological symptoms of patients infected with toxoplasma encephalitis are local signs superimposed on encephalopathy. The course of the illness is usually subacute, over 1-2 weeks. The lesions are usually identified as multiple ring-enhancing lesions with oedema on imaging and usually they are found in the basal ganglia. The diagnosis of *T Gondii* is not always straightforward and the CSF findings may be non-specific. It is difficult to distinguish between active and chronic toxoplasma infection with western blot methods and the only definitive means of establishing a diagnosis is a brain biopsy demonstrating tachyzoites on histological examination. These need to be excision biopsies as needle biopsies may be negative. Due to this, several authors recommend that a trial of anti-toxoplasma therapy is commenced in these patients and if therapy fails a brain biopsy is then performed. Current therapy for toxoplasma is a combination therapy with Sulfadiazine and Pyrimethamine.

Herpes viruses

These include the *Herpes Simplex virus*, the *Varicella Zoster virus*, *Epstein-Barr virus* and *Cytomegalo virus*. Human herpes viruses usually infect people early in their lives. In patients with normal immune function, they don't usually cause any complications but in immuno-compromised patients they come to the fore. The *Herpes Simplex virus type 1* is usually acquired through non-sexual activities during early childhood whereas type 2 is usually sexually transmitted. *Herpes Simplex virus type 1* encephalitis is an acute haemorrhagic necrotising encephalitis with severe morbidity. The CSF is non-specific showing a mostly mononuclear leukocytosis. The CSF may be tested for the virus specific antigens. The current management is to treat these patients empirically with Acyclovir rather than performing a brain biopsy. Therefore the treatment plan is immediate treatment with Acyclovir performing a polymerase chain reaction and, if this is negative, performing a brain biopsy. Whereas the *Herpes Simplex virus type 1* usually causes encephalitis, *Herpes Simplex type 2 viruses* usually cause meningitis and the treatment for this is Acyclovir.

Epstein-Barr virus

This is the infective agent for infectious mononucleosis and the central nervous complications of this disease are meningo-encephalitis, transverse myelitis, transcending myelitis and acute encephalitis. The outcome of Epstein-Barr virus encephalitis is usually favourable. This virus also causes Bell's palsy.

Cytomegalovirus

Cytomegalovirus is also a human herpes virus that is transmitted sexually, oral to oral or via respiratory transmission. There is both a congenital and an acquired form and treatment is with Acyclovir and Foskarnet.

Prion disease
Creutzfeld-Jacob disease

Prions are particles without nucleic acid and without detectable antigenicity but retain a clear capacity for infectivity. There are three distinct manifestations of this disease. There are sporadic cases; familial cases and cases of iatrogenic transmission. Clinical presentations include dementia and deficits of higher cortical function as well as myoclonic jerks and the disease is invariably fatal although some patients have survived as long as five years. On magnetic resonance imaging, the patient demonstrates cerebellar atrophy with increased signal intensity on T2 weighted images in the region of the basal ganglia. Diagnosis is made by brain biopsy. This is a highly infective agent and the use of disposable instruments is the only way to prevent disease transmission.

Parasitic diseases
Cysticercosis *(Taenia solium)*

This is the most common parasitic disease. It is caused by the tapeworm *T solium*. Humans are the definitive host for the parasite *T solium* with pigs being the intermediate host. Patients develop cysticercosis by ingesting fertilised eggs containing the scolex of the tapeworm carrier. These eggs are digested and embryos penetrate the blood stream and pass to the brain to form cysticerci. Cysticerci are vesicles with an invaginated scolex. Cysticercosis can have a variable presentation and may appear as cysts in the parenchyma, which can lead to seizures or encephalitis but may also present in the subarachnoid space, intraventricular space or inside the cerebellum. Spinal disease is rare but has been described. Imaging reveals variable presentations of this disease. Small granulomas and calcifications depict dead parasites. Hypodense, non-enhancing lesions represent viable cysticerci and hypodense lesions that enhance are demonstrated in the encephalitic phase and this may sometimes be combined with diffuse brain swelling. In making the diagnosis, CSF is invaluable and complement-fixation test is sensitive in 80% of cases and IGM antibody in ELISA testing has 95% specificity. The management includes medical therapy, stereotactic drainage and macroscopic, open excision. Medical management is with Albendazole. Some authors have reported a chemical meningitis and encephalitis if there is spillage of the daughter cysts during surgery and some surgeons advise using steroids to cover against this eventuality.

Echinococcosis *(Echinococcus granulosus)*

E granulosus causes hydatid disease, and humans are the intermediate host with dogs being the definitive host. Sheep and pigs are also intermediate hosts. Humans ingest the eggs along with food and liquids, and embryos freed from the eggs enter the intestinal mucosa and the vascular system. The CNS manifestation is usually that of a single large cyst in the area of the middle cerebral artery territory and the presentation is usually of a young patient presenting with symptoms and signs of increased intracranial pressure. Imaging reveals a non-enhancing, cystic lesion. Serological tests are used to diagnose the condition. At surgery, the cyst should be delivered without spillage as this could result in anaphylactic shock. Many authors report using a method of saline irrigation at the cyst-brain interface.

Granulomatous disease of the central nervous system
Mycobacterium tuberculosis

M tuberculosis is an acid fast bacillus and causes systemic infection (pulmonary, gastro intestinal tract) as well as meningitis. Infection with *M tuberculosis* is mostly a disease of the developing world. Intracranial tuberculomas form following infection in another systemic location with haematogenous spread of the organism. When a tuberculoma is formed intracranially, a thick capsule forms around it secondary to the host's main reaction and these non-caseating tuberculomas may be single or multiple. The organism frequently causes a basal arachnoiditis and meningitis (especially in the paediatric population) which can lead to communicating or non-communicating hydrocephalus. CSF analysis reveals increased protein with leukocytosis and a normal glucose. On imaging, the target sign is pathognomonic of a tuberculoma and this consists of a central calcification or nidus surrounded by a ring of enhancing material. Lesions may also be cystic. These lesions respond to chemotherapy with anti-TB drugs and it is only occasionally necessary to remove the lesions to relieve mass effect. In the case of meningitis and hydrocephalus, treatment with Diamox is used to reduce CSF production. In cases of obstructive hydrocephalus, treatment is CSF diversion with ventriculoperitoneal shunting or third ventriculostomy. These patients are frequently immunocompromised or in a poor systemic state with poor nutrition and low body weight and have a high incidence of post procedural shunt infections.

Spinal infection
Osteomyelitis
Vertebral osteomyelitis can develop from haematogenous spread, direct involvement from adjacent infection, penetrating trauma or from iatrogenic introduction of infectious agents. The onset may be quite insidious but the presentation is usually that of increasing spinal pain, accentuated by movement and may associated with radicular signs and symptoms. On examination, the spine is usually tender to palpation. *Staphylococcus Aureus* and gram negative organisms predominate as causative organisms. Concomitant epidural abscesses lead to cord or cauda equina compression and may result in neurological compromise. Blood cultures may be positive and the ESR and CRP are usually elevated, but the white cell count may not be elevated. Radionuclide scans are very sensitive for diagnosing these infections and are positive a long time before plain films show changes. CT scanning is also very sensitive, showing hypodensity at the site of the infected discs and vertebrae as well as showing gas within the vertebrae. When healing occurs of the lesions in the chronic phase, they become denser on CT. On MRI scan there are low intensity changes on T1 WI and high intensity changes on T2 WI because of the increased water content and the lesions frequently enhance with contrast. Most cases of purely bony osteomyelitis can be treated with antibiotics, bed rest and analgesia. If the organism has not been identified with blood cultures, a CT-guided needle biopsy may be necessary. If this fails, an open surgical biopsy might be indicated and if no organism is grown then empiric antibiotics should be administered. Authors differ in opinion about the length of antibiotic therapy but it is generally accepted that at least six weeks of IV antibiotics should be given. This should be monitored by testing inflammatory markers regularly and serial scanning and there should be an improvement of both parameters. Oral antibiotics may be instituted when there is a continued downward trend in the inflammatory markers and the imaging characteristics have stabilised. Because the bone becomes weak during infection, external bracing should be used for mobilisation and, after a period of mobilisation, repeat imaging should be performed. Surgery is reserved for cases that do not respond to antibiotic therapy or where there are definite mass lesions and compromise of nervous structures. This frequently requires an anterior approach with bony grafting and fusion. Permanent morbidity is related to vascular thrombosis secondary to sepsis and to neural compromise secondary to compression.

Epidural empyema (abscess)
The mode of infection is the same as for osteomyelitis. There are several predisposing factors in both of these conditions namely diabetes mellitus, immuno-incompetence, alcoholism, malignancies and chronic systemic diseases. The signs and symptoms are very similar to those of osteomyelitis as a spinal epidural abscess is frequently an extension of the

osteomyelitic disease. Back pain with focal tenderness is the hallmark and this is associated in the lumbar spine with radicular compromise and conus medullaris/cauda equina syndrome when there is significant compromise of the theca. The presentation of epidural abscesses in the thoracic and cervical spine is different. Myelopathic signs predominates and the plain films might show some bony erosion or disc space changes, but these are rare. MRI scanning of the spine is the imaging of choice showing a hypointense lesion on T1 WI which is hyperintense on T2 WI and enhances with contrast. Radionuclide scans are extremely sensitive and are usually the first imaging modality that diagnoses these lesions. These conditions are medical emergencies due to the permanent morbidity that they cause if not aggressively treated. Morbidity is secondary to vascular thrombosis or to neural compromise by direct compression. Immediate surgical decompression with concomitant antibiotic therapy is the treatment of choice. At surgery the most usual finding is that of organised infected tissue although liquid pus might also be found. The pathogen most frequently involved is *Staphylococcus Aureus and Streptococci*. In cases where the neurological deficit is secondary to vascular thrombosis the prognosis is extremely poor.

Subdural abscess (empyema)

The same risk factors and mode of spread and dissemination for this holds true as for the two previous conditions and the clinical presentation and infecting organisms are much the same. At surgery these tend to have a less granulation tissue and a more fluid consistency. Treatment is complete evacuation and broad-spectrum antibiotics.

Intramedullary abscess

These are rare lesions but have the same aetiology, presentation and management as the previous lesions. They usually appear as hypointense lesions on T1 WI and hyperintense lesions on T2 WI and enhance strongly with contrast in the intramedullary space. Treatment is with drainage and long term IV antibiotics.

Discitis

Spontaneous discitis

Spontaneous haematogenous spread or spread from nearby infection may result in discitis, as with osteomyelitis. The blood supply of the cartilage is restricted to the periphery and it is a relatively avascular structure but this does not preclude infection from occuring in an intervertebral disc. Discitis presents in a similar fashion as osteomyelitis and also has the complication of an epidural abscess. Treatment is with broad-spectrum antibiotics, bed rest and analgesia. The diagnosis is made by demonstrating raised inflammatory markers and isolating the organism from either blood culture or a direct needle aspiration biopsy.

Iatrogenic discitis

Iatrogenic discitis following spinal surgery can either be an irritant chemical discitis or infective discitis. Patients with infective discitis tend to have a higher level of inflammatory markers. The inflammatory markers usually stay elevated for about two weeks post surgery but should return to normal thereafter in cases not complicated by infection. On imaging the infected disc appears hypointense on T1 WI and hyperintense on T2 WI, demonstrating a higher fluid content and may enhance with Gadolinium contrast administration. Treatment is bed rest and antibiotics following isolation of the organism and, in cases where there is an associated fluid collection, complete drainage of the collection producing neural compromise should be performed.

Tuberculosis of the spine

Mycobacterium Tuberculosis infection of the spine is endemic in some parts of the developing world but is now also spreading to the developed world. Infection with *M Tuberculosis* starts off in the vertebra or adjacent endplate and its hallmark is destruction of the vertebra and gibbus formation with collapse of the vertebra whilst the integrity of the disc is maintained until quite late in the disease. Spinal TB can cause the destruction of several contiguous levels or can result in skip lesions and in some cases can cause epidural abscesses. The disease usually begins within the metaphyseal bone and then spreads underneath the anterior longitudinal ligament. The patient may present with the effects of pulmonary TB or with spinal pain and neurological deficit. On X-ray, vertebral involvement with erosion kyphosis with mostly involvement of the vertebrae, sparing the posterior elements, is seen. There is frequently some soft tissue involvement with calcification. CT scans are quite useful in delineating the extent of the disease and skin testing is usually positive. In the developing world the treatment of spinal TB is ambulatory chemotherapy and, in the case of severe paraparesis, bed rest and chemotherapy. The cornerstone of treatment is chemotherapy rather than surgery. Surgery is reserved for cases of severe kyphosis. Deformity following chemotherapy frequently is equal to or is better than in cases of surgery. In the developed world, the movement towards surgery is more aggressive and a combination of surgery (for gibbus formation and deformity) with chemotherapy is used. It is important to understand that the correction of deformity will deteriorate over time and therefore external bracing is important whilst the patient is ambulant. In cases where there are epidural pus collections, surgery is indicated to drain the collections. The patient should be on chemotherapy for at least 6 months.

14

DEGENERATIVE CONDITIONS

W Adriaan Liebenberg

Contents

Rheumatoid Arthritis
Intervertebral disc disease
Spondylolysis and spondylolisthesis
Spinal canal stenosis

Rheumatoid Arthritis

Rheumatoid arthritis is a chronic, relapsing inflammatory arthritis. Inflammatory pannus in the synovium of the facet joints lead to destruction of cartilage, ligaments and bone. The clinical manifestations include early morning stiffness, fatigue and a myriad of extra-articular manifestations including pericarditis, myocarditis, pulmonary nodules, pleural effusions, kerato-conjunctivitis, scleritis and many others. The cervical spine is commonly involved due to the large number of synovial joints and the disease has a predilection for the craniocervical junction. Atlanto-axial subluxation is initiated by the loss of the retaining power of the transverse ligament, inflammatory changes in the joints and changes in the quality of the odontoid process (softening and osteoporosis). Softening and loss of bone in the lateral mass of the atlas leads to basilar impression (basilar invagination refers to the congenital variety and basilar impression to the acquired variety) and upward migration of the ondotoid relative to the skull base. The combination of atlanto-axial subluxation and basilar impression leads to anterior compression of the spinal cord and ventral medulla. The radiological findings include excessive mobility on dynamic imaging, evidence of pannus formation, ventral spinal cord compression and upward migration of the peg. Patients present with pain and myelopathy and in cases of compression of the medulla oblongata, present with brainstem dysfunction. Treatment is with atlanto-axial fixation. Severe cases of anterior pannus formation might require transoral resection of the pannus.

Intervertebral disc disease

The intervertebral disc is made up of a central, soft nucleus pulposus made up of a protein-polysaccharide mix and a retaining fibrous annulus fibrosus. Degeneration and trauma can lead to damage of the annulus fibrosus and herniation of the soft nuclear material into the intraspinal space.

There are 4 stages of disc herniation, see figure 1:

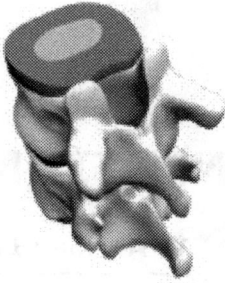

Figure 1. *Intervetebral disc herniation.*

Stage 1 (degeneration, annular tear, bulge): There are chemical changes in the disc and it appears black on T2 WI (MRI). There disc bulges but the nucleus pulposus does not breach the annulus.

Stage 1

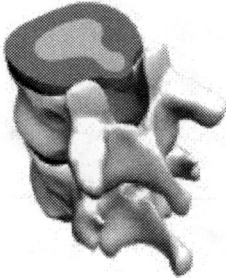

Stage 2

Stage 2 (protrusion, prolapse): The nucleus pulposus of the disc breaks through some of the annular fibres but does not extend beyond the anatomical space usually occupied by the disc.

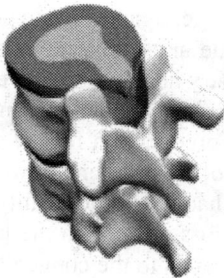

Stage 3

Stage 3 (extrusion): The nucleus pulposus of the disc breaks through the annulus and extends beyond the anatomical space usually occupied by the disc and into the spinal canal.

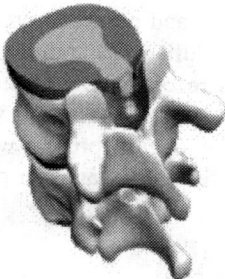

Stage 4

Stage 4 (sequestered fragment, migrated fragment, free fragment): The disc fragment breaks off and loses continuity with the rest of the disc and lies loose in the spinal canal.

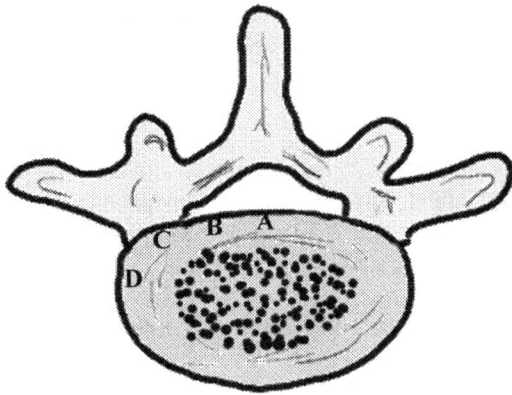

Figure 2. *The possible anatomical positions of a disc herniation is demonstrated A: Central disc herniation; B: Lateral disc herniation; C: Foraminal disc herniation and D Extraforaminal (far lateral) disc herniation.*

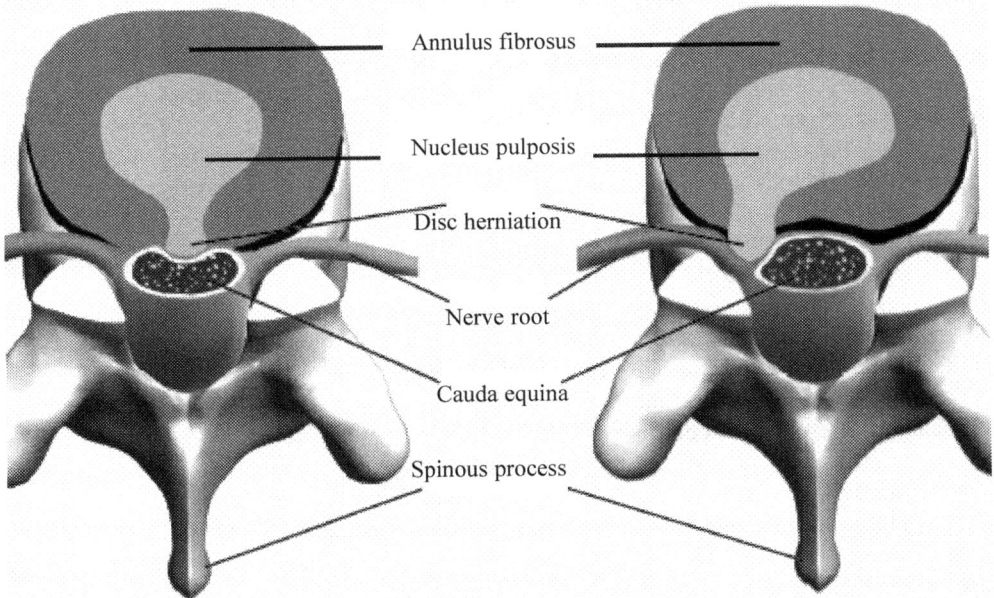

Annulus fibrosus

Nucleus pulposis

Disc herniation

Nerve root

Cauda equina

Spinous process

Figure 3. *The image on the left demonstrates a central disc herniation and the image on the right demonsrates a foraminal disc herniation. In these cases the herniations are in the lumbar spine and the effect of the foraminal herniation is that of a radiculopathy and in the central herniation it may be that of a cauda equina syndrome or radiculopathy. If the herniation was in the thoracic or cervical spine, the central herniation would lead to myelopathy and the foraminal herniation to a radiculopathy.*

Depending on the size, level and whether the disc is central, lateral, foraminal or far lateral, several possible clinical syndromes can ensue. Centrally herniated discs can compromise all the nerves below the level that they are located at if they are very large. The nerve roots leave the spinal canal by curling around and beneath the pedicle of the same named level in the thoracic and lumbar spines. For instance, the L4 nerve root curls around the pedicle of L4 vertebra, which is quite laterally situated and just above the disc space, therefore a central and lateral disc prolapse at L4/5 will not normally affect the L4 nerve root but the nerve roots lower down. In cases where the L4/5 disc prolapse is foraminal or extraforaminal the L4 nerve root on that side will be compressed.

Patients with early stages of disc disease may present initially with lower back pain (LBP) alone and this is thought to occur because of stretching of pain fibres in the annulus fibrosus. When the nuclear material herniates through the annulus fibrosus and compresses the nerve roots, this irritation, which is thought to be both mechanical and chemical, leads to radicular signs. Radicular signs can be lancing pain, paresthesia and motor weakness. The examination of lumbar disc disease includes the findings of a positive straight- leg raising test, the presence of sensory abnormalities or motor deficits.

See the chapter on history and examination for the dermatomes and myotomes affected by each level of disc prolapse. The examination of a patient with a prolapsed cervical disc herniation relies on the same principles and depending on the area of the paresthesias, sensory deficit and motor findings; the level of the prolapse can be fairly accurately defined. Remember that in the cervical spine a named root emerges above the pedicle of the same named vertebra - for example the left C6 nerve root passes through the left C5/6 intervertebral foramen. The obvious exceptions to the rule above is the C8 nerve roots which transverse the C7/T1 foramina. The distribution of the paresthesia in the affected dermatome is frequently the best indicator for the level of the pathology. There is a definite place for conservative management of prolapsed discs as some of them will resolve spontaneously. This is because the herniated nuclear matter, which is mostly made up of water, may dehydrate and shrink.

The accepted indications for lumbar discectomy are:
Massive midline prolapses with resultant cauda equina syndrome.
Significant motor dysfunction and weakness of a specific myotome.
Radicular pain that persists despite conservative management.
Relapses of acute LBP and sciatica that prohibits a patient from having a normal lifestyle, especially if these tend to be progressive with shorter symptom-free periods.

The possible complications of lumbar disc surgery include the following:
Damage to the cauda equina and paralysis or paresis of bladder and bowel function and variable dysfunction of the motor fibres below the level of the surgery. Also CSF leaks, post operative infection including discitis, empyema and superficial infection and post operative wound haematomas. Post operative residual or recurrent disc fragments can be differentiated from scar tissue by virtue of the fact that on T1 WI (MRI) with Gadolinium contrast enhancement, the scar tissue enhances and the disc material does not. It may however be very difficult to make the diagnosis.

Indications for a cervical discectomy:
Myelopathy (spasticity secondary to cord compression)
Muscle weakness and atrophy
Progressive radicular pains
Persisting radicular pains that prohibit a patient from having a normal lifestyle.
Foraminal cervical disc herniations can in some instances also be relieved by posterior foraminotomies which are less invasive and have been performed as day cases. Possible com-

plications following anterior cervical discectomy include damage to the recurrent laryngeal nerve with resultant vocal cord dysfunction and hoarseness, CSF leak, damage to the spinal cord, damage to the trachea, oesophagus and carotid artery (or dislodging an intra-arterial cholesterol plaque), infection and wound haematoma. A complication of a left anterior approach is damage to the thoracic duct.

Spondylolysis and spondylolisthesis

Spondylolysis is a defect in the pars interarticularis between the vertebrae of the lumbar spine and this leads to a forward slip or spondylolisthesis of one vertebra on another. Severe cases of spondylolisthesis may require fusion and the decision is usually based on the demonstration of a change in the degree of slip on dynamic flexion and extension lateral spine images. There are 5 grades which are based on the percentage of slippage of the superior vertebral body in relation to the inferior vertebral body:

Grade 1: 25%
Grade 2: 25-50%
Grade 3: 50-75%
Grade 4: 75-100%
Grade 5: greater than 100%

There are several types of spondylolisthesis:

Type 1 - Congenital: Facet dysplasia and abnormal orientation of the facet with secondary elongation of the pars interarticularis is the hallmark of this type and age of onset is usually before the age of 20.

Type 2 - Isthmic: A stress fracture of the pars interartricularis is responsible for this type. There is an association with contact sports and with the congenital type due to the biomechanical stresses placed on the pars by the orientation of the facet joints.

Type 3 - Degenerative: This is spondylolisthesis without a pars defect and is secondary to hyper mobility of the facet joints and disc pathology and results in lateral recess stenosis. Following decompression a decision to fuse should be made on a case for case basis.

Type 4 -Traumatic: Severe traumatic forces, especially hyper flexion forces can lead to fractures of the pars interarticularis.

Type 5 - Pathological: This is associated with pathological fractures of the pars.

Type 6 - Post surgical: Laminectomy carries the definite risk of spondylolisthesis and some surgeons try and limit the extent of their surgical procedures as much as possible for this reason. Posterior instrumentation subjects adjacent motion segments to endure added biomechanical stresses and the development of para fusion-segment spondylolisthesis is well known.

Spinal canal stenosis

Cervical stenosis

Spinal stenosis is either congenital or acquired and is narrowing of the spinal canal diameter due to several factors. Congenitally narrow canals and cases of acquired stenosis with canal diameters of less than 14mm are a risk factor for developing cord compression and myelopathy. The purest form of congenital spinal stenosis occurs in achondroplasia. This condition is characterised by increased periosteal bone formation and patients have abnormal vertebrae with trapezoidal shapes, shortened and thick pedicles and hypertrophied laminae. Acquired spinal stenosis can be caused by anterior compression from herniated discs, osteophytic bars, ossification of the posterior longitudinal ligament, subluxation of the vertebrae and vertebral compression fractures. Posterior and lateral compression may be caused by hypertrophy of the ligamentum flavum and the facet joints.

The clinical syndrome depends whether there is purely radicular compromise with lateral recess and neural foramina stenosis which produces a radiculopathy (pain, paresthesia, lower motor neurone motor weakness and decreased reflexes) or whether there is compression of the cord with resultant myelopathy (spasticity, upper motor neurone weakness). Myelopathic patients have a spastic quadriparesis and problems with fine motor control of the upper limbs and a spastic gait. These patients may present with a central cord syndrome where they have greater impairment of their arm function than their leg function if they suffer a hyperextension injury. This is because of the critical narrowing of the spinal canal which leads to the spinal cord being contused in such a fall, with damage to the central cord (see chapter 12). Treatment is by decompression and the approach is dictated by the pathology with the rule generally being that anterior compression needs anterior surgery and posterior compression, posterior surgery. Anterior surgery includes anterior cervical discectomy and vertebral corpectomy and posterior surgery would include laminectomy, laminotomy and foraminotomy.

Lumbar spinal canal stenosis

This is characterised by a clinical syndrome of radicular complaints, neurogenic (spinal) claudication and symptoms of cauda equina compression secondary to direct mechanical compression and indirect vascular insufficiency. Patients with lumbar spinal canal stenosis report reduced walking distances and decreased ability to stand for long periods. The spinal claudication is typically an aching pain in their calves that is reduced with rest but even more so with a change in posture and patients will report that sitting down or squatting is helpful. The condition is manifested by a decreased canal diameter on imaging with associated facet joint hypertrophy and ligamentum flavum hypertrophy. Treatment for this condition is spinal decompression with generous fenestrations (laminotomies) or laminectomy without or with fusion. The decision on fusion is based on demonstrating instability (movement) on flexion and extension images.

15

CONGENITAL NEUROSURGICAL CONDITIONS

W Adriaan Liebenberg

Contents

Spine
Spinal dysraphism
Spina bifida aperta (Spina bifida cystica)
Myelomeningocele, myeloschisis and meningocele
Spina bifida occulta
Diastematomyelia (split cord malformation)
Neurenteric cysts
Lipomas
Dermoids and dermal sinus tracts
The tethered cord syndrome

Craniocervical junction
Chiari malformation
Syringomyelia
Basilar invagination
Assimilation of the atlas
Atlantoaxial instability
Anomalies of the odontoid process
Aplasia/hypoplasia of the dens
Os odontoideum
Subaxial spine
Klippel-Feil syndrome

Brain
Disorders of neural tube closure
Cephaloceles
Disorders of structural development
Holoprosencephaly
Malformation of the corpus callosum
Leptomeningeal malformations
Lipomas
Arachnoid cyst
Posterior fossa malformations
Dandy-Walker malformation
Mega cisterna magna

Spine

Congenital spinal conditions are associated with maternal diabetes and exposure to teratogens in pregnancy. The presence of congenital spinal conditions is frequently associated with other neural tube defects and systemic defects such as cardiac and renal abnormalities

Spinal dysraphism (failure of closure of the primary neural tube)

The abnormal development of the spinal cord and spine is due to anomalous fusion of the embryonic midline structures.

Open lesions - Spina bifida aperta (Spina bifida cystica)

This condition is associated with maternal hyperthermia, deficiencies in folate and Vitamin A, and excessively high levels of Vitamin A. There is an increased incidence in families with a previous case of spina bifida.

Myelomeningocele, myeloschisis and meningocele

These develop between 2 and 7 weeks after conception. The basic deficit is that of an unfolded neural tube that presents as a placode. If the defect develops before 28 days, then the neural placode presents open and is referred to as myeloschisis. After 28 days the unfolded neural placode can present within a meningocele and is referred to as a myelomeningocele or there can be a meningocele separate from the spinal cord within the subarachnoid space and this is referred to as meningocele. Spina bifida can reliably be detected in the pre natal period on ultrasound and on maternal serum alpha-fetoprotein testing, although the sensitivity for skin-covered lesions is somewhat lower.

The management of this condition requires early surgical closure. Surgery within 24 to 48 hrs carry the potential benefits of preservation of neurological function, the prevention of infection of the CNS and has the benefits of cosmesis and easier nursing care. Surgery after 48 hours reduces the likelihood of such benefits and increases the risk of infection. There is an association with hydrocephalus requiring shunting in approximately 80% of cases. Approximately 20% of all patients with myelomeningoceles have significant hydrocephalus at birth; another 60-70% of patients develop it after closure of the myelomeningocele. There is a near complete association with Chiari II malformation with or without syringomyelia. The incidence of syringomyelia has been reported to be as high as 80% and up to a third of patients will become symptomatic from their Chiari malformation. There is an association with tethered cord and up to a third of patients may become symptomatic. Some patients are born with congenital scoliosis. Acquired scoliosis can also develop and the incidence is dependant on the level of the lesion with 100% of thoracic lesions and 10% of sacral lesions developing it. It is thought to be secondary to a muscle imbalance. There are a multitude of systemic and nervous system anomalies associated with myelomeningocele. Therefore a full neurological and systemic work up is required in these patients and anaesthesia can be challenging.

Hidden lesions - Spina bifida occulta

This is a developmental abnormality of the dorsal neural arch structures and may be an incidental finding or associated with other underlying abnormalities as described below.

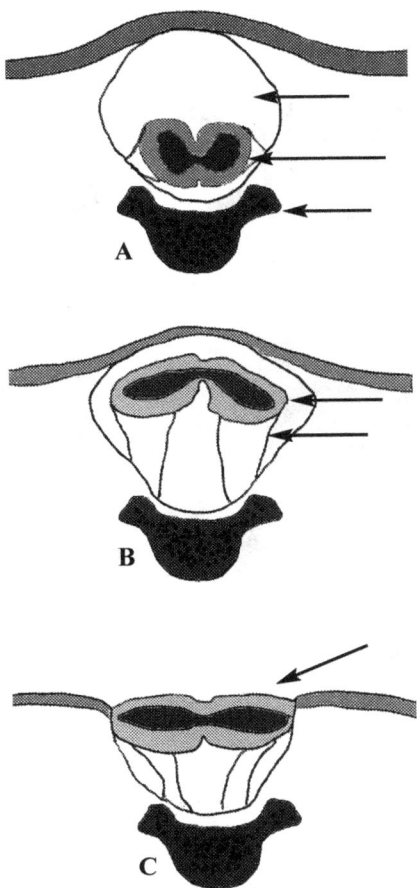

Figure 1. *A: Depicts a meningoele (top arrow), note how the spinal cord is normal (second arrow) and the third arrow demonstrates the associated spina bifida; B: This image depicts a myelomeningocele. Note the unfolded placode (top arrow) covered by thinned and abnormal skin and how the nerve roots descend from the placode (bottom arrow); C: This image depicts myeloschisis. Note how the unfolded neural placode (arrow) is exposed to the air.*

Diastematomyelia (split cord malformation)

There are two types, type I is associated with a bony septum and type II is a split cord malformation without a septum. These lesions are caused by adhesion between the ectoderm and endoderm in the embryonic period which leads to the formation of an accessory neurenteric canal and resultant split cord. The spinal cord above and below the lesion is usually normal. In cases with a septum the dura may also be split. These lesions are mostly found in the lumbar spine. Patients usually present in the first decade of life with symptoms and signs of spinal cord traction that include back pain and radicular pain, paresthesia and other sensory abnormalities as well as motor deficits. There may be associated cutaneous manifestations such as skin discoloration, a hairy patch, a dimple or dermal sinus, lipoma or meningocele. These lesions should be promptly treated if they are symptomatic with surgical release of the tethered cord.

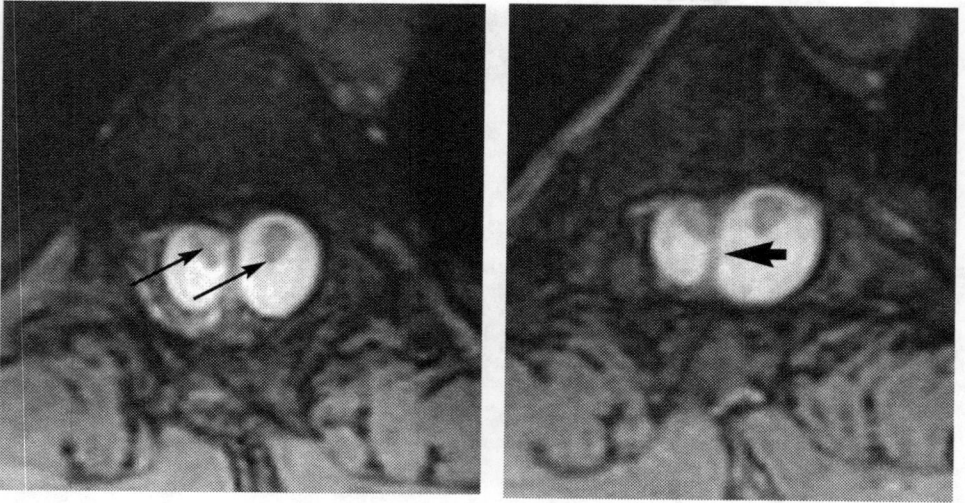

Figure 2. *Diastematomyelia. These axial T2 WI demonstrate a split cord malformation with a bony spur. Note the two halves of the cord (black arrows), and the bony spur indicated by the thick black arrow.*

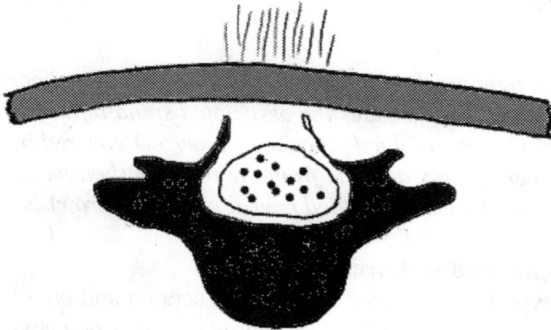

Figure 3. *This image depicts spina bifida occulta. Note how the lesion is skin covered. There may be associated cutaneous manifestations such as skin discoloration, a hairy patch, a dimple or dermal sinus or lipoma.*

Neurenteric cysts (enterogenous cyst, enteric cyst, gastrocytoma, dorsal enteric fistula, split notochord syndrome, teratoid cyst)

These cystic structures are from retained fragments of foregut (endoderm) and are most commonly found in the thoracic and cervical spine and most commonly to the right of the midline. Neurenteric cysts are not confined to the spinal column and may be found in the mediastinum, brain, abdomen and pelvis. The enterogenous cyst may be located ventral or dorsal to the cord and may be intramedullary, attached to the meninges or to the vertebrae. They may be associated with vertebral abnormalities and become symptomatic if they cause spinal cord compression.

Lipomas

These fatty masses may be associated with a myelomeningocele (lipomyelomeningocele) or occur alone as inclusion tumours. They present with symptoms and signs of spinal cord tethering or the mass effects of the lipoma on the neural tissues. There may be a palpable fatty mass or other dermal marker indicating an underlying lipoma. Current management is to treat these surgically as soon as they are diagnosed.

Dermoid cysts, epidermoid cysts and dermal sinus tracts

In a congenital dermal sinus, an epithelium lined channel connects the spinal canal with the skin of the back. These lesions are most frequently in the lumbar spine but can occur anywhere in the spine. They are not associated with spina bifida and are thought to arise because of adhesion and failed separation between the cutaneous ectoderm and the neural tube. The dermal sinus may be associated with an epidermoid or dermoid cyst. Patients usually present with infection due to migration of organisms down the tract or due to mass effects of the associated epidermoid or dermoid cyst. Treatment is surgical excision.

The tethered cord syndrome

Many conditions such as a split cord malformation, lipoma, tight filum terminale, dermal sinus and myelomeningocele are associated with cord tethering. In this syndrome, the cord is fixed in an abnormally low position below L1/L2 and mechanical stresses on the cord causes neurological dysfunction. There can be sensory, motor or sphincteric dysfunction. This condition may be associated with a dermal abnormality. Some patients are asymptomatic and some become symptomatic during growth spurts. A tethered cord should be managed surgically and the current approach is not to wait for asymptomatic patients to become symptomatic before surgically intervention.

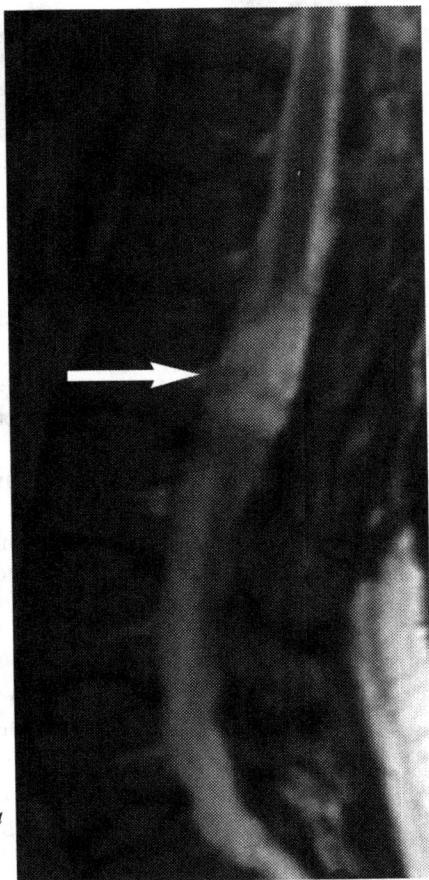

Figure 4. *This sagittal T2 WI demonstrates a dermoid cyst of the conus medullaris.*

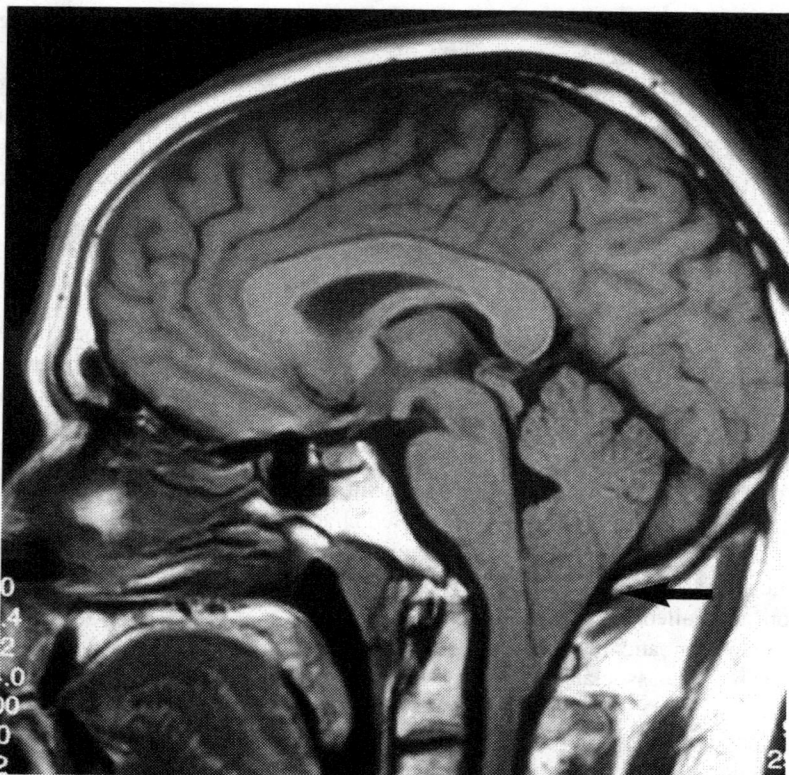

Figure 5. *This sagittal T1 WI demonstrates a Chiari 1 malformation. The arrow demonstrates the posterior border of the foramen magnum. There is obvious herniation of the tonsils of the cerebellum past this point.*

Craniocervical junction (CCJ)

Chiari malformation

Definition:

Type 1 – Downward displacement of the cerebellar tonsils for more than 5mm past the edge of the foramen magnum.

Type 2 – Displacement of the tonsils, vermis and fourth ventricle past the edge of the foramen magnum.

Type 3 - High cervical or occipitocervical hernia containing cerebellum.

Type 4 - Hypoplasia of the cerebellum sometimes associated with encephalocele.

Features:

Type 1 – Onset of symptoms is usually in the fourth and fifth decades. Cough and strain headaches are the salient feature. Myelopathy, sensory abnormalities of the face, upper limbs and trunk as well as dysaesthetic pain are also features. A large proportion of patients develop ocular manifestations and horizontal nystagmus with a downbeat component is associated specifically with this condition. Imaging for this condition includes MRI of the CCJ as well as the whole spine as these patients may develop syringomyelia and syringobulbia. Cranial imaging is performed to exclude hydrocephalus. In cases of hydrocephalus, CSF diversion may relieve the symptoms. The standard treatment for Chiari 1 malformation is posterior fossa decompression. This may be limited to a bony decompression (craniectomy) but usually includes a duraplasty. Some surgeons open the arachnoid and resect and apply diathermy to the cerebellar tonsils to shrink them.

Type 2 – These are associated with congenital defects and all infants with myelomeningocele have associated Chiari 2 malformation. More than 90% of these children also develop hydrocephalus which may require CSF diversion. The infants may present with respiratory distress and impaired swallowing, weak or absent crying, weakness and spasticity of the limbs and nystagmus. Children may present with spastic quadriparesis, nystagmus, syncopal episodes, recurrent pneumonia due to aspiration and deficient cough response and a gradual loss of function due to cervico-medullary compression. Cases with hydrocephalus, as in adults, need CSF diversion and cases with persistent symptoms, should undergo posterior fossa decompression.

Syringomyelia
Syringomyelia is the development of a fluid filled cavity in the spinal cord and hydromyelia is the dilatation of the central canal of the spinal cord. The mechanism of the formation of syringomyelia is incompletely understood and there are several postulated mechanisms. The mainstay of most theories is that there is an abnormality of CSF flow and that this is central to the mechanism of syringomyelia. Whether it is due to a pressure gradient, a ball valve mechanism or some other mechanism is unknown. The clinical presentation of syringomyelia is variable and includes both motor and sensory deficits but the hallmark is spinothalamic sensory abnormalities. As temperature and pain fibres cross the midline from the one side of the spinal cord to the other side, they are compromised by the centrally sited cavity of the syrinx. These patients frequently have decreased temperature appreciation and dysaesthetic pains. The main causes of syringomyelia are tonsillar herniation in Chiari malformation, mass lesions at the cranio cervical junction, basilar invagination or impression, trauma with spinal cord damage, chronic arachnoiditis and intramedullary tumours. It is known that the spinal cord is permeable to CSF and that draining the cavity of the syrinx either with a syringotomy or a drainage device is less successful than restoring the flow of CSF by removing adhesions and obstruction to the flow of CSF. Therefore surgery is aimed at restoring CSF flow. The prognosis following surgery is difficult to predict with some patients having improvement, a small number becoming worse and most patients remaining stable. It is important to point out to patients pre operatively that the aim of surgery is to stop them from getting worse and that it is a bonus if they become better.

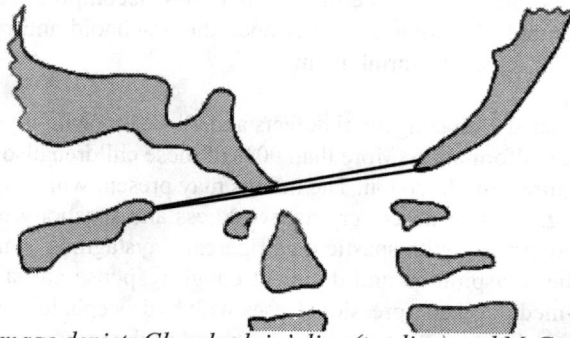

Figure 6. *This image depicts Chamberlain's line (top line) and McGregor's line (bottom line)*

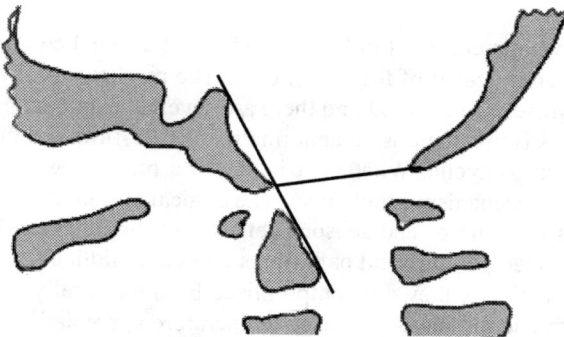

Figure 7. *This image depicts McRae's line and Wackenheim's clivus-canal line.*

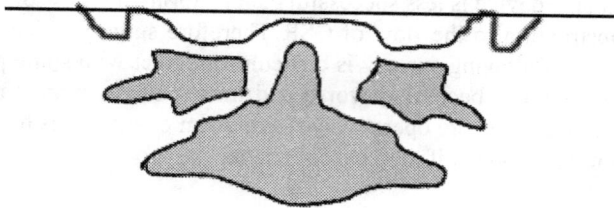

Figure 8. *This image depicts Fischgold's digastric line. This line is drawn through the apices of both digastric fossae.*

Basilar invagination

This term is reserved for the congenital elevation of the occipital bone which is frequently associated with platybasia. This condition leads to a smaller volume of the posterior fossa. Basilar impression is a term reserved for acquired basilar impression secondary to softening of the occipital bone due to pathological processes such as Paget's disease and rheumatoid arthritis. Patients present with spastic quadriparesis, bulbar symptoms or symptoms and signs from associated conditions such as Chiari malformation. The diagnosis is made by radiological evaluation of the craniocervical junction. There are several reference lines that are used to evaluate the position of the dens in relation to the base of the skull (see fig 6 to 9). The tip of the dens should not be elevated more than 1 cm above a line drawn through inferior edge of both mastoid processes and should not be above a line drawn through both digastric fossas.

Name	Anatomical points	Limits
Chamberlain's line	From the posterior edge of the hard palate to the anterior edge of the foramen magnum.	The tip of the dens should be below this line.
McGregor's line	From the posterior edge of the hard palate to the to the most inferior point of the caudal curve of the occipital bone	The tip of the dens should be less than 4.5mm above this line
McRae's line	From the anterior edge of the foramen magnum to the posterior edge of the foramen magnum	The tip of the odontoid process should be below this.
Wackenheim's clivus-canal line	This line runs along the base of the clivus and along the anterior edge of the spinal canal.	The tip of the odontoid process should not cross this line.
Fischgold's digastric line	This line joins the superior aspect of both digastric fossas	The tip of the odontoid process should not cross this line.

Figure 9. *Radiological criteria for diagnosing basilar invagination/impression.*

Assimilation of the atlas (fusion of the atlas with the occipital bone)
This is due to a segmentation defect and is frequently associated with other spinal defects such as Klippel-Feil syndrome and there are a large number of patients who also have C2-C3 fusion. This condition leads to atlanto-axial instability and basilar invagination with compromise of the medulla and upper spinal cord. Reduction of the instability and subsequent fusion is the treatment of choice.

Atlantoaxial instability
This can be due to congenital defects in the dens, laxity or rupture of the transverse ligament or may occur in cases of assimilation of the atlas as seen above. The C1/C2 joint is inherently unstable in this condition and excessive movement across this joint compresses the upper spinal cord. This condition is also associated with Klippel-Feil syndrome, Down's syndrome and can be acquired in rheumatoid arthritis. The instability is measured on a lateral X-ray by the atlanto dens interval which should be less than 3mm in adults and less than 4mm in children. Anything more than that suggests disruption of the transverse ligament. The treatment is reduction and occipito cervical fusion.

Anomalies of the odontoid process
Aplasia/hypoplasia of the dens
This condition may be seen in Down's syndrome and in association with os odontoideum. The abnormality of the dens leads to atlanto-axial instability and surgical fusion should be performed.

Os odontoideum
This is an independent ossicle of bone found in relation to the tip of the dens and may be seen in association with hypoplasia or aplasia of the dens. There are two types, the orthoptic and the dystopic type (see fig 10). In the orthoptic variety, the ossicle is in close relation to the position of the dens and in the dystopic variant; it is in close relationship to the basion (anterior border of the foramen magnum). The latter variant is more likely to cause neurological compromise but both variants lead to atlanto-axial instability and in symptomatic cases requires fusion.

Subaxial spine
Klippel-Feil syndrome
This syndrome is characterised by congenital fusion of the cervical spine with or without a short neck and low dorsal hairline. Up to two thirds of patients have associated scoliosis and another quarter of patients have associated renal abnormalities. These patients usually present secondary to spinal cord compression at the levels adjacent to the fused segment due to an unstable segment. These patients may require decompression and fusion of unstable segments.

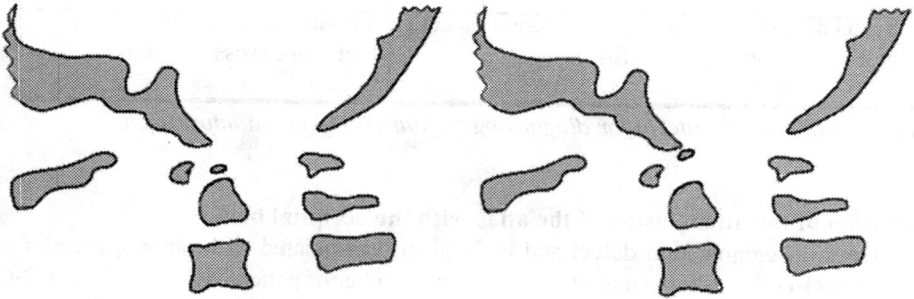

Figure 10. *Os odontoideum. The image on the left is of the orthoptic type and the image on the right of the dystopic type.*

Brain
Disorders of neural tube closure
Cephaloceles
These lesions are formed by hernias of intracranial tissue through the dura and bone into the extra cranial space. Meningoceles contain leptomeninges and CSF and encephaloceles contain brain tissue as well. Associated abnormalities such as abnormalities of the corpus callosum and Dandy-Walker malformation are common. They are usually, but not exclusively, located in the midline and there are 4 major types, occipital, parietal, frontoethmoidal and sphenoidal. Treatment is surgical resection of non-functioning brain, intracranial transposition of functioning brain and closure of the dural defect.

Disorders of structural development
Holoprosencephaly
This is a spectrum of disorders of differing severity characterised by hypoplasia or aplasia of the most rostral sections of the neural tube and premaxillary segment of the face. The associated facial abnormalities are most commonly of the eyes, nose and maxillae. The brain defects range from the absence of an interhemispheric fissure, falx cerebri, corpus callosum and septum pellucidum, with a single large crescent shaped ventricle and hypoplastic brain as a single fused mass that lies in the periphery of the cranial vault to minor midline fusion abnormalities with some areas of the most ventral and rostral cerebral hemispheres being fused.

Malformation of the corpus callosum
This is frequently associated with conditions such as Dandy-Walker malformation, Chiari II, cephaloceles and midline facial developmental abnormalities. MRI is excellent for diagnosing this abnormality and longitudinal callosal fibres can usually be seen adjacent to the interhemispheric fissure. These are the fibres that would normally have crossed in the corpus callosum. Other useful features are widening of the third ventricle and extension of the third ventricle superiorly between the bodies of the lateral ventricles. The lateral ventricles, not being supported by the white matter tracts of the corpus callosum frequently expand superiorly and laterally. The condition is usually asymptomatic.

Leptomeningeal malformations
Lipomas
These lesions are collections of fat included during abnormal embryological development of the leptomeninges and subarachnoid space and are usually found in the midline in the pericallosal area/interhemispheric fissure, quadrigeminal cistern and suprasellar cistern. They can also be found in the cerebellopontine angle and the Sylvian fissure. These lesions are frequently found in association with other intracranial abnormalities such as abnormalities of the corpus callosum and cephaloceles. The blood vessels and cranial nerves of the subarachnoid space frequently run through, rather than around these lesions. Resection is indicated in cases of mass effect.

Arachnoid cyst
These lesions are formed in the same manner as the lipomas above and are made up of encysted areas lined with normal arachnoid mater. They contain fluid with similar composition to CSF and some authorities believe that they communicate with the CSF spaces in a type of ball valve mechanism whilst others believe that it is an osmotic process. They present in many areas of the brain and more commonly in the Sylvian fissure, cerebellopontine angle and suprasellar areas. They have the same characteristics as CSF on imaging and may be difficult to distinguish from epidermoid tumours. The main differentiation is that epidermoid cysts do not suppress on FLAIR images, whereas arachnoid cysts do. Haemorrhage following trauma has been reported and intracystic vessels can sometimes be seen. In the Sylvian fissure they may present with seizures or increased intracranial pressure. Other cysts may present with other symptoms and signs depending on their location.

Posterior fossa malformations
Dandy-walker malformation
This condition is characterised by a large posterior fossa with superior elevation of the tentorium cerebelli and venous sinuses secondary to a large cystic fourth ventricle and cerebellar dysgenesis. This condition is associated with intracranial and extracranial developmental abnormalities. The extracranial abnormalities include facial abnormalities and systemic

abnormalities of different organ systems. Two thirds or more of patients develop hydro-cephalus and this was thought to be due to obstruction of the outlet foramina of the fourth ventricle but it has been shown to be untrue in over 80% of cases. The mechanism is more likely to be aqueduct stenosis with resultant obstructive hydrocephalus. Treatment is with CSF diversion with a ventriculoperitoneal shunt plus or minus a cysto peritoneal shunt.

Mega cisterna magna

This is a benign developmental variant where the cisterna magna is larger than normal and is thought to occur secondary to a delayed development of the foramen of Magendie. The cere-bellum is normal in these cases and there is no associated hydrocephalus, unlike the Dandy-Walker malformation. Another cystic condition that may present in the posterior fossa is an arachnoid cyst. These are usually distinctly separate from normal subarachnoid and cisternal spaces and may be off the midline.

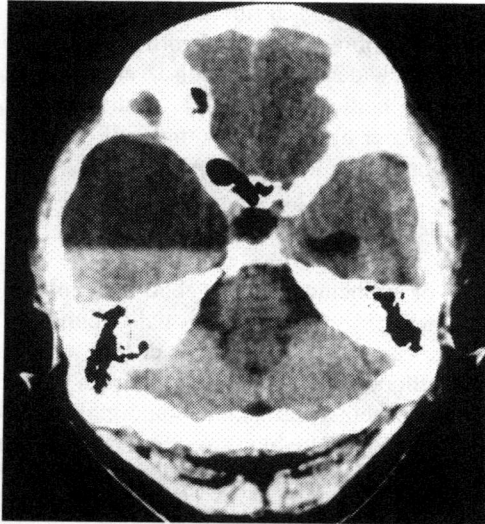

Figure 11. *This axial CT scan demonstrates a large right temporal arachnoid cyst with intra-cystic haemorrhage.*

16

MONITORING AND TREATMENT IN THE NEUROSURGICAL ICU

W Adriaan Liebenberg

Contents

Monitoring
Intracranial pressure monitoring
Measurement of cerebral blood flow
Transcranial Doppler Ultrasonography (TCD)
Jugular Venous Oximetry (JVO)
Near infrared spectroscopy (NIRS)
EEG and Bispectral analysis (BIS)
Brain tissue oxygen tension monitoring
Microdialysis
Evoked potentials

The injured brain
ICP and CPP
Management of ICP
Brain herniation
Status epilepticus

Monitoring
Intracranial pressure monitoring
Measurements are currently performed invasively. Devices are either catheter based or non-catheter based. In catheter based systems the intracranial pressure is measured with the aid of an external ventricular drain. This can either be done by transducing/measuring the height of the fluid column of the catheter or by incorporating a solid state/fibre optic transducer within the catheter. Non-catheter based systems are solid state/fibre optic transducers that are left intracranially at the time of surgery or inserted via a twist drill and bolt system. The transducer tip can either be placed subdurally or in the parenchyma of the brain. The most reliable way and the gold standard for intracranial pressure monitoring is intraventricular pressure monitoring via an external ventricular drain. The ICP readings are the most accurate reflection of intracranial pressure of any of the systems and intracranial hypertension may be treated by CSF drainage. Transducers in the parenchyma and those located subdurally can only account for the pressures of the parenchyma directly adjacent to the sensor. The advantage of the non catheter based systems is that they have a lower infectious potential. The *Codman* system is a silicon chip solid state system and the *Camino* system a fibre optic system.

The ICP is measured continuously via a monitor and a wave pattern is seen. The normal wave demonstrates slow fluctuations due to respiration with superimposed biphasic cardiac generated fluctuations. Usually the cardiac fluctuations are relatively small compared to the respiratory fluctuations. These can be imagined as large ocean waves (respiratory waves) with ripples on them (cardiac oscillations). In cases of reduced brain compliance the cardiac fluctuations become more pronounced.

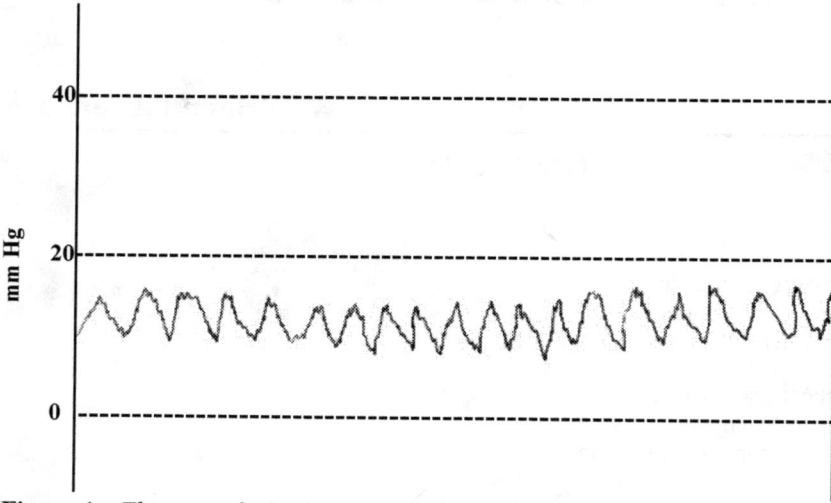

Figure 1 - *The normal ICP breathing curve.*

Reduced compliance and elevated ICP can lead to pathological waves as described by Lundberg:

Lundberg A (plateau waves) - These waves have a continued increase in the baseline ICP of 50 mm Hg or more and have a duration of 5 – 20 minutes. When they terminate, the baseline ICP is reset to a higher value. These waves are a poor prognostic sign and indicate that there is severely reduced intracranial compliance.

Lundberg B waves - These are less severe, last for 2 minutes or less and have lower amplitudes than A waves, and are commonly in the region of 10-20 mm Hg. They may be either sinus-like or ramp-like.

Lundberg C waves (Herring-Traube-Mayer waves) - These are of very limited pathological significance and are caused mainly by physiological fluctuations with low amplitudes and can be superimposed on the normal pattern.

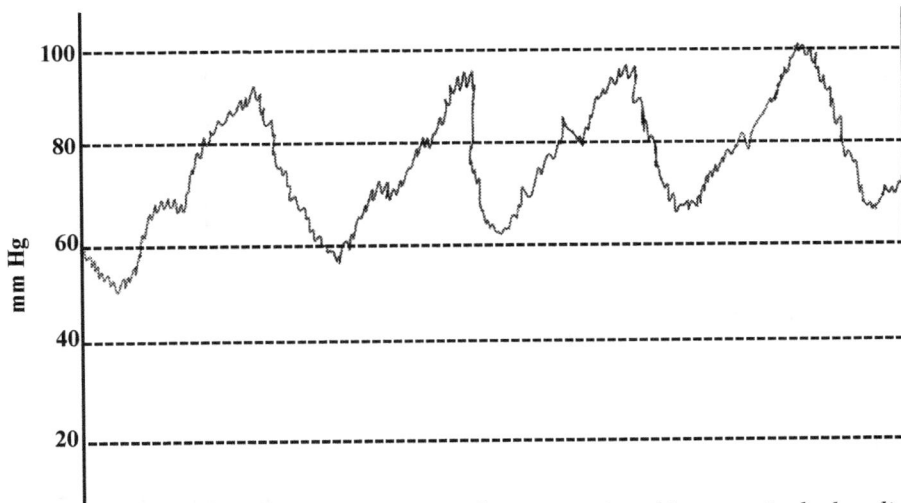

Figure 2 - *Lundberg A wave. These waves have a continued increase in the baseline ICP of 50 mm Hg or more and have a duration of 5 – 20 minutes.*

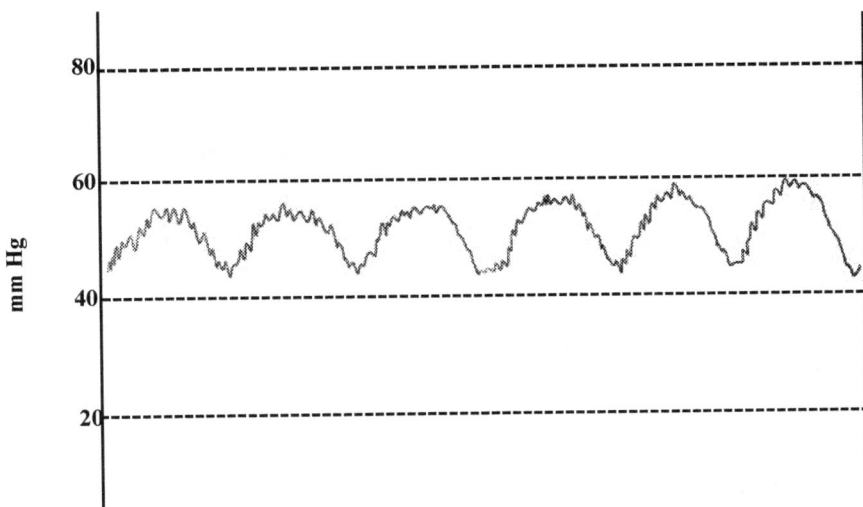

Figure 3. *Sinus-like B-waves. These are independent of changes of blood pressure, breathing, or CO2 level.*

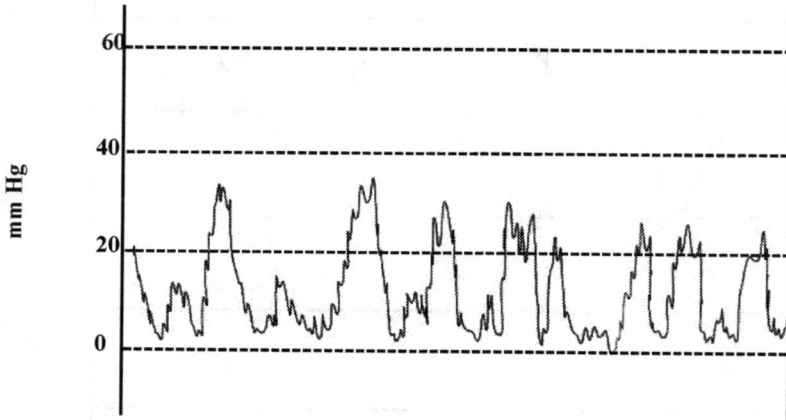

Figure 4. *Ramp-like B-waves. These are produced by snoring and concomitant pCO2 increases*

Measurement of cerebral blood flow

Transcranial Doppler Ultrasonography (TCD)

This is a non invasive method to indirectly measure the blood flow by measuring the velocity of intracranial blood flow. This is done by monitoring the shift in frequency spectra of the Doppler signal. By using a 2 MHz probe and using the natural windows to the intracranial space, the temporal bone, orbital foramen and the foramen magnum, signals are obtained that have proven to be clinically useful. The most common route is to measure the middle cerebral artery through the temporal bone. There is a proportional change in velocity and blood flow if the diameter of the blood vessel stays unchanged. A rise in flow velocity means that either the blood flow has increased or that the vessel diameter has decreased. To be able to tell whether a patient is hyperaemic or has vasospasm, the hemispheric index is used. This is the flow velocity of the middle cerebral artery divided by the flow velocity of the ipsilateral extracranial internal carotid artery. A value of greater than 3 indicates vasospasm. TCD is useful for monitoring CBF non invasively, diagnosing vasospasm and monitoring the response of treatment of vasospasm.

Jugular Venous Oximetry (JVO)

This is an indirect measurement of the cerebral blood flow (CBF) based on the fact that the cerebral metabolic rate of oxygen (CMRO2) is equal to the CBF multiplied by the difference in the arterial and venous oxygen concentration ((A-V)DO2)

$$CMRO2 = CBF \times (A-V)DO2.$$

Both the cerebral arterial oxygenation and the CMRO2 is usually constant , therefore any decrease in the venous oxygen saturation is usually an indication that the blood flow is reduced and that the tissue is extracting more oxygen out of the slow flowing blood. The measurement is done with a catheter placed in a retrograde fashion into the jugular bulb via the internal jugular vein. The tip of the catheter must be in or within 1 cm of the bulb to stop the blood from becoming mixed with extracranial blood. Three indices can be obtained from JVO monitoring:

SVJO$_2$ (The saturation of the JVO)

A normal value is between 60-80%, and a value of 90% or more indicates hyperemia, and a value of 50% or less, indicates hypoperfusion (there is very little time for oxygen to be

312

extracted from fast flowing blood).

CEO$_2$ (The cerebral oxygen extraction)
This is the difference between the arterial and jugular venous oxygen content. A normal value is between 24% and 40% with values lower than this range indicating hyperemia and higher values indicating hypoperfusion (there is a higher extraction of oxygen in slow flowing blood).

(A-V)DO$_2$ (The difference in the arterial and venous oxygen concentration)
Normal values are 5-7.5 vol % and lower values indicate hyperemia and higher values hypoperfusion.

Therefore a high SVJO$_2$ with low CEO$_2$ and (A-V) DO$_2$ indicates hyperemia and vice versa. It has been proven with the aid of JVO monitoring that patients suffer from episodes of decreased cerebral perfusion despite and adequate cerebral perfusion pressure. There is good outcome in patients who have JVO monitoring. The criticism of JVO monitoring is that it only supplies a global picture of brain perfusion and cannot identify focal areas of ischaemia.

Near infrared spectroscopy (NIRS)
This is a non invasive method for measuring regional blood flow. Light in the near infrared range can penetrate skin, bone and soft tissue up to a depth of 8cm and is absorbed at different spectra by oxygenated haemoglobin, deoxygenated haemoglobin and cytochrome aa$_3$. Changes in absorption can be measured and in infants this is done with transillumination and in adults it is measured from reflected light due to the thickness of the skull. Different equations can derive measurements for regional blood flow, cerebral oxygen saturation, cerebral metabolism and cerebral blood volume. In the clinical setting this technology is still hampered by the confounding effects of extracranial blood flow. Intracranial haematomas also skew measurements. A cerebral oxygen saturation of higher than 75% suggests adequate CPP and values lower than 55% suggest inadequate CPP. Current clinical experience has proven that, in adults, cerebral blood flow and cerebral blood volume are significantly underestimated. It may prove a very useful tool in the future.

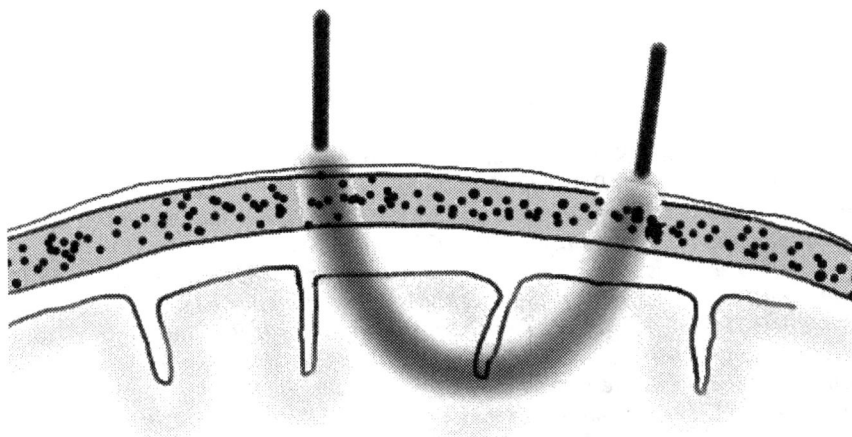

Figure 4. *Near infrared spectroscopy. The beam traverses the skull and soft tissue and is measured by the receiving probe.*

EEG and Bispectral analysis (BIS)

This is a tool that us used in both theatre and ICU to monitor the level of anaesthesia. Automated EEG processing has allowed bispectral analysis to become possible. A combination of different EEG processing parameters, obtained from a monitoring electrode strip with adhesive backing placed on the forehead, are used to make up the bispectral analysis. The bispectral index has been developed from a large amount of EEG data gathered from both volunteers and patients under different levels of sedation and ranges from a numerical value of 0 to 100. A value of 100 means that there is no sedation, 70 indicates a light hypnotic state, 60 indicates a moderate hypnotic state, 40 indicates a deep hypnotic state and 0 indicated EEG suppression. This value has been established in patients without brain damage and its use in patients with head injury is not validated. It is also important to realise that electromyogenic activity will give a falsely high number and therefore non paralysed patients could be over sedated. This is also true for the new BIS*xp* monitor.

Brain tissue oxygen tension monitoring (PbtO$_2$)

Direct regional measurements of the oxygenation of brain tissue can be performed using miniature Clarke's electrodes. There are two skull bolt systems currently available, the *Licox* system that measures brain tissue oxygen tension and temperature and the *Neurotrend* monitor that measures brain tissue oxygen tension, carbon dioxide tension, pH and temperature. The *Licox* device has two separate probes with sensors and the *Neurotrend* has one probe with four different sensors arranged along its 2 cm length. Normal values for PbtO$_2$ are 20-40 mmHg and there is increased risk of death for any period that the value is below 15 mmHg. Jugular venous oxygen monitoring correlates well with brain tissue oxygen tension monitoring and a SVJO$_2$ value of 50% correlates with a PbtO$_2$ value of 8.5 mm Hg. A combination of the global measurement of SVJO$_2$ and the local measurement of PbtO$_2$ is useful in the management of patients with brain injury.

Microdialysis

This is an invasive direct monitoring modality for the substrate and metabolites of the brain and is used to measure glucose, lactate, pyruvate, neurotransmitters and the levels of therapeutic agents. The catheter is very fine with a diameter of 0.5 mm and is perfused by a physiological solution at low flow rates. This is still mostly used for research activities and is quite labour intensive.

Figure 5. *The BIS monitor. See image on opposite page. There are several indices that are displayed on the monitor. The BIS value is indicated in the top left hand corner. In the right hand corner, the following 3 indices are displayed:* **The Signal Quality Index (SQI)** *Bar Graph is an indication of the quality of the EEG signal and optimal signal quality is indicated when the bar extends to the right side (+) of the graph.* **The Electromyograph (EMG)** *Bar Graph shows muscle activity. A low level of EMG is indicated when the bar is not present or at the left side of the graph.* **The Suppression Ratio (SR)** *Number is a calculated parameter to indicate when an isoelectric (flatline) condition may exist. Suppression ratio is the percentage of time over the last 63-second period that the signal is considered to be in the suppressed state. For example: SR=23 (isoelectric over 23% of the last 63 second review). The SR is displayed in the upper right corner of the screen. .*
The Electroencephalogram (EEG) Waveform Display is also on the top right-hand side. The main monitor demonstrates the trend. The bottom figure on the opposite page demonstrates the EEG slowing seen in progressively lower BIS values.

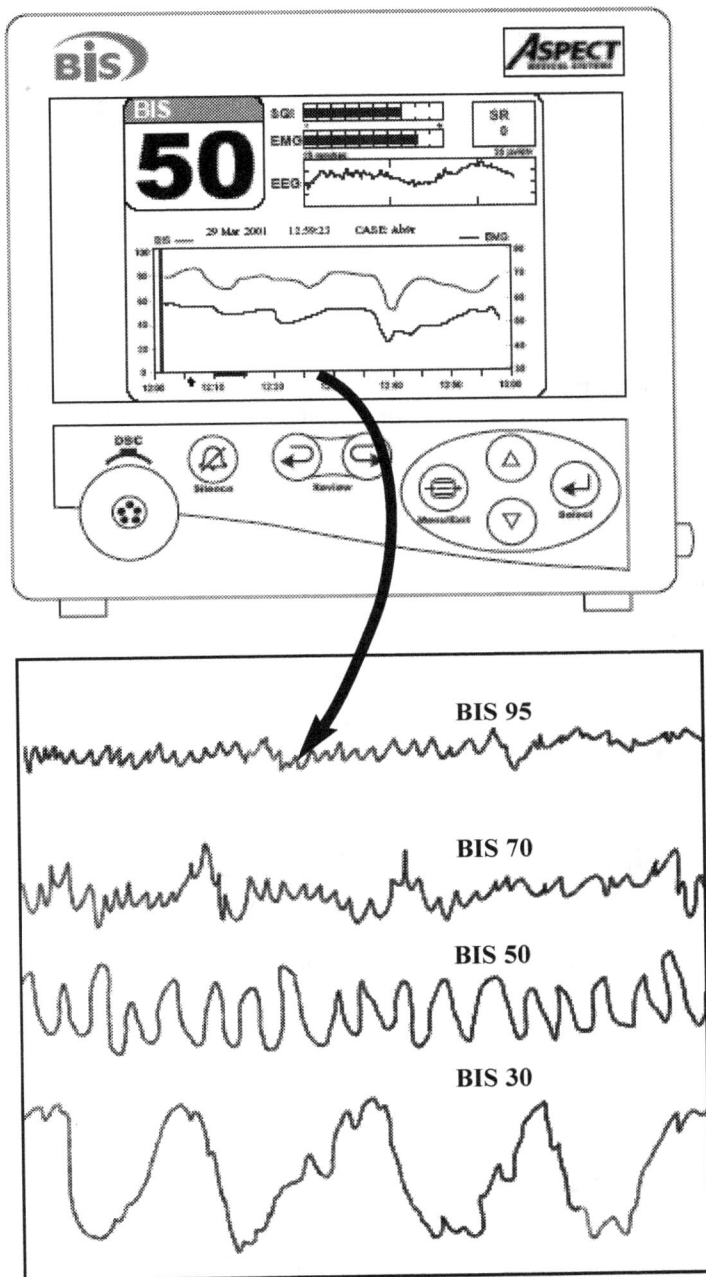

Figure 5. *The BIS monitor. See legend on opposite page.*

Evoked potentials

These potentials are generated by external stimulation of the nervous system and the potentials generated are then recorded. These potentials are much smaller that the normal background electrical activity and therefore a large number of impulses are generated and they are then averaged to account for the background noise. There are two basic types of evoked potential, sensory and motor.

Sensory evoked potentials – these are brainstem auditory evoked potentials (BAEP) which are generated by stimulating the eighth cranial nerve and recording the response by brainstem nuclei; visual evoked potentials (VEP) which is the response of the occipital cortex to visual stimulation by diodes during surgery and somatosensory evoked potentials (SSEP) which is the brain and spinal cord's response to the stimulation of a peripheral nerve. In the lower limb it is usually the posterior tibial nerve and in the upper limb it is usually the median or ulnar nerve.

Motor evoked potentials (MEP) – These are generated by transcranial stimulation of the cortex and the impulses can be measured in the epidural space, the peripheral nerves or in the muscles.

BAEP is used in surgery of the cerebellopontine angle, VEP is used for surgery around the optic nerves and optic chiasm and SSEP and MEP are used for spinal surgery.

The injured brain

Whatever kind of injury the brain receives, it is essential that the brain tissue is properly perfused. The cells of the brain do not have the capacity to store energy and if they are not constantly perfused, they die. When they die, the patient dies. The brain cannot be perfused if the blood pressure is too low for blood to flow through the brain or if the pressure is too high inside the cranium for blood to be able to flow through it. Therefore management of intracranial pressure and cerebral perfusion pressure is central to the management of the patient with brain injury.

ICP and CPP

The Monroe – Kelly doctrine is central to understanding the pathophysiology of raised intracranial pressure, compliance and elastance. It states that the fixed space contained within the skull is composed of brain, CSF and the blood contained in the vascular system. If either one of these increases then it does so to the detriment of the other two. An intracranial mass lesion has a deleterious effect on all three components. The two concepts that describe the effects of the Monroe - Kelly doctrine are elastance and compliance.

Intracranial elastance is the change in intracranial pressure as a function of a change of volume.

Intracranial compliance is the change in volume as a function as a function of the change in pressure.

Elastance describes the effect that added intracranial volume will have on the intracranial pressure. The elastance as can be seen from the elastance curve is the change in pressure over the change in volume or dP/dV. As elastance increases, a smaller change in volume results in the same amount of change in pressure. Compliance is exactly the opposite of that and is the change in volume due to a change in pressure or dV/dP. The practical effect of increased elastance is that intracranial haematomas, oedema, hyperemia, hydrocephalus and tumours increase the intracranial pressure to a critical level. There is capacity for the brain to accommodate some increased volume by displacing CSF up to a point. After this the pressure increases dramatically for a very small increase in volume.

The reason that a raised ICP has a deleterious effect on the brain is that it has a negative effect on the cerebral perfusion pressure (CPP). The equation that demonstrates the relationship between mean blood pressure (MAP), ICP and CPP is as follows: CPP = MAP – ICP.

The cerebral vasculature has the ability to autoregulate the blood flow by vasoconstriction and vasodilatation. This is intact for MAP's between 50 mmHg and 140 mmHg. Outside of these values autoregulation cannot function and the relation between blood flow and MAP becomes linear. In brain injured patients the autoregulation mechanism is frequently dysfunctional and the linear relationship takes over. When the relationship between MAP and blood flow becomes linear a drop in the MAP leads to a drop in the intracerebral blood flow and vice versa. If blood flow falls below a certain level, brain cell ischaemia follows and if the levels are low enough, there is failure of the transmembrane pumps and the associated influx of calcium leads to cell death. It is known that in patients with head injury the outcome is significantly worse if the CPP falls to below 60 mmHg. When CPP falls below 40 mmHg, a vasopressor response increases the MAP through a massive release of catecholamines, This is called the Cushing response which is typified by an increase in the systemic blood pressure and if there is associated central herniation (coning), bradycardia.

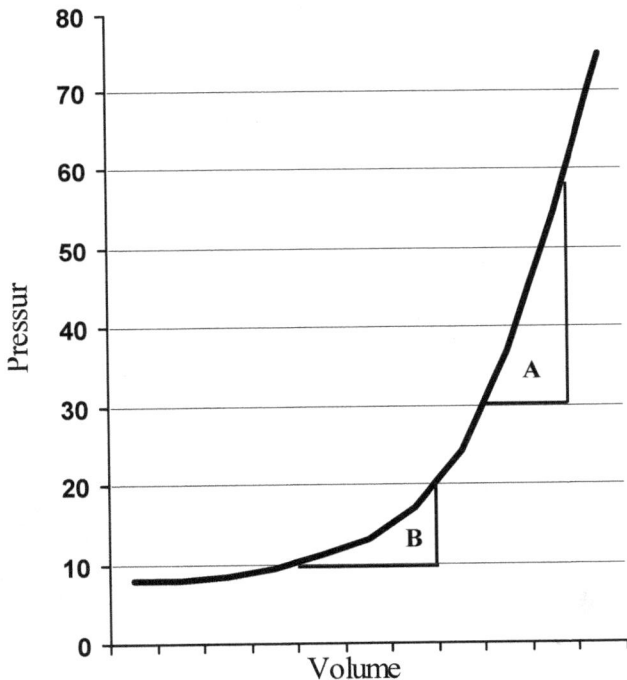

Figure 6. *The elastance curve. The elastance as can be seen from the curve is the change in pressure over the change in volume or dP/dV. Note that on the steeper part of the curve (A) , a small increase in volume, leads to a greater increase in pressure compared to on the less steep part of the curve (B).*

Management of ICP and CPP in brain injury

Medical therapy

Primary principles

The aim is to perfuse the brain (with well oxygenated blood containing the right concentration of glucose) by increasing the CPP to above 70 mmHg (some say 60 or 65 is acceptable) by either decreasing the ICP, increasing the MAP or both. An ICP consistently above 25 mmHg (some say 20 mmHg) is the threshold that requires treatment.

Position

Placing patients in a 10 – 15% head up position assists in venous drainage and helps to lower the ICP.

Ventilation

Normoventilation or slight hyperventilation is the current approach. Hyperventilation was used previously as it was though that the lowered $PaCO_2$ would lead to beneficial vasoconstriction with subsequent decreased ICP (Monroe – Kelly). However this lead to ischaemia in brain tissue already starved of perfusion. Keeping the $PaCO_2$ around 4.5 kPa or slightly lower is the current approach. Short periods of hyperventilation with FiO_2 of 100% can be used in conjunction with mannitol for sudden acute rises in ICP such as patients with traumatic extra axial collections on their way to theatre.

Temperature

It is important to maintain normothermia. Hyperthermia leads to increased metabolic work and subsequent increases in ICP. It was thought that hypothermia might decrease the ICP and have a neuroprotective effect. No definite benefit of induced hypothermia was found in adults and increased infection, coagulopathy and arrhythmias have complicated this treatment. There is thought to be some benefit in children.

Electrolytes

Sodium is the most important electrolyte for the neurosurgeon and neurosurgical intensivist.

Hyponatremia leads to brain swelling and lowers the seizure threshold. Hyponatremia is frequently found in SAH. It is associated with high volume infusions of sodium poor fluids, cerebral salt wasting (CSW) and the syndrome of inappropriate ADH secretion (SIADH). It can be difficult to discern between SIADH and CSW. Both these conditions lead to low serum sodium, CSW does so because there is a loss of salt and SIADH does so because of water intoxication. In SIADH vasopressin is secreted despite volume overload. A low CVP or pulmonary capillary wedge pressure (PCWP) with increased hematocrit is typical of CSW. As a broad distinction, cases with CSW are dehydrated, and cases with SIADH are fluid overloaded (water intoxication). It is important to distinguish between these two as the treatment for CSW is fluid and sodium replacement which can be fatal in cases of SIADH. Conversely the treatment of SIADH is fluid restriction which can be fatal in cases of CSW, especially when occurring in SAH.

Hypernatremia may lead to restlessness, confusion and coma. It may be caused by over zealous administration of normal saline. Another more sinister cause is diabetes insipidus (DI) due to insufficient vasopressin (ADH) which leads to large amounts of fluid and electrolytes being lost as urine output dramatically increases. Central DI may be caused by any damage to the hypophysis or hypothalamus following transsphenoidal surgery, trauma, vascular infarct and compression from sellar tumours. The diagnosis is made by noting large volumes of dilute urine, more than 250 ml/hr in three consecutive hours with a low specific gravity (S.G) in the range of 1.001 to 1.005. Care must be taken not to confuse this with the patient who is having a diuresis due to a large fluid load. This is frequently seen in patients returning from theatre that have had large amounts of fluid infused. It is always helpful to look at the total fluid balance. In cases of DI the large urine output will be associated with raised serum osmolality and serum sodium. The urine will also be dilute macroscopically. Treatment is with desmopressin and fluid replacement. In the awake patient oral intake may be all that is required but in the comatose patient IV fluid needs to be infused or water may be given via the nasogastric route. It is important to use sodium-poor fluid and also to restrict dietary intake of sodium by low-sodium diet or nasogastric feed. DI may be temporary or permanent.

Magnesium has neuroprotective qualities and should be supplemented if levels are low.

Glucose control and nutrition

Hyperglycemia leads to lactate build up which mediates cell damage. Hypoglycemia leads to energy failure of the cells. It is imperative that patients are on a very tight glucose control and all patients should be on an insulin sliding scale. Feeding should be instituted as early as possibly, preferably within 24 – 48 hours to provide for both the energy needs of the injured brain and also to combat stress ulcers. The patient with an injured brain needs 1.5 times the normal amount of calories. H_2 receptor antagonists, proton pump inhibitors or sucralfate should also be used to combat stress ulcers.

Seizures

Phenytoin is effective in reducing early seizures, although it has no effect on the long term development of epilepsy. Convulsions increase the metabolic activity of the brain and may also cause muscle activity which can increase the ICP. Both Phenytoin and Phenobarbitone can be loaded IV and are effective in terminating seizures.

Blood pressure

Adequate MAP prevents reflex intracranial vasodilatation with resultant hyperemia as part of cerebral autoregulation when autoregulation is intact. When autoregulation is intact an adequate MAP leads to an adequate CPP. When the autoregulation is not functioning, a MAP that is too high will lead to intracranial hyperemia. To sustain the MAP, adequate intravascular filling and the use of inotropic support, when the blood pressure is still low despite adequate filling, is used. When the systolic pressure rises above 200 -210 mmHg, this may lead to intracranial haemorrhage. Control of blood pressure should be done carefully as a sudden drop of filling pressure in cases where the brain is already ischemic, may lead to infarction. Therefore a short acting agent that can be titrated is recommended. Labetalol is a short acting beta blocker which is frequently used and titrated as an IV infusion.

Hyperosmolar therapy

Mannitol is an osmotically active compound that is used as the mainstay of treatment of raised ICP. It acts by osmotically drawing fluid from the brain parenchyma and excreting this fluid as part of a general osmotic diuresis. It also has the properties of being able to decreases CSF production; lowers blood viscosity and leads to improved rheology; it reduces brain swelling and oedema and is a free radical scavenger. It is usually used in 0.25g/kg boluses. Serum osmolality should be kept below 320 mosmol. It may be administered in conjunction with, and is potentiated by, loop diuretics (frusemide). Mannitol however can have a detrimental effect on patients with raised ICP secondary to hyperemia due to its effect on rheology. Hypertonic saline is being evaluated currently as a promising new treatment modality to reduce ICP and improve intracranial blood flow.

Sedation

Patients should always be deeply sedated to control ICP. Agents that are commonly used are propofol, fentanyl and midazolam. Propofol is used as an infusion and has the advantage that it does not accumulate and has a very short wash out period. Consequently patients can be roused very quickly following cessation of propofol infusion. It is also a very potent agent and can be used to provide burst suppression in salvage ICP management and intractable epilepsy.

Ventriculostomy

Draining CSF through an external ventricular drain is the most effective way of controlling the ICP. Drains are commonly set at the level of pressure that is acceptable or desired and any rises above that pressure will then produce CSF drainage and reduce the ICP (Monroe – Kelly). The zero mark is usually set at the external auditory meatus and the reservoir at 10 or 15 mmHg.

Neuromuscular blockade

Atracurium is non cumulative, not associated with myopathy and is commonly used in the intensive care to paralyse patients to reduce the ICP by reducing movement, coughing and straining and decrease muscle tone. Other agents are also used.

Barbiturates

The use of barbiturates is reserved for refractory ICP management. Barbiturates and their metabolites take a long time to be eliminated from the body and therefore patients have prolonged periods in ICU following termination of the infusion before they can be assessed neurologically. Hypotension and loss of pupillary constriction complicates barbiturate therapy. Inducing barbiturate coma is often the final therapeutic manoeuvre available for cases with intractable intracranial hypertension and consequently signifies a poorer prognosis.

Surgical management
Mass lesions

All significant mass lesions must be removed as soon as they are diagnosed.

Decompressive craniectomies

Traditionally this has been used as salvage therapy but it is being used more frequently in the aggressive and early management of malignant ICP. The aim is to relieve the constraints of the skull by doing wide craniectomies. Some surgeons do a duraplasty. and leave the dura open. This procedure is associated with a poorer prognosis since the procedure is reserved for patients with refractory raised ICP.

Brain herniation

There may be supratentorial and infratentorial herniation of the brain depending on the nature of the pathology causing the raised intracranial pressure and also the location of that pathology. There are 3 supratentorial herniation syndromes and one infratentorial herniation syndrome:

Subfalcine or cingulate herniation
When the pathology is restricted to a single cerebral hemisphere, the cingulate gyrus may herniate underneath the free edge of the falx cerebri and thus cause midline shift. It is this midline shift that we look for on a trauma CT scan to evaluate whether an extra axial haemorrhage needs to be evacuated. The ventricular system is also displaced and obstructive hydrocephalus may be caused by obstruction of the foramen of Monroe. The anterior cerebral artery or its continuation, the pericallosal artery may be compressed by the edge of the falx cerebri and lead to infarction of the medial cerebral hemispheres.

Uncal herniation (lateral transtentorial herniation)
The uncus is the inferomedial point of the temporal lobe. Masses in the middle fossa cause the temporal lobe to be displaced medially away from the temporal bone. The uncus is compressed against the brainstem and herniates downward into the posterior fossa past the free edge of the tentorium. As the uncus pushes against the brainstem it compresses the ipsilateral oculomotor nerve with resultant ipsilateral pupil dilatation, it also compresses the cerebral peduncle directly and the descending corticospinal tracts (which cross lower down in the medulla) leading to a contralateral hemiparesis.

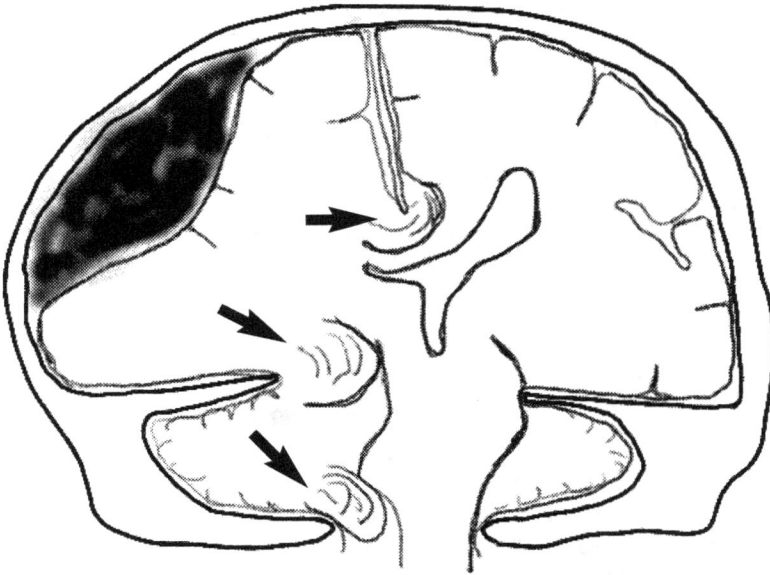

Figure 7. *Brain herniation syndromes. The top arrow demonstrates subfalcine (cingulate) herniation, the middle arrow demonstrates uncal herniation and the last arrow demonstrates tonsillar herniation.*

In Kernohan's paralysis, the brainstem which is being displaced by the uncus is pushed up against the contralateral tentorial edge, causing a notch to form in the brainstem – Kernohan's notch. The contralateral cerebral peduncle is compressed and because the fibres cross lower down, leads to an ipsilateral hemiparesis. The reticular activating system which is located in the brainstem is also compressed leading to impaired consciousness. The posterior cerebral artery may also be compressed at the posterior edge of the tentorial hiatus, causing an occipital lobe infarct.

Central transtentorial herniation
Lesions outside of the middle fossa may cause the diencephalon and midbrain to be pushed through the tentorial hiatus. This leads to patients becoming comatose/obtunded, develop loss of upward gaze, have small reactive pupils and Cheyne-Stokes breathing.

Tonsillar herniation
When there is increased pressure inside the posterior fossa from swelling of the cerebellum or due to a space occupying lesion, the cerebellar tonsils may herniate into the upper spinal canal and thus compress the medulla. This leads to depressed consciousness but also compression of the cardiac and respiratory centres of the midbrain. Hypertension, arrhythmias and abnormal breathing patterns may be seen. Cheyne-Stokes breathing or neurogenic hyperventilation may occur.

Status epilepticus

There are a myriad of causes for epilepsy in a neurosurgical patient. Status epilepticus is associated with severe morbidity and mortality. Status epilepticus can be:

Convulsive status or major motor status is defined as 3 convulsions expressed by major motor twitches with depressed conscious level without patient resurfacing into consciousness, or a single ongoing seizure of more than 30 minutes.

Myoclonic status is when there is a reduced consciousness with myoclonus (shock like contractions of a muscle or muscle group).

Complex partial (temporal lobe seizures with reduced consciousness and automatisms) or absence status is when there is a prolonged period of reduced consciousness that is diagnosed on EEG to be ictal activity.

Subtle status is manifest by minor events such as myoclonic twitches, roving eyes and depressed consciousness.

Epilepsia partialis continuans is focal motor status that does not lead to reduced consciousness.

Overall mortality for status epilepticus is between 10 – 15%. If status persists beyond 4 hours, mortality may be as high as 50% and if it persists beyond 12 hours the mortality is as high as 80%. It is important that all patients with depressed levels of consciousness are intubated to protect their airway. Intravenous access should be established immediately, blood taken for anticonvulsant levels and a 50 ml bolus of 50% dextrose administered. Remember that most anticonvulsants are most effective quite close to or over the toxic level. Epileptic activity should be stopped with a short acting drug and followed by a longer acting drug to control seizures in the longer term (see fig 8).

```
┌─────────────────────────────────────────────────┐
│   INTRAVENOUS ACCESS, TAKE BLOODS FOR           │
│        ANTICONVULSANT LEVELS                    │
└─────────────────────────────────────────────────┘
                      ▼
┌─────────────────────────────────────────────────┐
│   ADMINISTER 50ML 50% D EXTROSE AS IV PUSH      │
└─────────────────────────────────────────────────┘
                      ▼
┌─────────────────────────────────────────────────┐
│   INTUBATE PATIENTS WHO ARE COMATOSE OR CANNOT  │
│        PROTECT THEIR AIRWAY                     │
└─────────────────────────────────────────────────┘
                      ▼
┌─────────────────────────────────────────────────┐
│   ADMINISTER 10 Mg DIA ZEPAM OR 4 Mg LORA       │
│        ZEPAM AS IV PUSH                         │
│        REPEAT IF IN EFFECTIVE                   │
└─────────────────────────────────────────────────┘
                      ▼
          ┌───────────────────────┐
          │   Ongoing seizures    │
          └───────────────────────┘
                      ▼
┌─────────────────────────────────────────────────┐
│   PHENYTOIN 15 – 18 Mg/Kg AS IV LOADING DOSE    │
│        AT RATE < 50 Mg/min                      │
│   BEWARE OF DYSRHYTHMIA AND HYPOTENSION         │
└─────────────────────────────────────────────────┘
                      ▼
          ┌───────────────────────┐
          │   Ongoing seizures    │
          └───────────────────────┘
                      ▼
┌─────────────────────────────────────────────────┐
│   PHENOBARBITAL 10 -15Mg/Kg IV LOADING DOSE     │
│        AT RATE < 100Mg/min                      │
└─────────────────────────────────────────────────┘
                      ▼
          ┌───────────────────────┐
          │   Ongoing seizures    │
          └───────────────────────┘
                      ▼
┌─────────────────────────────────────────────────┐
│   THIOPENTONE – 250 Mg BOLUS AND THEN           │
│        2 -5 Mg/Kg/hr                            │
│        OR                                       │
│   PROPOFOL – 2Mg/Kg BOLUS AND THEN 5 -10Mg/Kg/hr│
└─────────────────────────────────────────────────┘
```

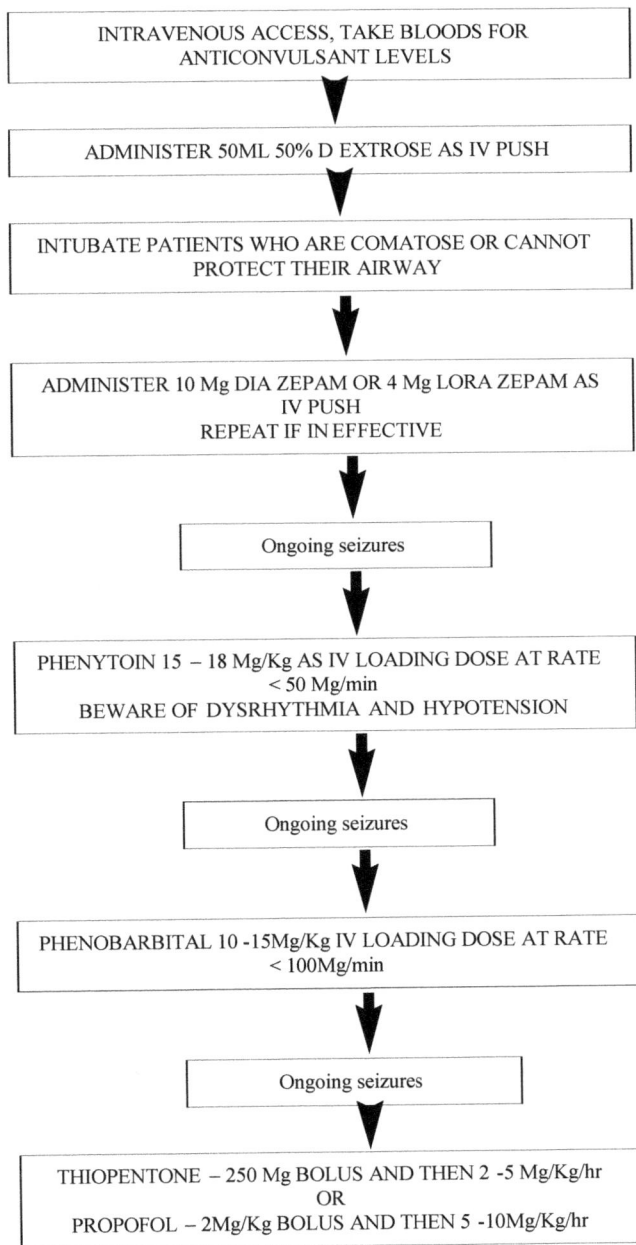

Figure 8. *This flow diagram demonstrates a suggested treatment plan for status epilepticus.*

17
COMMONLY USED DRUGS IN NEUROSURGERY

Andreas K Demetriades

Contents

Anticonvulsants
Carbamazepine
Phenytoin
Sodium Valproate
Keppra
Phenobarbitone

Anti-inflammatories (incl Steroids)
Dexamethasone
Methylprednisolone
Ibuprofen
Diclofenac

Analgesics
Paracetamol
Codeine phosphate
Pethidine
Opioids

Antiemetics
Cyclizine
Granisetron
Stemetil

Anti-vasospasm
Nimodipine
Papaverine
ReoPro (abciximab)

Intensive Care
Mannitol
Propofol
Thiopentone
Lorazepam
Haloperidol
Labetalol
Atracurium

Anticoagulants
LMW Heparin
Warfarin
Aspirin
Clopidogrel

Anticonvulsants

There are several drugs used to treat seizures, whether partial or generalised. The commonest are carbamazepine, phenytoin and sodium valproate. There are no prospective placebo controlled randomised trials for antiepileptic monotherapy in generalised epilepsy but the choice of drugs comes from widespread consensus. Furthermore, systematic reviews have not shown any good evidence on which to base a choice among these drugs in seizure control. Similar data on choice lacks in monotherapy for partial epilepsy. In drug resistant epilepsy, adding a second line drug has been shown in systematic reviews to be effective with gabapentin, levetiracetam, lamotrigine, oxcarbazepine, tiagabine, topiramate, vigabatrin and zonisamide. However, trials again are lacking as to the differences amongst the choices of medication.

Changes in the dosage should be considered in the face of side effects. Should a side effect be suspected, patients are advised to stop the medication while contacting their physician. Stopping abruptly may cause seizures. Life-threatening complications are rare but immediate presentation of patients to a hospital should be advised in cases of asthma, severe rashes, anaphylactic symptoms (swelling of lips, face, hands, throat, tongue), bruising, jaundice or symptoms of overdosage.

Carbamazepine
Other names: Tegretol
Indications: Epileptic seizures, especially partial seizures; trigeminal neuralgia; glossopharyngeal neuralgia, peripheral nerve pain.
Time to work: stable body concentration after 1-2 weeks. Serum levels are used to ensure appropriate concentrations in the body. First level check done at around one month.
Dosage: 200mg TDS to maximum of 1200mg per day.
Drug interactions: Alcohol, aspirin, anticoagulants, anti-depressants, paracetamol, among others, may affect the level of the drug in the body
Side effects: Allergic symptoms, breathlessness, rash, blood disorders (thrombocytopaenia and bruising; anaemia from bone marrow depression), liver failure, foetal defects, confusion, drowsiness, overdose (drowsiness, confusion, slurred speech, difficulty walking).
Cautions: Pregnancy, heart disease, kidney disease, liver disease, prostate disease, porphyria, glaucoma, hypotension, blood and platelet disorders.

Phenytoin
Other names: Dilantin
Indications: Epileptic seizures. Pain syndromes. Abnormal heart rhythm.
Time to work: The plasma half-life in patients after oral administration of phenytoin averages 22 hours, stable body concentration after 1 week. Serum levels are used to ensure appropriate concentrations. First level check done at one week.
Dosage: Maintenance dose is 300mg a day. In seizures, IV loading dose 18-20mg/kg (50mg/min maximum infusion rate); oral loading, 15-20mg/kg in doses of 400mg or less at 4 hr intervals.
Side effects: Allergic symptoms, breathlessness, rash, gum hypertrophy, coarse facial features, liver failure, osteomalacia, overdose (nausea, vomiting, visual acuity deterioration,

drowsiness, confusion, slurred speech, difficulty walking).
Cautions: pregnancy, heart disease, kidney disease, liver disease, porphyria, hypotension.

Sodium Valproate
Other names: Epilim
Indications: Epileptic seizures, including petit mal and grand mal seizures.
Mechanism of action: Increases the concentration of the inhibitory neurotransmitter GABA thereby inhibiting signal transmission in neurons and preventing the spread of seizure activity.
Time to work: stable body concentration after 3 days and a week is commonly needed to get the dose correctly adjusted. Serum levels are used regularly to ensure appropriate concentrations in the body. First level check done at around one week.
Dosage: 300mg BD, with 200mg daily increments to a maximum of 1000mg per day.
Drug interactions: Alcohol, aspirin, anticoagulants, among others, may affect the level of the drug in the body
Side effects: Allergic symptoms, breathlessness, rash and severe skin reactions, hair loss blood disorders (thrombocytopaenia and bruising), liver failure, nausea , vomiting, foetal defects, overdose (drowsiness, confusion, slurred speech, difficulty walking).
Cautions: pregnancy, heart disease, kidney disease, liver disease, hypotension, blood and platelet disorders.

Levetiracetam
Other names: Keppra.
Indications: adjunctive treatment of partial seizures with or without secondary generalisation.
Dosage: initially 500mg BD, adjusted in increments 500mg per dose every 2-4 weeks to a max of 1500mg BD.
Side effects: drowsiness, dizziness, asthenia, rash, diplopia, anorexia, diarrhea, dyspepsia, nausea, ataxia, amnesia, depression, emotional lability, insomnia, anxiety, psychosis, aggression, tremor, vertigo, headache, leucopaenia, pancytopaenia, thrombocytopaenia.
Cautions: pregnancy, breast feeding, kidney disease, liver disease, avoid sudden withdrawal.

Phenobarbitone
Other names: Phenobarbital, elixir.
Indications: all forms of epilespsy except absence seizures; status epilepticus.
Dosage: PO, 60-180mg nocte; child 5-8mg/kg daily.
Status epilepticus: 10mg/kg iv infusion at a rate of no more than 100mg/minute. Maximum 1g.
Acute seizures: 200mg im (15mg/kg child) repeated after 6 hours.
Drug interactions: lowers plasma concentration of carbamazepine, clonazepam, lamotrigine, phenytoin, tiagabine and valproate, and ethosuximide.
Side effects: lethargy, drowsiness, mental depression, ataxia, allergic skin reactions, restlessness and confusion in the elderly, hyperkinesias in children, megaloblastic anaemia (responsive to folic acid).
Cautions: pregnancy, breast feeding, kidney disease, liver disease, respiratory depression, porphyria, elderly, children, debilitated, avoid sudden withdrawal.

Anti-inflammatory drugs

Dexamethasone
Other names: dexamethsone.
Indications: In brain tumours it is used to reduce the surrounding oedema. In sciatica or

brachialgia it is sometimes used to reduce the swelling around the compressed cord or nerve. In pituitary disease it may be used as a hormone replacement.

Mechanism of action: A synthetic steroid. In brain tumours it reduces the fluid leakage by blood vessels affected by the tumour. In sciatica it reduces inflammation of the nerve involved. In pituitary disease it is a hormone replacement.

Time to work: 24 hours.

Dosage: 4mg QDS in brain tumours with reduction regime post-operatively. In sciatica 1.5-3 mg per day for a few weeks until symptoms improved. It is stopped not abruptly but slowly.

Side effects:

Short term treatment: hypertension, pro-diabetic, hiccoughs, risk of infection, high appetite, confusion, acute psychosis.

Long term treatment: diabetes, gastric ulceration, rectal bleeding, cataract, glaucoma, proximal myopathy, osteoporosis, immunosuppression, hypertension, fluid retention, obesity, Cushing's syndrome.

Cautions: pregnancy, heart disease, kidney disease, liver disease, hypertension, peptic ulcer, infection, ankle swelling.

Methyl prednisolone

Other names: medrone, depomedrone, solumedrone.

Indications: Traumatic spinal cord injury.

Nota Bene: Published in 1990, NASCIS II (National Acute Spinal Cord Injury Study)did not prove a beneficial neurological effect from methylprednisolone compared to naloxone or placebo. However, post-hoc subgroup analysis identified that those who received the drug within 8 hours of injury had better motor scores at 6 and 12 months. NASCIS III (1997) showed than methylprednisolone given for 48 hours was not better than 23 hours. Post-hoc subgroup analysis showed that in those treated within 3-8 hours after injury, 48 hours of treatment were associated with improved motor scores at 6 weeks and 6 months when compared to 23 hours of therapy. These results have led to a widespread use of methylprednisolone, only to come under increasing scrutiny for methodological flaws. At present, the role and effectiveness of corticosteroids in spinal cord injury is still unclear and a matter of dispute.

Mechanism of action: A corticosteroid which experimentally reduces inflammatory changes, oedema, excitotoxicity, cytoskeletal degradation and lipid peroxidation associated with spinal cord injury.

Time to work: When instituted less than 8 hours after traumatic spinal cord injury, methyl prednisolone sulphate was associated in two clinical trials with statistically significant improvement in the motor scores at 6 and 12 months. However, these results and their clinical relevance remain under dispute.

Dosage: Based on the NASCIS II and III studies, the regimens depend on time after injury. For Spinal Cord Injury less than 3 hours: 30mg/kg iv, then 5.4mg/kg/hour for 23 hours. For Spinal Cord Injury 3-8 hours: 30mg/kg iv, then 5.4mg/kg/hour for 48 hours.

Side effects: Gastrointestinal: peptic ulceration, rectal bleeding, acute pancreatitis, oesophageal ulceration and candidiasis. Musculoskeletal: proximal myopathy, osteoporosis, vertebral and long bone fractures, tendon rupture, avascular osteonecrosis. Endocrine: diabetes, adrenal suppression, Cushing's syndrome, amenorrhoea or other menstrual upset, weight gain hirsutism, increased appetite. Neuropsychiatric: confusion, acute psychosis, depression, insomnia aggravation of epilepsy and schizophrenia. Ophthalmic: cataract, glaucoma, papilloedema in children, corneal or scleral thinning, fungal or viral disease. Other: Immunosuppression, hypertension, skin atrophy, bruising, decreased healing, fluid and electrolyte imbalance, hypersensitivity reactions, thromboembolism, nausea, malaise, hiccups.

Cautions: pregnancy, heart disease, kidney disease, liver disease, hypertension, peptic ulcer, infection, ankle swelling.

Ibuprofen

Other names: brufen, nurofen.
Indications: Pain and inflammation in arthritic and other musculoskeletal disorders; postoperative analgesia; mild to moderate pain; migraine.
Mechanism of action: A proprionic acid derivative with anti-inflammatory, analgesic and anti-pyretic properties.
Time to work: pain relief starts soon after first dose and full analgesic effect reached within a week. Anti-inflammatory effect up to three weeks.
Dosage: 1.2-1.8g per day in 3 doses.
Drug interactions: Other anti-inflammatories, aspirin, antibacterials (eg increased tendency for convulsions with quinolones), anticoagulants, phenytoin, diuretics, antidepressants.
Side effects: gastrointestinal discomfort and bleeding, peptic ulceration, nausea and vomiting, analgesic nephropathy, rash, angioedema and bronchospasm (as in asthmatics), liver damage, aseptic meningitis (rarely in connective tissue disorders).
Cautions: elderly, pregnancy, asthmatics, renal/cardiac/hepatic impairment, peptic ulceration.

Diclofenac

Other names: voltarol, motifene, diclomax, voltaren.
Indications: Pain and inflammation in arthritic and other musculoskeletal disorders; postoperative analgesia, acute gout.
Mechanism of action: similar to proprionic acid derivatives with anti-inflammatory, analgesic and anti-pyretic properties.
Time to work: pain relief starts soon after first dose and full analgesic effect reached within a week. Anti-inflammatory effect up to three weeks.
Dosage: Maximum daily by any route 150mg. Orally 75-150mg per day in 2-3 doses; intramuscular injection 75mg once or twice daily, intravenously 75mg in between 6 hours for a maximum of 2 days; suppositories 75-150mg daily in 1-2 doses.
Drug interactions: other anti-inflammatories, aspirin, antibacterials (eg increased tendency for convulsions with quinolones), anticoagulants, phenytoin, diuretics, antidepressants.
Side effects: gastrointestinal discomfort and bleeding, peptic ulceration, nausea and vomiting, analgesic nephropathy, rash, angioedema and bronchospasm (as in asthmatics), liver damage, aseptic meningitis (rarely in connective tissue disorders).
Cautions: elderly, pregnancy, asthmatics, renal/cardiac/hepatic impairment, peptic ulceration.

Analgesic drugs

Paracetamol

Other names: panadol, disprol.
Indications: mild to moderate pain, pyrexia (NB. No anti-inflammatory activity).
Time to work: pain relief starts soon after first dose.
Dosage: 1g QDS po
Drug interactions: anticoagulants, domperidone, metoclopramide.
Side effects: rarely rashes, blood disorders. Liver damage on poisoning.
Cautions: hepatic/renal impairment, alcohol dependence.

Opioids

Examples:
Codeine phosphate- or cocodamol, kapake, solpadol tylex (in mixture with paracetamol).
Dihydrocodeine-or DF118, DHC Continus.

Tramadol-or zamadol, zydol, dromadol.
Fentanyl-or actiq, durogesic.
Pethidine.
Morphine.

Indications: Codeine phosphate in mild to moderate pain. Dihydrocodeine is similar in analgesic effect to codeine phosphate. Doubling the dose to 60mg may provide some extra analgesia but at the expense of nausea and constipation. Tramadol is used in moderate to severe pain. Fentanyl is used for intra operative analgesia by injection or postoperatively by a transdermal patch. Pethidine gives prompt but short-lasting analgesia and is weaker than morphine. Morphine is the most useful opioid in severe pain, although it often causes nausea and vomiting.
Mechanism of action: via opioid receptors .
Time to work: analgesic effect soon after dosage.
Dosage: Codeine phosphate and dihydrocodeine: 30-60mg QDS orally or by intramuscular injection (3mg/kg in divided doses). Tramadol: 50-100mg QDS orally or by intramuscular or intravenous injection. Fentanyl: a patch may last up to 72 hours releasing 25 mcg per hour. Pethidine: 4-hourly dosages of 50-150mg by mouth, or 25-100mg intramuscular or subcutaneous injection, and 25-50mg intravenously. Morphine: 4-hourly injection of 10mg subcutaneous or intramuscular injection, or in the form of oral solutions (oramorph, sevredol, MST continus).
Drug interactions: alcohol, antidepressants, antiepileptics, anticoagulants, cardiac glycosides, domperidone, metoclopramide.
Side effects: nausea, vomiting, constipation, drowsiness, respiratory depression and hypotension in larger doses, ureteric/biliary spasm, dry mouth, sweating, headache, facial flushing, arrhythmia, postural hypotension, rash, pruritus.
Cautions: children, hypotension, hypothyroidism, asthma, decreased respiratory reserve, pregnancy, epilepsy, dependence.

Antiemetic drugs

Cyclizine
Other names: valoid
Indications: nausea, vomiting, vertigo, motion sickness, labyrinthine disorders.
Mechanism of action: an antihistamine.
Time to work: effective soon after dosage
Dosage: 50mg TDS iv/im/po.
Drug interactions: alcohol, antacids, antidepressants, anti-arrythmic, anti-bacterials, antimuscarinics, beta blockers, diuretics.
Side effects: arrythmias, hypersensitivity, extrapyramidal effects, sleep disturbance, blood disorders, liver dysfunction, anti-muscarinic effects, drowsiness.
Cautions: heart failure, hepatic disease, renal impairment, epilepsy, children, elderly, porphyria.

Granisetron
Other names: kytril.
Indications: nausea or vomiting related to cytotoxics or radiotherapy; postoperative symptoms.
Mechanism of action: 5HT3 antagonist for CNS and gastrointestinal tract receptors.
Time to work: effective soon after dosage.
Dosage: 1-2mg orally or intravenously within an hour of treatment, then 2mg daily in divided doses. Maximum 9mg daily.

Side effects: constipation, headache, rash, transient rise in hepatic enzymes, hypersensitivity.
Cautions: pregnancy and breast-feeding.

Prochlorperazine
Other names: stemetil.
Indications: severe nausea and vomiting associated with neoplastic disease, radiation sickness, opioids, anaesthetics and cytotoxics; vertigo, labyrinthine disorders.
Mechanism of action: a phenothiazine which acts as a dopamine antagonist centrally by blocking the chemoreceptor trigger zone.
Time to work: soon after administration.
Dosage: Orally: 20mg initially then 10mg two hours later. Intramuscular injection: 12.5mg, followed by an oral dose 6 hours later. Rectally: 25mg, followed by an oral dose at least 6 hours later.
Side effects: extrapyramidal symptoms including, parkinsonian tremor, dystonia, dyskinesia, akathisia; hypotension, temperature dysregulation, drowsiness, agitation, insomnia, convulsions, dizziness, confusion, anti-muscarinic symptoms, neuroleptic malignant syndrome, endocrine disturbance like galactorrhoea, dysmenorrhoea, gynaecomastia, impotence.
Cautions: children, elderly, hepatic/renal/cardiac impairment, Parkinson's disease, epilepsy, depression, myasthenia gravis, glaucoma, prostatic hypertrophy, jaundice, blood dyscrasias.

Subarachnoid Haemorrhage and Anti-Vasospasm

Nimodipine
Other names: nimotop.
Indications: prevention and treatment of ischaemic neurological deficits following aneurysmal subarachnoid haemorrhage.
Mechanism of action: Calcium-channel blocker.
Dosage: Prevention: orally 60mg four-hourly, starting within 4 days of subarachnoid haemorrhage and continuing for 21 days.
Treatment: intravenous infusion via central line, initially 1mg/hour, increased after 2 hours to 2mg/hour if no severe hypotension, and continued for 5 days. If treated by intervention during treatment, continue for a minimum of 5 days before changing to oral administration. Total length of treatment is 21 days.
Drug interactions: calcium-channel blockers, alcohol.
Side effects: arrhythmia, hypotension, headache, flushing, sweating, nausea, gastrointestinal disorders including ileus, thrombocytopaenia.
Cautions: severely raised ICP, cerebral oedema, hypotension, other calcium-channel blockers, beta-blockers, renal impairment, hepatic impairment, grapefruit juice may affect metabolism.

Contra-indicated within 1 month of myocardial infarction and in unstable angina.

Papaverine hydrochloride
Other names: Pavabid
Indications: prevention and treatment of ischaemic neurological deficits following aneurysmal subarachnoid haemorrhage.
Mechanism of action: smooth muscle relaxant.
Dosage: 1 to 4 ml IV every 3 hours as needed
Drug interactions: should not be added to Lactated Ringer's Injection, because precipita-

tion would result
Side effects: general discomfort, nausea, abdominal discomfort, anorexia, constipation or diarrhea, skin rash, malaise, vertigo, headache, intensive flushing of the face, perspiration, tachycardia, and slight hypertension.
Cautions: children, pregnancy, glaucoma

Abciximab
Other names: ReoPro
Indications: percutaneous angiography and endovascular coiling of intracranial aneurysms.
Mechanism of action: a glycoprotein IIbIIIa inhibitor.
Dosage: IV bolus of 0.25 mg/kg
Side effects: bleeding manifestations, nausea, vomiting, hypotension, bradycardia, backpain, chest pain, headache, puncture site pain, pyrexia, hypersensitivity, adult respiratory distress, thrombocytopaenia.
Cautions: measure baseline PT, APTT, platelet count, haemoglobin and haematocrit; monitor haemoglobin and haematocrit 12 and 24 hours after commencement of treatment, and platelet count at 2-4 and 24 hours. Concomitant drugs that may predispose to bleeding. Hepatic and renal impairment; pregnancy. Stop usage in event of serious bleeding.
Contra-indications: major surgery, stroke, intracranial neoplasm, active internal bleeding, vasculitis, thrombocytopaenia, hypertensive or diabetic retinopathy.

Critical care

Mannitol
Indications: cerebral oedema, rising ICP. A drug that is potentially life-saving in situations when time needs to be 'bought' to facilitate the transfer of a head injured patient to a neurosurgical centre. Generally should be given only after the advice from a neurosurgeon and, in acute cases, if surgery is to take place within about 4 hours.
Mechanism of action: osmotic diuretic.
Time to work: 24 hours.
Dosage: 1g/kg of a 20 percent solution given intravenously.
Side effects: pyrexia, chills.
Cautions: thrombophlebitis and inflammation due to extravasation. Limited repeated use due to rising hypernatraemia and osmolality.

Contraindicated in pulmonary oedema or congestive heart failure.

Propofol
Other names: propofol-lipuro, diprivan.
Indications: intravenous anaesthetic agent with rapid recovery and without hangover effect. Used for the induction of anaesthesia; maintenance of anaesthesia; sedation in intensive care.
Mechanism of action: Uncertain but is believed to work on GABA-A receptor
Time to work: seconds.
Dosage:
For a 1 percent injection:
Induction: 1.5-2.5mg/kg at a rate of 20-40mg per 10 seconds
Maintenance: 4-12mg/kg/hour
Sedation in intensive care: 0.3-4mg/kg/hour
For a 2 percent injection:
Induction: 1.5-2.5mg/kg at a rate of 20-40mg per 10 seconds
Maintenance: 4-12mg/kg/hour
Sedation in intensive care: 0.3-4mg/kg/hour

Side effects: pulmonary oedema, pyrexia, pain on intravenous injection, muscle movements, seizures, anaphylaxis, bradycardia, delayed recovery.
Cautions: pregnancy; monitor blood-lipid concentration if risk of fat overload or if sedation more than 72 hours.
Contra-indications: Use in those less than 17 years old may cause cardiac failure, metabolic acidosis, hepatomegaly, rhabdomyolysis, hyperlipidaemia.

Thiopental
Other names: thiopentone.
Indications: induction of general anaesthesia; short duration anaesthesia; reduction of intracranial pressure in controlled ventilation.
Mechanism of action: a barbiturate.
Time to work: seconds.
Dosage: 100-150mg over 10-15 seconds, followed by further amount up to 4mg/kg depending on response after 30-60 seconds.
Interactions: anaesthetic agent.
Side effects: arrythmia, myocardial depression, cough, sneeze, laryngeal spasm, rash, hypersensitivity.
Cautions: cardiorespiratory depression, hepatic impairment, pregnancy, tissue necrosis and severe pain if extravasation occurs. While awakening from a moderate dose is rapid due to redistribution to other tissues, metabolism is slow and sedative effects may persist for over 24 hours. It has no analgesic effect.
Contra-indications: porphyria.

Lorazepam
Indications: sedation with amnesia; premedication; anxiolytic.
Mechanism of action: a benzodiazepine
Time to work: minutes.
Dosage: Sedation dose involves a slow intravenous infusion of the drug diluted with an equal volume of normal saline infusion or water for injections 50mcg/kg.
Drug interactions: anxiolytics and hypnotics.
Side effects: amnesia, persistent drowsiness after end of infusion, confusion, ataxia, dependence, paradoxical aggression, headache, vertigo, hypotension, salivation changes, visual disturbance, dysarthria, tremor, thrombophlebitis, incontinence, urinary retention, gastrointestinal disturbance.
Cautions: respiratory depression, acute pulmonary insufficiency, muscle weakness, drug or alcohol abuse, pregnancy, hepatic or renal impairment, porphyria, chronic psychosis.

Haloperidol
Other names: Haldol, dozic, serenace.
Indications: agitation and restlessness, severe anxiety, intractable hiccup.
Mechanism of action: a butyrophenone antipsychotic.
Time to work: minutes.
Dosage:
Oral administration:
Mania, psychomotor agitation or psychosis: 1.5-3mg 2-3 times daily, or 3-5mg 2-3 times daily if resistant.
Agitation and restlessness in the elderly: 0.5-1.5mg once or twice daily.
Severe anxiety: 500mcg twice daily.
Intractable hiccups: 1.5mg TDS.
Intravenous administration: 2-10mg every 4-8 hours, to a maximum of 18mg daily.
Drug interactions: consult formulary as several, eg. effects reduced by muscarinics; avoid

with clozapine; exacerbation of extra-pyramidal side effects with dopaminergics.
Side effects: extrapyramidal symptoms especially dystonia and akathisia; hypoglycaemia, weight loss, inappropriate anti-duiretic hormone secretion, photosensitivity. Less sedating and fewer muscarinic or hypotensive symptoms compared to other antipsychotics like chlorpromazine.
Cautions: subarachnoid haemorrhage, hypokalaemia, hypocalcaemia, hypomagnesaemia, pregnancy.
Contraindications: Comatose states, CNS depression, phaeochromocytoma, breast feeding.

Labetalol
Other names: trandate.
Indications: controlled hypotension under anaesthesia; hypertension; hypertension with angina or after myocardial infarction.
Mechanism of action: a beta-blocker with also an arteriolar vasodilating action, thus lowering peripheral vascular resistance.
Time to work: minutes.
Dosage: 2mg/minute until satisfactory response, then stopped. Usual total dose 50-200mg.
Side effects: postural hypotension, headache, weakness, tiredness, nausea, vomiting, rash, difficulty in micturition, epigastric pain, scalp tingling, liver impairment.
Cautions: liver damage; interferes with laboratory tests for catecholamines; stop in case of jaundice or liver damage.
Contra-indicated in asthma, severe bradycardia, uncontrolled cardiac failure, sick sinus syndrome, second or third degree heart block, peripheral arterial disease, cardiogenic shock, phaeochromocytoma.

Atracurium
Other names: tracrium
Indications: muscle relaxation for surgery or during intensive care.
Mechanism of action: a non-depolarising muscle relaxant, of the benzylisoquinolinium group, with slower onset of action than depolarizing muscle relaxants like suxamethonium, and reversed by anticholinesterases such as neostigmine. Non-depolarising muscle relaxants have no analgesic or sedative effects. Atracurium is suitable in intensive care as its long term muscle relaxation is via non-enzymatic metabolism and not dependent on hepatic or renal elimination.
Duration of action: 30-40 minutes.
Dosage: 300-600mcg/kg initially followed by 4.5-29.5mcg/kg/minute.
Side effects: histamine release causing hypotension, bradycardia, bronchospasm, anaphylaxis, skin flushing.
Cautions: pregnancy, hypothermia, myasthenia gravis, burns.

Anticoagulants

Anticoagulants are used to prevent deep vein thrombosis (DVT) or extension of existing thrombus, and thrombus formation on prosthetic cardiac valves. Overdosage may lead to haemorrhage and neurosurgeons are often faced with such complications as intracerebral haemorrhage, chronic subdural or acute subdural haematoma. The special case of prosthetic heart valves is still an unresolved matter, for there are no agreed international guidelines on how long after a neurosurgical procedure the anticoagulation should be started. The balance between preventing re-bleeding and avoiding thromboembolism is best discussed between neurosurgeons, cardiologists and haematologists at each institution.
In addition, neurosurgical patients are commonly treated with anticoagulants after interventional neuroradiology procedures.

Low Molecular Weight Heparins

Examples: dalteparin (fragmin), enoxaparin (clexane), tinzaparin (innohep).

Indications: prevention of venous thromboembolism, with longer duration of action than unfractionated heparin and no need to closely monitor the clotting profile (APTT) as in unfractionated heparin. Some are also used in the treatment of pulmonary embolism, unstable angina, peripheral artery occlusion, haemodialysis and cardiac bypass circuits. In the event of haemorrhage protamine is used to reverse unfractionated heparin but is less effective on low molecular weight heparin.

Mechanism of action: acts on the intrinsic clotting cascade, inactivating factor Xa, but not thrombin. Half-time is 2-4 times longer than standard heparin so response is more predictable and administration is only necessary once or twice daily.

Duration of action: minutes.

Dosage: for prophylaxis of DVT): dalteparin 2500 units SC daily (or double if high risk of DVT); enoxaparin 20mg SC once daily, tinzaparin 4500 units once daily.
If DVT or PE proven doses vary.

Side effects: bleeding at operative site and intracranially.

Cautions: pregnancy, elderly, hepatic and renal impairment.

Contra-indicated: uncontrolled bleeding; endocarditis.

Warfarin

Other names: coumarin

Indications: long-term oral anti-coagulation as prophylaxis against embolisation in atrial fibrillation, rheumatic heart disease, prosthetic heart valve; prophylaxis against and treatment for DVT and pulmonary embolism.

Mechanism of action: antagonizes the effects of vitamin K by inhibiting the reductase enzyme responsible for regenerating the active form of the vitamin.

Time to work: 48-72 hours.

Dosage: 10mg once daily for two days as loading, then maintenance (3-9mg) depending on target INR (2-2.5 for prophylaxis or treatment of DVT/PE; 2-3.5 if recurrent).

Side effects: haemorrhage, hypersensitivity, rash, diarrhea, hepatic impairment, pancreatitis, skin necrosis, nausea, vomiting.

If there is severe bleeding the warfarin should be stopped, and its action reversed by vitamin K (5mg by slow iv injection, prothrombin complex concentrate (factors II, VII, IX, X) 30-50mg/kg; or fresh frozen plasma 15Ml/kg.

Cautions: elderly, previous GI bleeds, recent surgery, renal or hepatic impairment, breast-feeding.

Contra-indicated: peptic ulcer, bleeding diathesis, severe hypertension, endocarditis, liver failure, intracranial aneurysm, pregnancy.

Aspirin (Acetyl salicylic Acid)

Other names: Angettes 75, Caprin, Nu-seals Aspirin.

Indications: primary and secondary prevention against cerebrovascular disease or myocardial infarction. Post endovascular interventional neuroradiology like stenting or coiling.

Mechanism of action: an antiplatelet agent, aspirin irreversibly acetylates cyclo-oxygenase, preventing thromboxane A2 production and inhibiting platelet aggregation and thrombus formation.

Dosage: initial dose is 150-300mg followed by a daily dose of 75mg orally or dispersed in water.

Side effects: bronchospasm, gastrointestinal haemorrhage, intra- and post-operative bleeding. Associated with chronic subdural haematomas.

Cautions: asthma, uncontrolled hypertension, previous peptic ulcers, pregnancy. Stop for a week before elective neurosurgery.
Contra-indicated: intracranial haemorrhage, breast-feeding, children under 16 years (Reye's syndrome), bleeding diathesis, active peptic ulcers.

Clopidogrel
Other names: Plavix.
Indications: prevention of atherosclerotic events in peripheral vascular disease; within 35 days of myocardial infarction and 6 months of ischaemic stroke; with aspirin in acute coronary syndrome without ST elevation on ECG.
Mechanism of action: a thienopyidine, it exerts an antiplatelet effect via unknown effect
Dosage: 75mg once daily.
Side effects: intracranial bleeding, headache, gastrointestinal bleeding diathesis, dyspepsia, gastritis, diarrhea, peptic ulcers, nausea, vomiting, leukopaenia, thrombocytopaenia, eosinophilia, rash, pruritus.
Cautions: avoid for the first week after ischaemic stroke or myocardial infarction; trauma; surgery; stop a week before elective neurosurgery, hepatic or renal impairment; pregnancy.
Contra-indicated: breast-feeding, active bleeding, intracranial haemorrhage.

18

TECHNOLOGY IN NEUROSURGERY

Deon Louw and Paul McBeth

Contents

From stone to silicone
Microscope
Neurosurgical navigation
Frame based stereotaxy
Frameless stereotaxy
Intraoperative imaging
Future directions
Robotics
Surgical simulation

From stone to silicone

Bipedalism liberated the human hand to experiment with increasingly sophisticated tools for healing the sick and wounded. Early attempts to drain the brain's demons were based on the use of sharpened stones to trephine the skull. Remarkably, some of these courageous patients survived the process, evidenced by bony ingrowth of the craniectomies. The Iron Age permitted more precise engineering of cranial perforators, but surgical localisation remained speculative. The Industrial Age entrained surgical headlights, anaesthesia, blood pressure monitoring and electrical cautery into the operating room. Coupled with new knowledge of the compartmentation of cortical function, the era marked a true inflection point in the care of neurosurgical patients. Most recently, the Information Age heralded the introduction of computers into the operating room. This permits image-guided surgery, facilitates intraoperative imaging and renders robotics possible. It has also enabled modernization of the microscope, the keystone to contemporary neurosurgical technology.

Microscope

In the latter half of the 17th century, Anton von Leeuwenhoek made significant technical advances in microscopy. An inventive linen draper, he devised secret techniques that allowed him to obtain magnification 270 times that of the naked eye. He was thus able to discover and describe protozoa, sperm, and bacteria. In the 18th century, Robert Hooke added various refinements to microscopes, such as fine and coarse adjustment, and invented the name cell to describe the compartmental structure of cork. It was up to Carl Zeiss and Ernst Abbe though to develop lenses of reproducible quality. This led much later to a Zeiss microscope being used to perform the first microneurosurgical procedure in 1957. Bombsite based beam-splitters were added, permitting twin stereoscopic binoculars. Yasargil and Contraves developed a multi joint electromagnetic braking system, which provided superb mobility and stability. Image-guided and robotic capabilities were recently added to these microscopes.

Microscopes offer tremendous advantages in minimal access surgery. Magnification and co-axial illumination permit narrow surgical corridors, minimizing the surgical 'footprint'. However, it is important to familiarize oneself with basic optic principles and the balancing mechanism of the neurosurgical microscope before assisting the principal surgeon. The student will appreciate that magnification is acquired at the expense of depth and breadth of field, and that the binocular eyepieces can be adjusted to accommodate interpupillary distance. They may also be manipulated to compensate for myopia or hyperopia if corrective lenses are not worn. It is crucial to ensure that the diopter setting on the binocular lenses is set at zero if correction is not required.

Neurosurgical navigation
The progression of neurosurgery has largely paralleled advances in lesion localisation. Traditionally, surgeons have used anatomical landmarks to plan cranial and spinal access. These techniques require precise knowledge of anatomical and functional structures of the brain and a highly developed sense of three-dimensional spatial perception. Together with the trend of decreasing surgical case volumes and smaller lesion size, resulting from earlier disease detection, there is a need for improved localisation. These problems have been alleviated by the introduction of computer-based systems used to navigate the three dimensional space of the brain. Coupled with the inventions of CT and MR imaging, neuronavigation has augmented preoperative lesion localisation, permitting in more precise craniotomies and surgical corridors. Surgeons now have a better understanding of trajectory planning and lesion margins, resulting in improved surgical treatment.

Frame based stereotaxy
Stereotaxy is based on the localization of a specific point in space using 3D coordinates and was first introduced in the early part of the 20th century by Clarke. These Cartesian coordinates are based on theoretical planes in the axial, sagittal and coronal orientations (X, Y and Z-axes) which intersect at orthogonal (right) angles. Any point in the cerebral volume within the coordinate system could then be defined, i.e. given a stereotactic 'address', by knowing its position along these three axes. Limitations in medical imaging technologies initially prevented widespread use of stereotaxic principles. The development of CT and MRI technology by the late 1970's, however, significantly increased the capabilities of stereotactic neurosurgery. These imaging modalities provide the ability to see abnormal pathology and to determine its three-dimensional location within the cranium. During this era new localisation frames were developed such as the BRW (Brown-Roberts-Wells) and the CRW (Cosman-Robert-Wells) frames. Stereotactic neurosurgery quickly became accepted for use in biopsy, craniotomy placement, abscess aspiration, endoscopy, and functional procedures. Despite the high accuracy and beneficial outcomes of these systems, they remain cumbersome to use and unable to provide real-time image-based positioning.

Frameless stereotaxy
Computers were first used in the operating room by Bertrand, Olivier and Thompson in the early 1970's to stereotactically locate deep brain structures. Kelly continued these developments in the early 1980's using frame-based techniques and by developing software programs for calculation of stereotactic coordinates in the operating room. These pioneering efforts paved the way towards frameless stereotaxy - a technique allowing real-time localisation of surgical instrumentation in corresponding images of the patient without the need of a stereotactic frame. Advances in computer power and 3D tracking hardware in the early 1980 have allowed this development. Since these early developments, frameless navigation has become widely accepted and has augmented the delivery of cranial and spinal surgery.

Frameless stereotactic devices provide navigational data by relating the location of instruments in the operative field to preoperative or intraoperative images (Figure 1). This information permits optimised cranial openings, accurate identification of surgical corridors or trajectories, localisation of eloquent structures, and depending on the degree of brain shift, a method of resection control. The result is less invasive surgical procedures allowing patients to return to normal activity sooner. Using frameless navigation techniques the conventional stereotactic head frame is replaced with a collection of small fiducial markers used to define the patient coordinate space during registration. Registration is the process by which the coordinate frame describing the patent's head on the operating table is transformed to the coordinate frame of the imaging volume or the 'virtual patient'. Absence of the stereotactic head frame provides increased flexibility and freedom during surgery. Despite the name 'frameless' navigation these systems still require the head to be secured in a head frame for stabilisation.

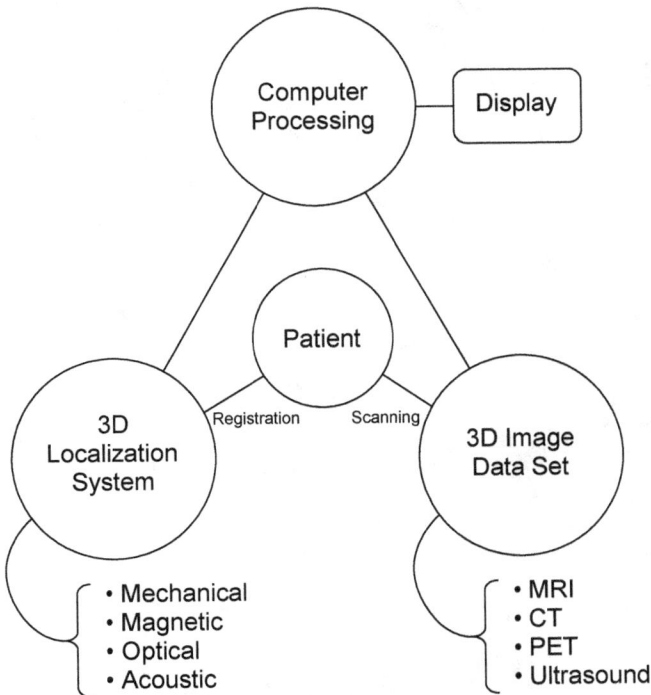

Figure 1. *Components required for image-guided neurosurgery.*

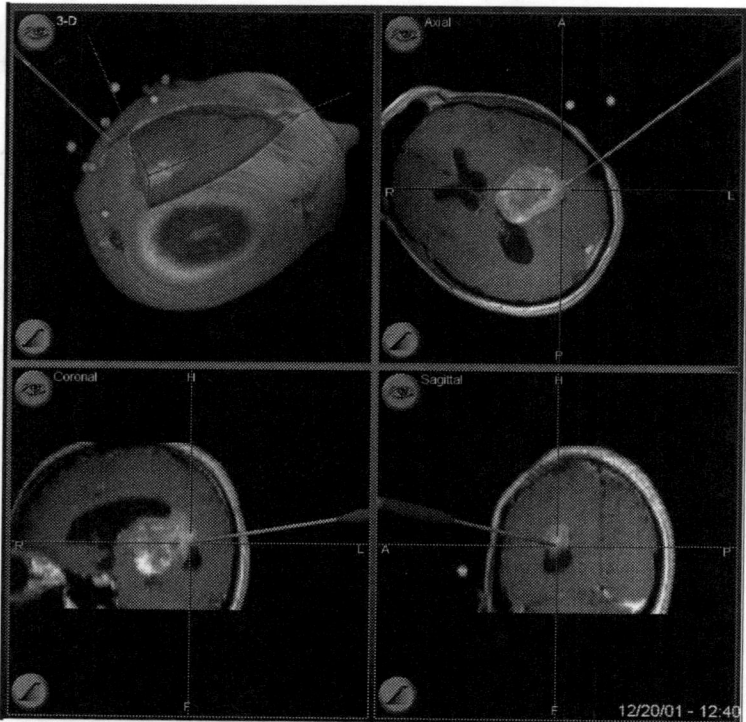

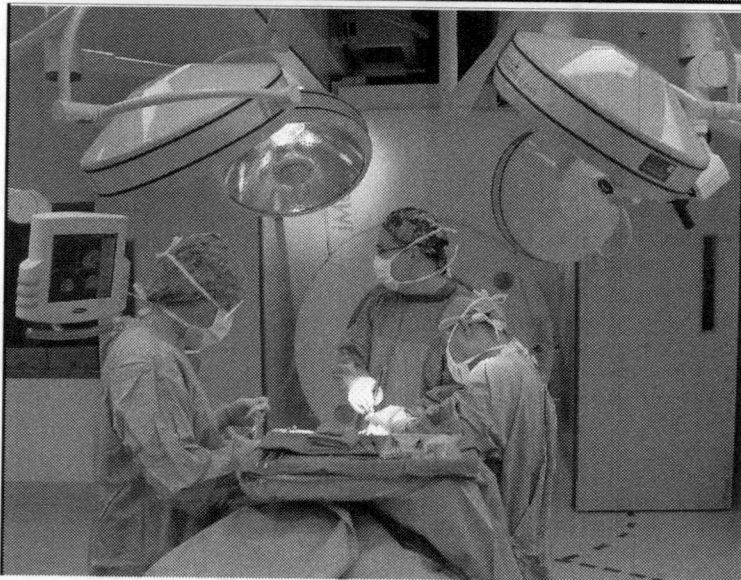

Figure 2. *(top) Example of a frameless navigation display. Display includes a touch-screen interface, a 3D reconstruction from MR imaging data and planar slices from the axial, coronal and sagittal views. (bottom) Example of a frameless navigation system in use. Notice that in this configuration the surgeon must look away from the surgical site to view the navigational display.*

Frameless navigation has been successfully applied in many clinical applications including biopsy, lesion resection, skull based procedures, epilepsy, endoscopy, functional procedures and radiosurgery (Figure 2). Using skull-mounted, guided tools, surgeons can accurately manipulate biopsy or drug delivery devices to exact targets within the brain. Lesion resection is enhanced though proper localization and identification of lesion boundaries, reducing the need for exploratory surgery and facilitating maximal resection.

Intraoperative imaging

Traditionally, neurosurgical navigation has relied on preoperative images and the assumption that anatomical structures of interest remain in the same position with respect to each other and the fiducials used for registration. During surgery, however, tissue deformation and shift disrupt the spatial relationship between the patient and the preoperative image volumes, resulting in errors of localisation. Intraoperative imaging techniques appear to be the best approach to counter these problems. Three-dimensional ultrasound, CT and MRI have been introduced to compensate for intra-operative changes, residual tumor and to update navigation registration.

The development and integration of intra-operative magnetic resonance imaging (iMRI) systems into the operating room has provided a major advance in neurosurgery. Surgeons no longer solely rely on preoperative diagnostic scans to navigate the brain. Instead intra-operative imaging provides surgeons with updated MR images allowing for assessment of brain shift, evaluation of tumor resection, exclusion of hematoma, and identification of ischeamic brain. The Harvard group, using a 0.5-Tesla vertical, open configuration system, pioneered these developments (Figure 3). The Calgary group has developed a system capable of providing high quality intra-operative images. They are produced using a mobile, 1.5-Tesla magnet. The magnet is mounted on ceiling rails and moves in and out of the operating room when required. It also permits the use of traditional, ferromagnetic surgical instrumentation. A popular low field-strength device is the Polaris, developed by Odin.

Future directions

Capitalising on the advances of medical imaging, computer power and surgical navigation the future of neurosurgery is to embrace surgical manipulators that will allow surgeons to move beyond current constraints of dexterity and stamina. Introducing image guidance into surgical robotics will allow targeting of specific anatomical or functional locations and potentially permit autonomous, image-guided surgery. Several groups have already developed robotic systems for stereotactic applications while others are working to develop microsurgical robots with image guidance and tele-operative capabilities.

Robotics

The majority of time in neurosurgical cases is spent on micromanipulation. However, most neurosurgical robotic systems perform only stereotactic procedures. The Robot Assisted MicroSurgery (RAMS) and the Steady Hand projects have, however, developed robotic systems for enhanced tool manipulation (Figure 4). RAMS was developed by NASA to provide a dexterous platform to perform surgery at increased precision. The system is based on master-slave control with the motion of a 6-DOF slave arm linked to the motion of a 6-DOF haptic hand-controller. RAMS is equipped with adjustable tremor filters and motion scalers to enhance dexterity. A feasibility study of microvascular anastomosis in neurosurgery was done by Le Roux. Carotid arteriotomies were performed in 10 rats, and subsequently repaired by surgeons, students, engineers and RAMS. Within the surgical group RAMS was as effective in achieving vessel patency, but took nearly twice the time.

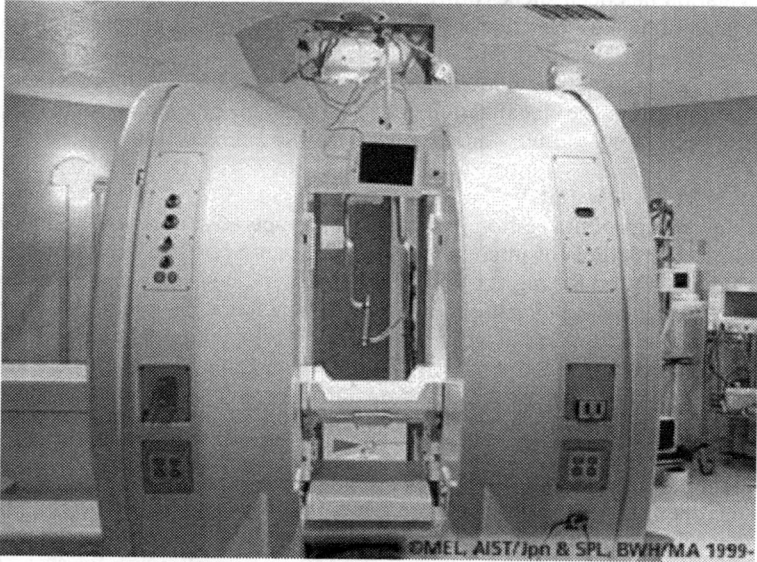

Figure 3. *Harvard intraoperative MRI (General Electric)*

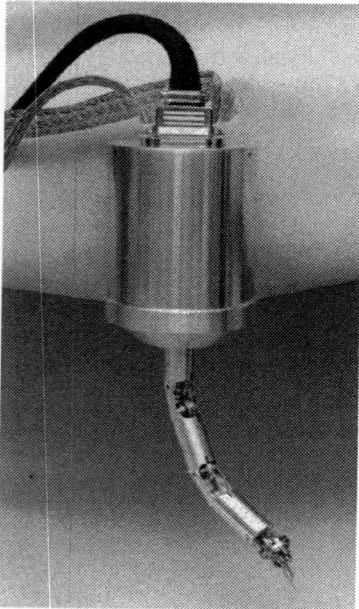

Figure 4. *RAMS microsurgical robot*

Goto's group from Japan has developed a robot platform for tele-controlled microneuro-surgery through the portal of an endoscope. The robot is based on a 10 mm endoscope equipped with twin tissue forceps, a camera, a light source, and a laser. Investigators performed neurosurgery on a cadaveric head and concluded the system facilitated more accurate, and less invasive, surgery. NeuRobot was subsequently used to remove a portion of a tumor from a patient with a recurrent, atypical meningioma.

Surgical robotic systems are also used for spinal applications. The SpineAssist robot developed by Mazor Surgical Technologies (Israel) was recently awarded FDA approval for spinal surgery. The system, no larger than a pop can, is designed to attach directly to the patient's spine - acting as a guide for tool positioning and implant placement. It includes sophisticated software for image guidance, permitting reduced invasiveness of surgical procedures. It also has non-spine orthopedic applications.

The neuroArm design consists of a robot, a controller, and a workstation (Figure 5). The system is based on master-slave control in which commanded hand controller movements are replicated by the robot arms. The workstation will provide visual, audio, and tactile feedback, creating an immersive environment with colocalisation of visuohaptics. Recreating the usual surgical environment in this way will aid adaptation to this new technology. A binocular display can provide stereoscopic views of the surgical worksite and desk-mounted displays provide MR images, robot parameter updates, and various views of the surgical worksite. Tools will be superposed on the MR images, providing real-time visual feedback for intracranial procedures.

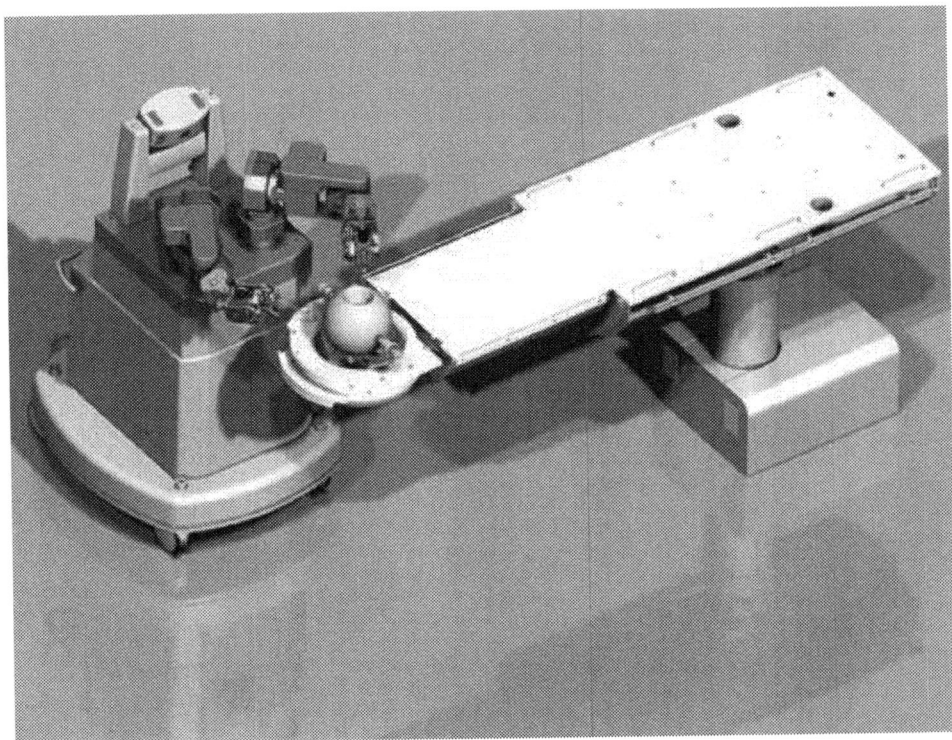

Figure 5. *NeuroArm in position for microsurgery*

Surgical simulation
Surgical training programs are moving towards a more structured curriculum in which physical models and simulators will play a more important role both in developing surgical skill and in evaluating and certifying trainees. Surgical simulation involves performing surgical procedures inside a virtual environment that may include visual, audio, tactile (hap-

tic), or other, feedback. It allows apprentice surgeons to practice routine procedures in a safe environment, permits performance evaluation, and provides senior surgeons a means to rehearse complex cases in a risk-free environment.

Robotic surgery workstations have the advantage of sharing the same platform as simulators, with dual-use capability as a sophisticated surgical simulator. Continually improving models of brain biophysical properties, tool-tissue interaction, realistic rendering of haemorrhage and co-registration with universal brain atlases and multimodal imaging will make virtual surgery performed at the workstation less distinguishable from reality. Patient-specific modeling and simulation can be done by importing MRI data into the simulation program. Haptic hand controllers will have removable end pieces structured after standard neurosurgical tools. For example, haptic-enabled forceps installed on hand controllers would be used to simulate the fine suturing of blood vessels.

In conclusion, in the tradition of Cushing, contemporary neurosurgeons continue to pioneer technological advances. Tremor-free, indefatigable robots are being coupled to intraoperative imaging, heralding a new era in the specialty. The data generated by this technological marriage will authenticate the virtual world of surgical simulation, providing promise of risk-free rehearsal for trainees and superior patient outcomes.

19

ETHICAL CONSIDERATIONS IN NEUROSURGERY

Deon Louw

Contents

Introduction
The basics
Some ethical frameworks
Deontological ethics
Hippocratic ethics
A practical approach
Conclusion

Introduction

There is always an implicit moral dimension to the patient-physician relationship, and to collegial interaction. This is perhaps more pertinent to the neurosurgeon than any other clinician. We deal with the moral and ethical distress provoked by the complexities of brain death, vegetative states, terminal cancers, competency, chronic pain management and consent, on a quotidian basis. This already difficult terrain has new obstacles of controversy: 'therapeutic' cloning, stem cell research and neuromodulation are some of the challenges facing us. Moreover, we are obliged to address these areas in a culturally sensitive and contextual manner. Despite the high drama and stakes for the patients, their families and caregivers, we are remarkably ill-trained for this vital role. However, some simple concepts, coupled to a fundamental ethical framework, can provide clarity and consistency to our approach.

The Basics

Ethics deal with the rules of what is right. A more formal definition for caregivers would be "the set(s) of values or principles (implicit and explicit) which govern the decision-making and practice of giving and receiving health care". The term ethics derives from *ethos* (Greek), for community spirit.

In contrast, morality is the application of these principles at the individual or personal level. Its etymology is *mores* (Latin), for custom. There may be circumstances where morality and ethics clash, such as a patient requesting referral from a pro-life caregiver, to an abortion clinic.

345

Some Ethical Frameworks
Virtue Ethics (Plato and Aristotle)
Natural Law Ethics (Aquinas)
Deontological Ethics (Kant)
Utilitarian/Consequentialist Ethics (Bentham and Mill)
Situation Ethics (Fletcher)
Distributive Justice Ethics (Rawls and Nozick)
Rights Ethics (Dworkin)

Deontological ethics and consequentialism
Although all these frameworks are pertinent to patient care, it is easiest to initially concentrate on just two fundamental pillars: deontology and consequentialism. The former is a moral framework and the latter an ethical one. Deontology would demand the best care for a particular patient, whereas consequentialism would favour the interests of the group.

Deontology subtends:
A fixed set of rules or principles, considered absolute
A stress on duty, balanced on the notion of fixed rights
A denial of any clash between private morality and public ethic
The primacy of the individual over the community
People must always be ends and never means

The Kantian ethos underpinning deontology is: "I ought never to act in such a way that I could not also will that my maxim should be a universal law". Kant's Universability Test reveals mandatory moral rules, such as the illegality of theft. He points out that if everybody stole from everybody else, then not only would society collapse, but the concept of theft would enter an irrational "black hole".

Strengths:
Simple to understand and operate
Capable of universal adoption
Good match with European and North American culture
Weaknesses:
Individualistic
Does not allow for variety, circumstances or complexity
May not work in non Judaeo-Christian contexts

Consequentialism subtends:
A denial that actions are intrinsically either good or bad
A requirement to compare the consequences of different decisions
The importance of the universal dimension – "the greatest good of the greatest number"
The need to calculate the consequences before acting

Strengths:
Reduces clash with personal moralities
Good for population and generalisability
Respects the variety, circumstances, individuality of the patient
Potentially more fair
Weaknesses:

Difficult (impossible) to predict or measure outcomes accurately
The weakness of the concept of utility – what is useful, good, beneficial?

Hippocratic Ethics
Always seeks the good of the individual patient
Never does harm
Never prescribes a deadly drug
Never gives advice that could lead to death
Never procures abortion
Acknowledges the duty of confidentiality

It is clear from the earlier descriptions that Hippocratic Ethics are largely duty-based, or deontological. Although they continue to form a core to much of modern medical morality, contemporary values require a more flexible approach. Beauchamp and Childress have responded by synthesizing four basic principles to underpin bioethics:

Autonomy - respect for individuals and their rights
Justice - the care for the just distribution of limited resources
Beneficence - always act for good
Non-Maleficence - do nothing that will harm

Under certain circumstances, these principles may be ranked in lexical ordering. In other situations, one principle may trump another. Typically, an individualistic society with access to private health care will favour the primacy of autonomy, whereas the delivery of a national health service will warrant careful scrutiny of distributive justice issues.

A practical approach

Michael McDonald has provided a framework for ethical decision-making, to be used as a guide rather than blueprint. It provides a pragmatic plan for dealing with complex ethical dilemmas in medicine, and can be downloaded in full from:

http://www.ethics.ubc.ca/mcdonald/conflict.html

We provide a précis here for brief review:
Collect information and identify the problem
Be alert; be sensitive to morally charged situations
Identify what you know and don't know
State the case briefly with as many of the relevant facts and circumstances as you can gather within the decision time available.
Consider the context of decision-making:

Clinical
What is the patient's prognosis?
Is the condition reversible?
What are the probabilities of success?
What are the plans in case of therapeutic failure?

Preferences
Has the patient been informed of benefits and risks; understood, and given consent?

Is the patient mentally capable and legally competent? Evidence of incapacity?
Has the patient expressed prior preferences, e.g. Advanced Directives?
If incapacitated, who is the appropriate surrogate? Is the surrogate using appropriate standards?

Quality of Life/Death
What are the prospects, with or without treatment, for a return to the patient's normal life?
What physical, mental, and social deficits is the patient likely to experience if treatment succeeds?
Are there any plans and rationale to forego treatment?
What are the plans for comfort and palliative care?

Contextual Features
Are there religious, cultural factors?
Are there problems of allocation of resources?
What are the legal implications of treatment decisions?
Is there an influence from clinical research or teaching?

Specify feasible alternatives
Use your ethical resources to identify morally significant factors in each alternative
Principles (e.g. Beauchamp and Childress)
Moral models (mentors)
Use ethically informed sources (e.g. institutional policies)
Personal judgments
Organised procedures of ethical consultation (case conference, ethics committee, ethicist)
Propose and test possible resolutions
Make your choice
Live with it
Learn from it

Conclusion

It is helpful to consider that all our interpersonal interactions have a moral aspect. In fact, they have a simple moral anatomy: the underlying motive or intention, the action itself, and the consequence. Reflective learning along these basic lines will provide insight into why disputations may have arisen, and usefully undermine our internal alibi's.

A final hint is not to always agonise over *what* decisions are to be made - it is often more important to consider *who* makes the decisions. In most circumstances this is clear, and the only difficulty is deciding whether those responsible have acted so unreasonably as to forfeit that privilege.

20

FURTHER READING

Andreas K Demetriades

Contents

Journals: Basic science
Journals: Clinical
Texts: Basic science
Texts: Clinical

We hope that you have enjoyed our book, however this "pocket survival guide" is an introduction only to more illustrious texts. Please find below a selection of excellent texts.

Journals: Basic science

Science
Nature
Nature Neuroscience
Nature Reviews in Neuroscience
Neuron
Cell
Trends in Neurological Sciences
Journal of Neuroscience
Neuroscience
Journal of Physiology
American Journal of Physiology
Proceedings of the National Academy of Science
Journal of Neurobiology
Journal of Comparative Neurology
Brain
Cerebral Cortex
Synapse

Journals: Clinical

Lancet
Lancet Neurology
New England of Medicine
British Medical Journal

Cochrane Reviews
Neurosurgery Clinics of North America
Journal of Neurosurgery
Neurosurgery
Acta Neurochirurgica
British Journal of Neurosurgery
Surgical Neurology
Neurosurgical Focus
Neurosurgery Quarterly
Clinical Neurology and Neurosurgery
Journal of Neurology Neurosurgery and Psychiatry
Journal of Neurosurgery: Pediatrics
Child's Nervous System
Pediatric Neurosurgery
Journal of Neurosurgery: Spine
Spine
European Spine
Journal of Bone and Joint Surgery
Minimally Invasive Neurosurgery
Strereotactic and Functional Neurosurgery
Movement Disorders
Journal of Neurooncology
Acta Neuropathologica
Neuroradiology

Texts: Basic science

Neuroanatomy
The Whole Brain Atlas at www.med.harvard.edu/AANLIB/home.html
Kandel ER, Schwartz JH, Jessell TM. Principles of Neural Science, 4th edition, McGraw-Hill/Appleton & Lange, 2000.
Martin JH. Neuroanatomy: Text and Atlas, McGraw-Hill/Appleton & Lange, 2003.
Haines DE. Neuroanatomy: An Atlas of Structures, Sections, and Systems, 5th edition, Lippincott Williams & Wilkins, 2002.
Hendelman WJ. Atlas of Functional Neuroanatomy, CRC Press, 2000.

Neurophysiology
Kandel ER, Schwartz JH, Jessell TM. Principles of Neural Science, 4th edition, McGraw-Hill/Appleton & Lange, 2000.
Carpenter RHS. Neurophysiology, 4th edition, Arnold Publishers, 2002.

Neuropathology
Greenfield JG, Lantos PL and Graham DI. Greenfield's Neuropathology (2 Volumes), 7th edition, Arnold Publishers, 2002.
Nelson JS. Principles and Practice of Neuropathology, 2nd edition, Oxford University Press, 2003.

Microbiology of the CNS
Osenbach RK and Zeidman SM. Infections in Neurological Surgery: Diagnosis and

Management, Lippincott Williams & Wilkins, 1998.
Hall WA and McCutcheon IC. Infections in Neurosurgery, Thieme Medical Publishers, 2000.

Texts: Clinical

History of neurosurgery
Greenblatt SH, Dagi TF and Epstein MH (eds). A History of Neurosurgery. In its scientific and Professional Contexts, The American Association of Neurological Surgeons, 1997.

General neurology
Patten JP. Neurological Differential Diagnosis, 2nd edition, Springer, 1998.
Greenberg D, Aminoff MJ and Simon RP. Clinical Neurology, 5th edition, McGraw-Hill/Appleton & Lange, 2002.
Jones Jr HR and Netter FH. Netter's Neurology, Novartis Medical Education, 2004.

General neurosurgery
Introductory texts:
Black PMcL and Rossitch E. Neurosurgery: An Introductory Text, Oxford University Press, 1995.
Lindsay KW and Bone I. Neurology and Neurosurgery Illustrated, 4th edition, Churchill Livingstone,
2004.
Kaye AH. Essential Neurosurgery, 3rd edition, Blackwell Publishers, 2005.
Liebenberg WA and Gunasekera L. Neurosurgery Lecture Notes: An International Curriculum, Vesuvius Books, 2005.
Liebenberg WA and Johnson RD. Neurosurgery for Basic Surgical Trainees, Hippocrates Books, 2004.

Specialised texts:
Greenberg MS. Handbook of Neurosurgery, 5th edition, Berlin: Thieme Publishers, 2001.
Winn RH (ed). Youman's Neurological Surgery, 5th edition, W. B Saunders, 2004.
Rengachary SS and Ellenbogen RG. Principles of Neurosurgery, 2nd edition, Mosby, 2004.
Awad I. Philosophy of Neurological Surgery, Thieme/AANS, 1995.

Operative Surgery
Rhoton Jr AL. Cranial anatomy and surgical approaches. Lippincott William & Wilkins/CNS, 2003.
Kaye AH and Black PMcL. Operative Neurosurgery, Churchill Livingstone, 2000.
Schmidek HH and Sweet WH. Schmidek & Sweet's Operative Neurosurgical Techniques: Indications, Methods, and Results, 4th edition, Elsevier, 2000.
Conolly ES, McKhann GM, Huang J and Choudhri TF. Fundamentals of Operative Techniques in Neurosurgery, Thieme Medical Publishers, 2002.
Day JD, Koos WT, Matula C and Lang J. Color Atlas of Microneurosurgical Approaches, Thieme Medical Publishers, 1997.
Fossett DT and Caputy AJ. Operative Neurosurgical Anatomy, Thieme Medical Publishers, 2002.
Sekhar L and de Oliveira E. Cranial Microsurgery: Approaches and Technique. Thieme Medical Publishers, 1999.

Yasargil MG. Microneurosurgery (Volumes 1-4), Thieme Medical Publishers, 1984-1996.

Trauma
Valadka AB and Andrews BT. Neurotrauma: Evidence-Based Answers to Common Questions. Thieme Medical Publishers, 2005.
Marion D. Traumatic Brain Injury. Thieme Medical Publishers, 1999.

Neuro-critical care
Andrews BT (ed). Intensive Care in Neurosurgery, Thieme, 2003.
Suarez JI (ed). Critical Care Neurology and Neurosurgery, Humana Press, 2004.

Neuroradiology/ Interventional neuroradiology
Osborn AG and Maak J. Diagnostic Neuroradiology, Mosby, 1994.
Kirkwood JR. Essentials of Neuroimaging, 2nd edition, Churchill Livingstone, 1995.
Byrne JV (ed). Interventional Neuroradiology: Theory and Practice, Oxford University Press, 2002.
Osborn A, Blaser S and Salzman K. Diagnostic Imaging: Brain, W.B. Saunders, 2004.
Hosten N and Liebig T (translated by Telger TC). CT of the Head and Spine, Thieme Medical Publishers, 2002.

Neurovascular
Byrne JV (ed). Interventional Neuroradiology: Theory and Practice, Oxford University Press, 2002.
Grand W and Hopkins LN. Vasculature of the Brain and Cranial Base. Thieme Medical Publishers, 1999.
Ojemann RG and Ogilvy CS. Surgical Management of Neurovascular Disease, 3rd edition, Williams & Wilkins, 1995.

Neuro-oncology
Berger MS and Prados M. Textbook of Neuro-Oncology, Elsevier/Saunders, 2004.
Apuzzo MJ. Benign Cerebral Gliomas, Volumes I and II, 1995, Thieme/AANS.
Fischer G and Brotchi J. Intramedullary Spinal Cord Tumors, Thieme Medical Publishers, 1996.

Skull Base
Dolenc VV and Rogers L. Microsurgical Anatomy and Surgery of the Central Skull Base, Springer, 2003.
Sen C, Chen CS and Post KD. Microsurgical Anatomy of the Skull Base and Approaches to the Cavernous Sinus. Thieme Medical Publishers, 1997.

Spine
Benzel EC. Spine Surgery, Churchill Livingstone, 2004.
Haher TR and Merola AA Surgical Techniques of the Spine, Thieme Medical Publishers, 2003.
Devlin VJ. Spine Secrets, Hanley & Belfus, 2003.
Vaccaro A, Betz RR and Zeidman. SM Principles and Practice of Spine Surgery, Mosby, 2002.
Benzel E. Biomechanics of Spine Stabilisation, Thieme/AANS, 2001.

Peripheral nerves
Maniker A. Operative Exposures In Peripheral Nerve Surgery, Thieme Medical Publishers, 2004.
Kline DG. Atlas of Peripheral Nerve Surgery, 2nd edition, W.B. Saunders, 2001.

Functional neurosurgery
Schulder M. Handbook of Stereotactic and Functional Neurosurgery, Marcel Dekker Ltd, 2003.
Gildenberg PL and Tasker RR. Textbook of Stereotactic and Functional Neurosurgery, McGraw-Hill, 1997.
Germano I. Neurosurgical Treatment of Movement Disorders, Thieme/AANS, 1998.

Pain
Burchiel K. Surgical Management of Pain, Thieme Medical Publishers, 2002.

Neuroendocrinology
Powell MP, Lightman SL and Laws Jr ER. Management of Pituitary Tumors: The Clinician's Practical Guide, 2nd edition, Humana Press, 2003.

Pediatric neurosurgery
Choux M, Hockley AD and Di Rocco C. Pediatric Neurosurgery, Churchill Livingstone, 1999.
McLaurin RL and McLone D. Pediatric Neurosurgery: Surgery of the Developing Nervous System, Saunders, 2000.
Albright AL, Pollack IF and Adelson PD (eds). Operative Techniques in Pediatric Neurosurgery, Thieme Medical Publishers, 2000.

Index

A

abbreviated mental test score 106, 108
abciximab 329, 336
abducens 40, 56, 57, 58, 66, 72, 73, 74, 77, 78
Abducens nerve 40, 57, 58, 72, 73, 74, 77
Abscess 124, 142, 160, 161, 283, 284, 285, 286, 290
acceleration–deceleration 134
Accessory meningeal artery 40
Accessory nerve 40, 59
acetazolamide 262, 263
ACTH 216, 232
Acyclovir 287, 288
adenohypophysis 70
adrenal gland 70
adrenocorticotropic hormone 70, 216
adrenocorticotropin 70
AICA 78, 80, 81, 82
ambient 130
ambient cistern 130
American Spinal Injury Association 280
amygdala 62, 66, 67
Anaplastic (malignant) astrocytoma 226, 241
Anaplastic (malignant) oligodendroglioma 227, 241
Anaplastic astrocytoma 123, 141, 142
Anaplastic ependymoma 228, 241
aneurysms 225
angiogram 188, 189, 190, 196, 197, 198, 199, 200, 205, 206, 207, 208, 211, 212, 213, 214, 215, 216, 217, 218, 219
angiography 188, 189, 190, 207, 209, 211, 212, 213, 214, 215, 216, 217, 219, 220
angular gyrus 48, 49, 52, 55
anhydrosis 112
annulus fibrosus 293, 296
anterior caudate veins 201, 202
anterior cerebral arteries 190, 192
anterior cerebral artery 53, 68, 69, 193, 196, 206
anterior choroidal artery 66, 68, 191, 197, 206
anterior clinoid 37, 38, 43, 44, 46, 53, 67, 68, 69, 71, 72, 76
Anterior clinoid process 37, 38, 43, 53, 67, 68, 69, 71, 72, 76
Anterior commissure 43, 63, 64
anterior communicating artery 68, 69, 189, 190, 192, 193, 196, 198, 206, 208, 212
Anterior cranial fossa 38
anterior inferior cerebellar arteries 192, 195, 207
anterior inferior cerebellar artery 77, 78, 80, 81, 197, 207

Anterior intercavernous sinus 44
Anterior medullary venous plexus 202
anterior meningeal artery 195
anterior ponto-mesencephalic vein 203
Anterior pontomesencephalic venous plexus 202
anterior radicular branch 204
anterior spinal artery 77, 192, 195, 204
Anterior spinal cord syndrome 280
anterior temporal arteries 193
anterior vertebral line 165, 167
anti-diuretic hormone 70
Antonio de Egas Moniz 26, 189
apoptosis 223, 224
aqueduct 51, 52, 56, 60, 61, 63, 64, 127
aqueduct of Sylvius 127
arachnoid 41, 42, 45, 68, 71
Arachnoid cyst 123, 147, 148, 164, 179, 299, 309, 310
arachnoid cysts 225, 237
Arachnoid mater 41, 42, 45, 71
Arterial infarct 124, 154
arteriovenous fistula 209, 218
Arteriovenous Malformation 124, 158, 159, 164, 183, 190, 209, 212, 216
Arteriovenous malformations 251
artery of Adamkiewicz 204
ASIA 280, 281
Aspirin 330, 331, 333, 340
Asterion 33
asterion. 34
astrocytoma 123, 124, 140, 141, 142, 152, 163, 177, 225, 226, 227, 239, 241, 245, 248
Astrocytomas 223, 225, 226, 227, 238
ataxia 115, 116, 118
atlanto – occipital dissociation 166
Atlantoaxial instability 299, 307
Atlanto-axial subluxation 293
atlanto-dens interval 166, 167
Atlanto-occipital dislocation 272
Atracurium 330, 338, 339
auriculotemporal nerve 32
autoregulation 83, 84, 85, 86, 87, 88, 96, 97, 102, 103
AVM 251, 252, 254

B

Bacterial meningitis 283, 284
BAEP 320
Barbiturates 324
Baron Larrey 19
Barrow's classification 210

basal cisterns 129, 130, 132, 136, 137, 139, 147, 155, 157, 158
basal vein of Rosenthal 201, 202, 208
Base of skull fractures 268
basilar 46, 64, 69, 76, 77, 78, 80, 81, 82
basilar arteries 207
basilar artery 69, 76, 77, 78, 80, 190, 192, 195, 196, 197, 199, 200, 207, 208, 216
Basilar invagination 299, 305, 306, 307
Basiocciput 38, 39, 74
Basisphenoid 37, 38, 39, 74
BAX 224
BBB 103
Benign intracranial hypertension 261, 263
Bernard de Montfauchon 15
beta HCG 233
Biceps 116
BIH 263
Bilateral facet dislocations 275
Bilateral transtentorial herniation 97
bilirubin 137, 254, 269
BIS 313, 318, 319
Bispectral analysis 313, 318
bitemporal hemianopia 109
blood brain barrier 83, 86, 88, 89, 90, 91, 92, 93, 99, 100, 103
blood-CSF barrier 92
Bony tumours 163, 170, 245
Borden's classification 210
brachiocephalic 190
brain abscess 283, 284, 285, 286
brain death 97
Brain herniation 97, 100, 102, 313, 324, 325
Brain oedema 99, 125, 154
Brain tissue oxygen tension 313, 318
brain tumours 123, 126, 140, 223, 224, 225, 228
brainstem 29, 41, 46, 56, 57, 68, 69, 74, 76, 77, 78, 79, 80, 81, 82, 115
brainstem auditory evoked potentials 320
bregma 35
Broca 55
Broca's area 55
Brown Séquard syndrome 280
Brown-Séquard syndrome 118
Burst fracture 273, 276, 278, 279
Burst fractures 276, 278

C

calcarine 195, 196, 199
calcarine fissure 51, 54
Caldwell's view 190
calloso-marginal arteries 193
callosomarginal artery 193, 197
calloso-marginal artery 193
Camino 314
Capillary endothelial cell 92
capsular artery of McConnell 191
Carbamazepine 329, 330, 331
carboplatin 238
carmustine 227, 237, 238
carotid artery 32, 38, 40, 48, 66, 67, 68, 69, 72, 73, 74, 188, 189, 190, 191, 193, 197, 198, 205, 208, 209, 212, 216
carotid cavernous fistula 209, 213
carotid cistern 53
cartilage producing tumours 163, 170
cauda equina 168, 170, 182
Cauda equina syndrome 280, 295, 296
caudate nucleus 61, 67
cavernoma 184
cavernomas 252
Cavernous angioma 164, 184
Cavernous angiomas 251, 252
Cavernous malformation 124, 159, 184
cavernous malformations 252
Cavernous sinus 29, 44, 46, 68, 71, 72, 73, 74, 78, 113, 191, 201, 202, 203, 209, 210
cavernous sinuses 202
CBF 84, 85, 86, 87, 88, 97, 102, 103, 316
CCF 209, 210
Central cord syndrome 280
Central neurocytoma 229, 241
Central neurocytomas 124, 149, 225
Central retinal vein 40, 67
Central sulcus 35, 36, 48, 49, 51, 54
Central transtentorial herniation 325
CEO2 317
Cephaloceles 299, 308, 309
cerebellopontine angle 29, 47, 74, 75, 76, 78, 80, 81
cerebellopontine fissure 74, 75, 80
cerebellum 29, 32, 42, 43, 46, 49, 51, 58, 59, 64, 74, 76, 80
Cerebral aneurysms 251, 252, 253
cerebral blood flow 84, 85, 89, 96, 97, 313, 316, 317
cerebral herniation 101, 103
cerebral metabolic rate of oxygen 316
cerebral oedema 83, 100, 103, 134
cerebral oxygen extraction 317
cerebral peduncle 66, 68, 77
cerebral salt wasting 322

Cerebritis 124, 160, 283, 284, 285, 286
Cerebrospinal fluid 83, 90
cervical spondylosis 169
Cervical stenosis 297
cervical sympathetic trunk 48
Chamberlain's line 306, 307
Chance fracture 278
Charles Sherrington 25
chemodectoma 235, 243
Chiari 1 malformation 304, 305
Chiari 2 261
Chiari II malformation 300
Chiari malformation 299, 300, 304, 305, 307
Chiari malformations 261
chiasm 109, 110
chiasmatic cistern 67
Chiasmatic sulcus 37, 38, 39
Chondrosarcoma 234, 235, 242, 243, 246
chondrosarcomas 225, 234, 237
Chordoma 124, 152, 163, 173, 235, 236, 243, 247
chordomas 225, 235, 237
Choriocarcinoma 233, 242
choriocarcinomas 233
choroid plexus 62, 64, 65, 66, 76, 77, 80, 83, 89, 90, 91, 92, 93, 101
Choroid plexus carcinoma 228, 241
Choroid plexus papilloma 228, 241
choroid plexus tumours 224, 225
choroidal fissure 62, 68
cingulate gyrus 46, 51
cingulate herniation 324
cingulate sulcus 51, 53, 54
circle of Willis 190, 192, 196, 206, 212, 252, 254, 255
Circular sulcus 53, 54
Cisplatin 238
Clay shoveller's fracture 276
Clivus 37, 38, 39, 46, 69, 71, 74, 76
Clopidogrel 330, 340
CMRO$_2$ 316

Coagulase-negative Staphylococci 285
Cochlear nerve 40, 66, 81, 113
Codeine phosphate 329, 334
Codman 314
Colloid cyst 123, 132, 134, 146, 147
comatose 105, 120
Comminuted fractures 268
common carotid artery 190, 205
common femoral artery 214
communicating hydrocephalus 132, 133, 157
compliance 314, 320

Compression fractures 276, 277
consensual light reflex 112
contrecoup 270
conus 175
conus medullaris 204, 303
Conus medullaris syndrome 280
corneal sensation 113
corona radiata 115
coronal suture 131
corpus callosum 43, 46, 51, 61, 63, 64
corticospinal tracts 102
Corticotropin releasing hormone 70
Coup 270
CPA 225, 237
CPP 85, 86, 87, 96, 97, 103, 313, 317, 320, 321, 322, 323
Cranial nerves 105, 108, 110, 111, 112, 113, 114
Craniocervical junction 299, 304, 307
Craniopharyngioma 231, 232, 242
Craniopharyngiomas 124, 149, 223, 225, 236, 237
Creutzfeld-Jacob disease 288
Cribriform plate 37, 38
Crista galli 37, 38, 39, 42, 43
Cryptococcus 286
Cryptococcus meningitis 286
CSW 256, 322
Cushing 25
Cushing's disease 232
Cushing's syndrome 232
Cyclizine 329, 334
Cysticercosis 288
Cytomegalo virus 287
Cytomegalovirus 288
Cytotoxic oedema 99, 102, 103

D

DAI 270
Dandy-Walker cyst 262
Dandy-Walker malformation 299, 308, 309, 310
DAVF 210
David Ferrier 22
DBI 134, 270
Decompressive craniectomies 324
deep cerebral veins 208
Deep tendon reflexes 117
Deltoid 116
Demyelination 126, 127
Denis 277, 278

Deontological ethics 349, 350
deoxyhaemoglobin 137, 254
Depressed fractures 268
dermatome 115, 118
dermatomes 119, 120
Dermoid cyst 123, 146, 164, 179, 181, 303
dermoid cysts 225, 230, 237
Dermoid tumours 125
dermoids 225, 237, 299
Desmoplastic infantile ganglioglioma 229, 241
Dexamethasone 329, 332
Dexamethasone suppression test 232
DI 322, 323
diabetes insipidus 322
Diamox 262, 263
Diaphragma sellae 45, 46, 67, 71
Diastematomyelia 299, 301, 302
Diclofenac 329, 333
diffuse axonal injury 270
Diffuse Brain Injury 123, 134, 137, 267, 269, 270
diplopia 111
Disc herniation 163, 166, 293, 294, 295, 296
disc prolapse 167, 168, 170, 296
Discitis 164, 181, 182, 185, 283, 290, 291
dominant hemisphere 105, 106
dopamine 70
Dorello's canal 74
dorsum sellae 38, 39, 41, 67, 71, 76, 135
Dura mater 29, 41, 42, 45
Dural arteriovenous fistula 164, 183
Dural arteriovenous fistulas 209
Dural AVF 209, 210
dysdiadocokinesia 116
Dysembryoplastic neuroepithelial tumor 229, 241
Dysplastic gangliocytoma of the cerebellum 228

E

E granulosus 288
EAA 103, 271
Ebers Papyrus 17
Echinococcosis 288
Echinococcus granulosus 288
echo time 126
Edinger Westphal nucleus 110
Edinger-Westphal 110, 111
EEG 313, 318, 326
elastance 320, 321

elastance curve 320, 321
embryonal carcinoma 233, 242
emissary veins 202
Empyema 124, 160, 283, 284, 290
Endodermal sinus tumour 233
endodermal sinus tumours 233
ependyma 66, 177
Ependymal cell tumors 227, 241
ependymal tumours 225
Ependymoma 123, 143, 163, 175, 177, 225, 227, 228, 241, 245, 248
ependymomas 177, 223, 224, 225, 228, 238
Epidermoid cyst 123, 146, 164, 179
epidermoid cysts 225, 237
epidermoids 225, 237
Epidural abscess 283, 284, 290
Epidural empyema 164, 182
Epidural haematoma 164, 185
Epidural haematomas 269
Epilepsia partialis continuans 326
Epstein-Barr virus 287, 288
Escherichia Coli 262
Eschericia Coli 285
esthesioneuroblastoma 229, 230, 241
esthesioneuroblastomas 225
ethmoid 37, 38, 39, 40, 71
ethmoid bone 38
Evoked potentials 313, 320
Ewing sarcoma 247
Excitatory amino acids 103
Extensor hallucis longus 116
external auditory meatus 190
External beam radiotherapy 237
external carotid artery 32, 188, 190, 197, 205, 209, 212, 216
external jugular veins 32
external occipital protuberance 31, 33, 34, 35, 36, 39, 43, 47
Extra axial 123
Extra-axial haemorrhages 269
Extradural haematomas 41
extradural haemorrhage 100
extrapyramidal 114, 115, 118

F

facial colliculus 58, 65, 66
Facial nerve 30, 32, 40, 57, 59, 66, 73, 74, 75, 77, 80, 81, 82
falciform ligament 67, 69
falx 41, 42, 45, 46, 51, 129, 130, 133, 144
Falx cerebelli 45

Falx cerebri 42, 133
femoral artery 214, 216
fentanyl 323
fetal posterior cerebral artery 205
Filum terminale ependymomas 248
Fischgold's digastric line 306, 307
Fisher grading scale 156
FLAIR 126, 142, 145, 146, 147
flow voids 183
flow-metabolism coupling 85, 86, 87
fluid attenuation inversion recovery 126
Focal injury 267, 269
follicle stimulating hormone 70
Folstein's Mini Mental Status Examination 107
foramen caecum 38
Foramen lacerum 37, 38, 40, 72
Foramen magnum 37, 38, 39, 40, 59, 76, 194, 195, 197, 203, 216
foramen of Magendie 61, 66
Foramen ovale 37, 38, 40, 75, 76, 78, 79
Foramen rotundum 37, 38, 40, 73, 75, 76, 78
foramen spinosum 37, 38, 40, 48, 73, 76
Fornix 43, 51, 61, 62, 63, 64
Fourth ventricle 43, 51, 60, 61, 64, 65, 66, 75, 127, 130, 132, 133, 143, 157, 158
Fractures of the atlas 273
Fractures of the axis 274
Fractures of the dens 274
Frankel grading system 280
Frontal air sinus 43
frontal bone 31, 32, 33, 38, 39, 43
frontal gyri 48
Frontal lobe 38, 45, 48, 51, 52, 53, 54, 135, 136
frontal nerve 32, 40
Frontal sinus 39
frontal sulci 48
Frontalis muscle 30
frontopolar artery 193
fronto-polar artery 193
Frontozygomatic suture 33
fundoscopy 109, 111, 114

G

gag reflex 113, 114
galea 29, 30
Galea aponeurotica 30
Gangliocytoma 228, 241
Ganglioglioma 229, 241
Gasserian 45, 73, 74, 75, 78

Gasserian ganglion 74, 75, 78, 191
GCS 120, 121
Genu 43, 51, 61, 63
germ cell tumours 225, 233, 238, 240, 242
Germinoma 124, 150, 233, 242
GFAP 224
Glabella 36
Glasgow Coma Scale 120
Glial fibrillary acidic protein 224
Glial tumours 125, 152
Glioblastoma 123, 141, 142
Glioblastoma Multiforme 123, 142, 225, 226, 241
glioblastomas 223, 226, 238
gliomas 224, 225, 226, 227, 228, 238, 241
Glomus jugulare tumour 236
Glossopharyngeal nerve 40, 57, 74, 113
Gradenigo's syndrome 74
gradient echo 126
Granisetron 329, 335
greater petrosal nerves 40
Group A Streptococci 285
Group B Streptococci 285
growth hormone 70, 232
Guide Catheters 213

H

habenular commissure 64
Haemangioblastoma 164, 178
Haemangiopericytoma 234, 242
Haemophilus Influenza 262, 284
Haemophilus Influenzae 285
haemorrhagic contusions 270
haem-oxygenase 254
Haloperidol 329, 338
Hangman's fracture 275
Harvey Cushing 24
head injury 102, 103
Hemangioblastoma 124, 151, 235, 240, 243
Heparin 330, 339
Herpes Simplex virus 287
Herring-Traube-Mayer waves 314
Heschl's gyrus 53, 55
HHH therapy 258, 259
hippocampus 62, 66, 67
Hippocratic ethics 349, 351
HISTORY 105, 106
HIV 287

Holoprosencephaly 299, 309
homonomous hemianopia 109
homunculus 53
Horner's syndrome 112
Hounsfield 125, 138
Hughlings Jackson 21
Human immunodeficiency virus infection 286
Hunt and Hess grading scale 254, 256
Hydrocephalic oedema. 100, 102
hydrocephalus 57, 64, 74, 83, 91, 96, 98, 100, 101, 102, 123, 127, 132, 133, 134, 143, 146, 147, 149, 150, 151, 156, 157, 256, 259, 261, 262, 263
hydrostatic pressure 133
Hyperglycemia 323
Hypernatremia 322
hyperreflexia 115
hypertensive haemorrhage 124, 158
Hyperventilation 322, 325
hypoglossal artery 197
hypoglossal canal 37, 39, 40, 59, 76
Hypoglossal nerve 40, 57, 59
hypoglossal triangle 65, 66
Hyponatremia 256, 322
hypoplasia of the dens 299, 308
hypothalamus 62, 63, 70
hypotonia 115

I

Ibuprofen 329, 333
ICA 191, 196, 197, 200, 205, 206, 210, 211, 213, 217
ICP 85, 87, 88, 93, 94, 95, 96, 97, 100, 101, 102, 103, 271, 313, 314, 315, 320, 321, 322, 323, 324
idiopathic intracranial hypertension 261, 263
Inferior colliculus 43, 51, 56, 58, 65, 68
inferior frontal veins 202
inferior hypophyseal artery 73, 191
inferior occipital gyri 51
inferior ophthalmic vein 202
Inferior petrosal sinus 44, 46, 188, 203, 216
Inferior petrosal sinus sampling 188, 216
inferior petrosal sinuses 39, 46, 72
inferior rectus 111
Inferior sagittal sinus 42, 45, 46, 201, 202, 208
inferior temporal sulci 52
Inferior vermian vein 202, 208
inferior vermian veins 203
infundibulum 208
inion 34

innominate artery 190
Insula 53, 54
interhemispheric fissure 41, 42, 45, 68
Internal acoustic meatus 37, 40, 73, 75, 76, 78, 80, 81
internal auditory meatus 38, 81
internal capsule 58, 67
internal carotid arteries 190
internal carotid artery 38, 40, 66, 67, 68, 69, 72, 73, 188, 190, 191, 193, 197, 198, 205, 208, 209, 212, 216
internal cerebral vein 201, 202
internal cerebral veins 201, 208
internal jugular vein 40, 46
internal jugular veins 202
internal occipital protuberance 34, 35, 37, 39, 42, 43, 45, 47
Interpeduncular cistern 43, 51, 52, 67, 68, 69
Interstitial radiotherapy 237
intervertebral disc 164, 165, 166, 168, 170, 182
Intracerebral haemorrhage 123, 136, 158
Intracranial compliance 314, 320
Intracranial elastance 320
intracranial pressure 83, 84, 85, 94, 95, 96, 97, 98
Intracranial pressure monitoring 313
intracranial volume 95, 96, 101
intramedullary 163, 171, 177, 179, 183, 184
intraparietal sulcus 48, 49
inversion recovery 126
isodense 125, 139, 142, 143, 146, 148

J

J.S. Billings 20
Jacopo Berengario da Capri 19
Jefferson fracture 273
Jefferson's fracture 273
John Caius 19
Jugular foramen 37, 38, 40, 44, 46, 74, 75, 76
jugular vein 203
Jugular Venous Oximetry 313, 316
JVO 313, 316, 317

K

K+ 87, 91, 93, 94, 99
Karnofsky score 226
Keppra 329, 331
Kernohan's paralysis 325
Keyhole 35, 36
Ki-67 224

Klippel-Feil syndrome 299, 307, 308

L

Labetalol 330, 338
labyrinthine artery 81, 82
Lacrimal nerve 40
Lambda 33, 34, 35
lambdoid 131
Lambdoid suture 33
lamina terminalis 51, 63, 64, 67
Lateral mass fracture 274
lateral medullary syndrome 76
Lateral mesencephalic vein. 202
lateral mesencephalic veins 201
lateral occipital artery 195, 196
lateral posterior choroidal artery 196
lateral rectus 111
lateral sacral arteries 216
lateral transtentorial herniation 324
lateral ventricle 129, 133, 134, 157, 161
lateral ventricles 127, 129, 132, 134, 156, 157
lesser occipital nerves 32
Lhermitte-Duclos disease 228
ligamentum flavum 166, 168, 169
Light touch 118
Liliequist's membrane 41, 68
linear fracture 267
Linear fractures 267, 268
Lipoma 234, 242
Lipomas 299, 303, 309
Listeria Monocytogenes 285
locus coeruleus 66
lomustine 238
Lorazepam 329, 337
lower motor neurone signs 115
Lundberg 314, 315
lutenizing hormone 70
lymphoma 123, 145, 163, 171, 247
lymphomas 223, 224, 232, 238, 242
Lymphoproliferative tumours 163, 171

M

Macroadenomas 124, 148
macula 54, 56
Magnetic Resonance Imaging 125
mamillary bodies 41, 51, 64, 66, 78

Mamillary body 43, 57, 63, 77
Mandible 30, 31
Mandibular nerve 30, 40, 73, 75, 78, 79
Mannitol 322, 323, 329, 336
MAP 85, 88, 97, 103
Marcus Gunn pupil 111
marginal ramus 51
Marginal sinus 44, 203
Marshall classification 136
Maxilla 39
maxillary artery 191
Maxillary nerve 40, 72, 73, 75
McAfee 278
McConnell's capsular arteries 73
McGregor's line 306, 307
McRae's line 306, 307
Meckel's cave 38, 45, 73, 74, 76, 78
medial eminence 66
medial lenticulostriate arteries 193
medial longitudinal fasciculus 56, 74
medial occipital artery 195, 196
medial-posterior-choroidal artery 196
median sacral arteries 204
median sacral artery 216
median sulcus 58, 59, 65, 66
Medulla 40, 43, 49, 51, 56, 57, 58, 59, 61, 64, 65, 66, 74, 76, 77, 81, 82
Medulla oblongata 43, 49, 51, 56, 59, 114, 115
medullary veins 201
Medulloblastoma 124, 151, 225, 242
medulloblastomas 223, 224, 225, 231, 238
mega cisterna magna 262, 300, 310
melanocyte stimulating hormone 70
membrane of Liliequist 67
Meninges 29, 40, 41, 42, 67, 71
Meningioma 123, 144, 145, 163, 174
meningiomas 176, 223, 224, 225, 231, 234, 248
Meningitis 283, 284, 286, 287, 288, 289
meningo hypophyseal trunk 191
meningocele 299, 300, 302
meningohypophyseal trunk 73
MEP 320
Metastatic 124, 127, 153
Metastatic tumours 163, 173, 245, 247
Methylprednisolone 329, 332
MIB-1 224
Microadenomas 123, 148
Microcatheters 209, 213
Microdialysis 313, 318
Microscope 341, 342

Microvilli 92
midazolam 323
middle cerebral artery 53, 66, 193, 194, 196, 197, 206
middle cranial fossa 38, 46, 48, 71, 73, 76, 78
middle fossa 35, 37, 38, 40
middle meningeal artery 34, 40, 48, 73, 191, 212, 215
mini mental state examination 106
Mixed germ cell tumour 233
Monroe 60, 61, 62, 63, 64
Monroe – Kelly 320, 322, 324
Motor evoked potentials 320
motor system 105, 114, 115, 117, 118
MRI 123, 124, 125, 126, 127, 130, 131
Multiple myeloma 163, 171, 172, 246, 247
mural nodule 178
muscle power 115
mycobacterium tuberculosis 182
Myelomeningocele 299, 300, 301, 303, 305
Myelopathy 293, 295, 296, 297, 298
myeloschisis 299, 300, 301
Myoclonic status 326
myosis 112
Myotomes 116, 118
Myxopapillary ependymoma 163, 175, 228, 241

N

Na+ 91, 93, 94
Na+/K+ ATPase 99
Nasal bone 39, 43
Nasion 36
Nasociliary nerve 40
navigation 341, 342, 343, 344, 345
Near infrared spectroscopy 313, 317
Neisseria Meningitidis 285
neo-vascularity 140
Nerve sheath tumours 245, 247, 248
Nervus intermedius 40, 81
Neural foramina 164, 165, 175
Neurenteric cyst 164, 179
Neurenteric cysts 237, 299, 303
neurilemoma 235, 243
neurinoma 235, 243
neuroangiography 219
NeuroArm 347
neurofibroma 175, 176, 235, 238, 243
Neurofibromas 247
Neurofibromatosis 223, 238

neurofilament 224
Neuron specific enolase 224
Neuronal tumours 124, 149
neuropeptide Y 86
Nimodipine 329, 335
NIRS 313, 317
Nitrosoureas 238
non-communicating 132
Normal pressure hydrocephalus 261, 263
NPH 263
nucleus pulposus 293, 294
nystagmus 116

O

Obstructive hydrocephalus 132, 134, 146, 147, 262, 263
occipital artery 32, 40
occipital bone 31, 32, 33, 34, 35, 38, 39, 42, 43, 46, 74
Occipital condyle fractures 272
Occipital lobe 51, 54, 61
occipital pole 51, 54
occipital sinus 45, 47, 202, 203
Occipitalis muscle 30
Octreotide 232
oculomotor 40, 56, 57, 66, 67, 68, 69, 72, 73, 77, 78
Oculomotor nerve 40, 57, 66, 67, 68, 69, 72, 73, 77
Odontoid 274
odontoid peg 166
olfactory bulb 52, 67
Olfactory nerve 40, 52
Olfactory neuroblastoma (esthesioneuroblastoma) 229, 241
Olfactory tract 52, 67
Oligodendroglial tumors 227, 241
oligodendroglial tumours 225
Oligodendroglioma 123, 143, 227, 241
oligodendrogliomas 223, 227, 229, 238, 248
oncogenes 223, 224
ophthalmic 31, 32, 40, 46, 67, 68, 72, 73, 75, 78, 79
ophthalmic artery 31, 40, 67, 68, 73, 191, 197, 205
ophthalmic nerve 72, 73, 75
Ophthalmic veins 40, 46, 72
ophthalmoplegia 112
Opioids 329, 334, 335
Opthalmic artery 191
Optic chiasm 38, 43, 51, 52, 63, 64, 67, 68, 69, 70
Optic nerve 40, 67, 68, 69, 71, 108, 109, 110, 111, 112
orbicularis oculi 30, 32
orbitofrontal artery 193

orbito-frontal artery 193
Os odontoideum 299, 308
Osmotic oedema 99, 100
Osteoblastoma 163, 171, 246
Osteochondroma 163, 171, 246
Osteoid osteoma 163, 170, 171, 245, 246
Osteomyelitis 164, 181, 182, 185, 283, 284, 289, 290
Osteosarcoma 246
Oxygen Extraction Ratio 84, 85
oxytocin 70

P

p21 224
p53 224
palatal function 114
Palatine bone 39
Panjabi and White 276
Papaverine 329, 336
papilloedema 67, 97, 98, 101, 111
paracentral lobule 51
Paracetamol 329, 330, 333, 334
Paraganglioma 163, 176, 178, 235, 236, 243
paragangliomas 225
Paramagnetic 125, 126
parietal bones 32
Parietal lobe 48, 51, 52, 54
parieto-occipital arteries 195, 196
parieto-occipital artery 199
parieto-occipital sulcus 51
Parinaud's syndrome 225
Pars marginalis 51
Particle beam radiotherapy 237
Paul Broca 16, 21
PCV 227, 238
pedicle 165, 173, 175, 177, 178
Penetrating head injuries 269
pericallosal artery 193, 197
Pericranium 29, 30, 41
Perineural cyst 164, 179
periventricular nuclei 62, 70
persistent trigeminal artery 197, 200
Pethidine 329, 334
petroclinoid ligament 74
Petrolingual ligament 191
petrosal sinus 188, 202, 203, 216
petrosal veins 203
Petrous apex 37, 42, 43, 45, 74, 76, 78

petrous bone 42, 74

Petrous ridge 29, 34, 35, 37, 38, 44, 46, 69, 73, 74, 75, 76

petrous temporal bone 33, 38, 40, 45, 46, 74

Phenobarbitone 329, 331

Phenytoin 323, 329, 330, 331, 333

Pia mater 41, 42, 66

PICA 76, 78, 199, 206, 208

Pilocytic astrocytoma 123, 142

pineal 43, 45, 51, 56, 58, 60, 63, 64, 78

pineal cysts 225, 230

Pineal gland 43, 51, 56, 58, 63, 64

Pineal parenchymal tumors 230, 242

Pineal parenchymal tumours 124, 150, 225

pineal recess 51, 60, 63, 64

Pinealoblastoma 151

Pinealocytoma 150

Pineoblastoma 231, 242

Pineoblastomas 230, 231

Pineocytoma 230, 231, 242

Pineocytomas 230

Ping pong fractures 268

pituitary 29, 37, 38, 39, 43, 45, 51, 62, 63, 64, 66, 67, 69, 70, 71, 72, 73

Pituitary adenoma 231, 232, 242

pituitary adenomas 225, 231, 232, 237

Pituitary apoplexy 231

Pituitary fossa 37, 38, 39, 45, 67, 71, 72

pituitary gland 29, 43, 45, 51, 63, 70, 71, 72, 73

pituitary hormones 70

pituitary lobe 62, 70

pituitary stalk 69, 70

placental alkaline phosphatase 233

Plasmacytoma 233, 242

pleomorphic xanthoastrocytoma 225, 227, 241

PML 286

PNET 231, 238

Porencephalic cyst 262

Postcentral gyrus 48, 49, 51

postcentral sulcus 48, 49

posterior auricular artery 32

posterior cerebral arteries 190, 192, 195, 196, 208

posterior cerebral artery 66, 67, 68, 69, 77, 195, 196, 205

posterior clinoid 37, 38, 41, 43, 44, 69, 71, 72, 73, 74, 76

posterior commissure 60, 63, 64

posterior communicating arteries 190

posterior communicating artery 66, 68, 69, 77, 191, 192, 195, 196, 197, 205, 206, 208, 212

posterior inferior cerebellar arteries 192, 195, 204

posterior inferior cerebellar artery 77, 78, 80, 82, 207

posterior inferior temporal arteries 196

Posterior intercavernous sinus 44, 203

posterior longitudinal ligament 166
posterior meningeal artery 195
posterior mesencephalic veins 203
posterior radicular branch 204
posterior spinal arteries 204
posterior spinal artery 77, 195, 204
posterior vertebral line 165, 167
Power's ratio 272
Pre medullary cistern 43
precentral cerebellar vein 202, 203, 208
Precentral gyrus 48, 49, 51, 53
precentral sulcus 48, 49
preoccipital notch 51
prepontine 130
Prepontine cistern 43, 64
Presenting complaint 105, 106
primary motor cortex 53
Primitive neuro-ectodermal tumour 151
primitive neuroectodermal tumours 231
Prion disease 288
Proatlantal intersegmental artery 197
Procarbazine 227, 238
prolactin 70
prolactinoma 70, 231
Prolactinomas 231, 232
propofol 323, 329, 337
proprioception 115, 118
Proton density 126
pseudotumour cerebri 261, 263
Pterion 33, 34
pterygo-maxillary sinus 202
ptosis 112
pulse sequences 126
pupil 111, 112
pupil constriction 111, 112
Pupillary constriction 110, 111, 112
pupillary dilatation 112
pyramidal system 114, 115

Q

Quadriceps 116
quadrigeminal 130, 195, 196, 201
Quadrigeminal cistern 43, 51, 52, 56, 62, 67, 69, 130

R

radicular arteries 204

radiculopathy 115, 295, 298
Raised intracranial pressure 83, 95, 97, 98
RAMS microsurgical robot 346
Rathke cleft cyst 236, 243
Rathke's cleft cysts 225
recurrent artery of Heubner 68, 193
reflex 110, 111, 112, 113, 114, 115, 117, 120
reflex arc 115
regma 36
repetition time 126
retinal fibers 109
Rheumatoid arthritis 163, 166, 293
rhomboid fossa 64
Richard Wiseman 19
Rinne's 113
Roberts Bartholow 21
Robotics 341, 345
Romberg 105, 118
Rostrum 43, 51, 61, 63, 64
Round cell tumours 245, 247

S

sagittal sinus 155
SAH 155, 156, 157, 251, 254, 256, 257, 258
Schwannoma 163, 175, 235, 239, 243
schwannomas 225, 235, 239, 247, 248
Secondary brain injury 267, 270, 271
Seizures 323, 326
sella turcica 38, 67, 71
sensory system 105, 118
septal vein 201, 202
septal veins 201
Septum pellucidum 43, 51, 61, 63, 133
short tau inversion recovery 126
SIADH 256, 322
Sigmoid sinus 34, 35, 40, 44, 46, 47, 76, 203, 208, 212
sigmoid sinuses 202, 203, 208
Signal Quality Index 318
Simpson grading 234
Skull fractures 123, 134, 267, 268
Snellen chart 108
sodium 91, 93, 95, 99
Sodium Valproate 329, 330, 331
Solitary plasmacytoma 163, 171, 247
somatosensory evoked potentials 320

Spetzler-Martin grading scale 251, 252
sphenoid 32, 33, 34, 35, 37, 38, 39, 40, 43, 53, 67, 69, 71, 72, 73, 76
sphenoid bone 33, 34, 38, 43, 71
Sphenoid sinus 39, 67, 71
Sphenoid wing 37, 38
Sphenoparietal sinus 44, 46, 72, 201, 202, 203
Spina bifida aperta 299, 300
Spina bifida cystica 299, 300
Spina bifida occulta 299, 300, 302
spinal accessory nerve 114
spinal arteries 204, 215
Spinal canal stenosis 293, 297, 298
spinal cord 164, 165, 166, 169, 174, 175, 184, 185
Spinal dysraphism 299, 300
Spinal stenosis 163, 166, 168
Spinal tumours 163, 170
spinolaminar line 165, 167
Splenium 43, 46, 51, 63
spondylolisthesis 293, 297
Spondylolysis 293, 297
squamous temporal bone 33, 34, 48
SSEP 320
Staphylococcus Aureus 264, 283, 284, 285, 289, 290
Staphylococcus Epidermidis 264
Status epilepticus 313, 326, 327
Stemetil 329, 335
Stereotactic radiosurgery 234, 237
stereotaxy 341, 342
sternocleidomastoid muscle 114
STIR 126, 146
Straight sinus 42, 43, 44, 46, 201, 202, 208, 211
Streptococcus Pneumonia 284
Streptococcus Pneumoniae 285
subarachnoid 124, 125, 130, 132, 136, 155, 157
Subarachnoid haemorrhage 83, 101, 124, 136, 251, 253, 254, 255, 257, 270
Subaxial fractures 276
subclavian artery 190, 194
subdural 134, 135, 137, 138, 139, 160
Subdural empyema 283, 284
subdural haematoma 135, 137, 138, 139, 164, 184
Subdural haematomas 269
subdural haemorrhage 134, 137
Subdural space 41, 42
subependymal giant cell astrocytomas 225
subependymal veins 201
Subependymoma 228, 241
subependymomas 225
subfalcine herniation 42, 97, 102
substance P 86

Subtle status 326
sulcus limitans 65, 66
superficial middle cerebral vein 201, 208
superficial middle cerebral veins 201
superficial sylvian vein 202
superficial temporal artery 31, 32
superior cerebellar arteries 192, 195
superior cerebellar artery 66, 68, 69, 77, 78, 79
Superior colliculus 43, 51, 52, 56, 58, 65, 110, 111
superior frontal gyrus 48, 49, 51
superior hypophyseal artery 191
superior intercostal artery 216
superior medullary velum 66
superior oblique 111
Superior orbital fissure 38, 40, 73, 74, 76, 78
superior petrosal sinus 34, 44, 45, 46, 74, 80
superior sagittal sinus 42, 43, 44, 45, 47, 201, 202, 208
superior temporal line 30, 31
Superior vermian vein 202, 203, 208
Suppression Ratio 318
supramarginal gyrus 48, 49, 53
supraorbital 31, 32
suprapineal recess 60, 63, 64
suprasellar 29, 34, 38, 41, 45, 64, 66, 67, 68, 69, 71
supratrochlear 31, 32
supreme intercostal arteries 216
SVJO2 317, 318
Sylvian cistern 53
Sylvian fissure 34, 35, 36, 38, 48, 52, 53, 54, 55, 67, 193, 194, 201
synaptophysin 224
syndrome of inappropriate ADH secretion 322
syndrome of inappropriate secretion of antidiuretic hormone 256
Synovial cyst 164, 179, 180
syringomyelia 178, 299, 300, 304, 305

T

T solium 288
Taenia solium 288
Tarlov cyst 164, 179
taste 113
TBI 267, 271
TCD 313, 316
Teardrop fractures 276
tela choroidea 63, 64, 66, 78
Temozolomide 227, 238
temporal bone 30, 31, 33, 34, 38, 40, 45, 46, 48, 74, 133, 135, 138
temporal gyri 52

temporal horn 133, 157
Temporal lobe 38, 46, 48, 51, 52, 53, 54, 64, 66, 68
Temporalis muscle 30, 31, 34, 35
Temporoparietal suture 33
tent 42, 43, 45, 66, 71, 74, 78
tentorial herniation 98
tentorial incisura 45
tentorium 41, 42, 44, 45, 46, 68, 69, 74
Tentorium cerebelli 42, 44, 46
Teratoma 233, 242
terminal vein 201, 202
tethered cord syndrome 299, 303
thalamostriate vein 201, 202, 208
thalamostriate veins 201
The Cerebellopontine Angle 74
The Scalp 29
Thiopentone 329, 337
Third ventricle 43, 51, 58, 60, 61, 62, 63, 64, 66, 67, 68, 69, 70, 78, 123, 127, 130, 132, 133, 134, 146, 147, 150, 156, 157
thyroid stimulating hormone 70
Tibialis anterior 116
Tibialis posterior 116
Tight junction 89
Tissue intensities 123, 126
Tonsillar herniation 325
torcular 35, 45, 46, 47
torcular herophili 45, 201, 202, 203
Towne's view 190, 207
Toxoplasma gondii 287
Transcranial Doppler 313, 316
Transcranial Doppler Ultrasonography 313, 316
transtentorial herniation 97, 98
Transverse pontine vein 202
Transverse sinus 34, 35, 44, 45, 46, 47, 201, 203, 208
transverse sinuses 202, 203, 208
transverse temporal gyri 52
Trapezius 114, 116
Traumatic brain injury 267, 271
Trepanation 15, 20
Triceps 116, 117
Trigeminal artery 197, 200
trigeminal ganglion 45, 73, 79
trigeminal nerve 32, 48, 58, 73, 74, 75, 77, 78, 79, 80, 81
trigone 129, 133
triple H 258
trochlear 40, 56, 57, 58, 65, 68, 69, 72, 73, 78
Trochlear nerve 40, 57, 58, 65, 68, 69, 72, 73
Tuber cinereum 51, 57, 64, 66, 67, 70, 77
Tuberculosis 164, 182, 283, 289, 291

Tuberculum sellae 39, 71
Tuberous sclerosis 227, 239
Tumour suppressor genes 224

U

uncal herniation 98, 324, 325
uncus 52, 66, 68, 138
Unilateral facet dislocations 275
upper quadrant hemianopia 109

V

vagal triangle 65, 66
vagus 40, 57, 59, 80, 81, 113
Vagus nerve 40, 57, 59
Varicella Zoster virus 287
Vascular anomalies 124, 158
Vascular malformation 188, 209
Vascular malformations 208, 209
vasoactive intestinal polypeptide 86
vasodilatation 86, 87, 96
Vasogenic oedema 99, 103
Vasospasm 251, 254, 256, 257, 258, 259
vein of Galen 201, 202, 203, 208, 209, 214
vein of Labbé 46, 201, 208
vein of Trolard 201, 208
veins of Trolard 201
Venous angioma 124, 159
venous angiomas 209, 251, 252
Venous infarct 124, 155
venous oxygen concentration 316, 317
Ventriculitis 283, 284, 286
Ventriculostomy 323
VEP 320
vermis 115
vertebral 40, 76, 77, 78, 82
Vertebral arteries 40, 76, 77, 78, 190, 192, 194, 195, 196, 204, 207
vertebral artery 195, 197, 199, 204, 205, 206, 207, 208, 213, 216
Vertex 36
vestibular nerve 113
Vestibular schwannoma 124, 130, 152
Vestibulocochlear nerve 57, 59, 73, 75, 77, 80, 81, 82, 113
vestibulocochlear nerves 74, 78, 80, 81
Victor Horsley 24
Vincristine 227, 238
Visual acuity 108, 109
visual confrontation testing 109, 110

visual evoked potentials 320
Visual fields 108, 109, 110
Vomer 39, 71
Von Hippel – Lindau 223, 235, 239

W

Wackenheim's clivus-canal line 306, 307
Wada test 188, 216
Walter Dandy 26
Warfarin 330, 339, 340
Water's view 190
Weber 113, 114
Wernicke's area 55
WFNS 254, 256, 259
WHO classification 223, 241
William Macewen 23
William Osler 24
World Federation of Neurological Surgeons 254

Z

zygomatic 30, 31, 32, 33, 34, 47
Zygomatic bone 33
zygomaticotemporal nerve 32

www.ingramcontent.com/pod-product-compliance
Lightning Source LLC
Chambersburg PA
CBHW052011230326
41598CB00078B/2466